This work sets out to show how tremendous progress was made in the treatment of wounded soldiers during the Great War which significantly improved chances of survival. It describes ground breaking advances in resuscitation, anaesthesia and surgery which established the foundations of modern war surgery. It stresses the importance of blood transfusion. In 1914, definitive management of wounds took place at base hospitals after a journey which sometimes took days. Resuscitation was practically non-existent, anaesthesia was poor and surgical methods were hopelessly inadequate. Many soldiers developed catastrophic wound infections and died as a result of overwhelming sepsis when they should have survived. During the Second Boer War, surgeons followed the teaching of Joseph Lister who had introduced antiseptic surgery in 1867. Antiseptic dressings were applied to prevent harmful organisms gaining access to wounds which were considered sterile. Results were satisfactory, but the Boer War was fought in dry grasslands of the Transvaal and Orange Free State and most wounds were caused by rifle bullets fired from long range and of relatively low energy. The Great War on the Western Front was fought in richly manured fields of France and Flanders and wounds were caused by high energy shell fragments or bullets carrying potentially lethal organisms into their depths. Many wounds were sutured, and antiseptic dressings applied in dressing stations of field ambulances, before patients were transferred to base hospitals for definitive surgery. Results were appalling. Two pioneering surgeons challenged established doctrine and introduced new surgical methods against much opposition and hostility from clinicians who lacked vision to see beyond existing methods of treatment. Resuscitation and anaesthesia were transformed as knowledge increased and by 1917 blood transfusion became very important in improving survival. From May 1918, Field Ambulance Resuscitation Teams were employed by Australian medical personnel to deliver resuscitation and surgery to wounded soldiers within a very short time, saving limbs and lives. When hostilities were over, it was hoped by many that lessons learned during the conflict would be applied subsequently to civilian practice. Professional jealousy and rivalry sometimes prevented this from happening.

I0894048

Tom Scotland graduated in Medicine from the University of Edinburgh in 1971 and became a Fellow of the Royal College of Surgeons of Edinburgh in 1975. He became Consultant Orthopaedic Surgeon with NHS Grampian and Honorary Senior Lecturer at the University of Aberdeen. He was lead clinician for the Scottish Sarcoma Managed Clinical Network for three years. He developed an interest in the Great War whilst a student, when there were still many veterans alive. His wife`s uncle was an 'Old Contemptible', one of the original small British Expeditionary Force which went to France in August 1914. He was killed in the Ypres Salient in 1915. Since retiring from the NHS, the author has kept in touch with former colleagues by leading cycling expeditions to the Western Front. He has pursued his interest of the Great War by making a particular study of Aberdonian surgeon Sir Henry Gray, who played a pivotal role in the development of orthopaedic surgery on the Western Front. In retirement he has re-invented himself as a cycling orthopaedic historian. He co-edited a book *War Surgery 1914-18*, and has co-authored four further works, *Wars, Pestilence and the Surgeon`s Blade*, *Understanding the Somme 1916: An Illuminating Battlefield Guide*, *Understanding the Ypres Salient: An Illuminating Battlefield Guide* and *Henry Gray, Surgeon of the Great War, saving lives in a theatre of destruction*.

A Time to Die and a Time to Live

Disaster to Triumph: Groundbreaking Developments in Care of the Wounded on the Western Front 1914–18

Tom Scotland

Helion & Company

Helion & Company Limited
Unit 8 Amherst Business Centre
Budbrooke Road
Warwick
CV34 5WE
England
Tel. 01926 499 619
Fax 0121 711 4075
Email: info@helion.co.uk
Website: www.helion.co.uk
Twitter: @helionbooks
Visit our blog http://blog.helion.co.uk/

Published by Helion & Company 2019
Designed and typeset by Mach 3 Solutions Ltd (www.mach3solutions.co.uk)
Cover designed by Paul Hewitt, Battlefield Design (www.battlefield-design.co.uk)
Printed by Lightning Source, Milton Keynes, Buckinghamshire

ISBN 978-1-911628-74-3

British Library Cataloguing-in-Publication Data.
A catalogue record for this book is available from the British Library.

This book is dedicated to Lyn and to Neil, Jennifer and Graham.

Contents

Acknowledgements

I would like to thank Stuart King, Derek (Surgeon) King, Gordon Stables, Kirsten Reilly and Lewis Taylor for their help with the preparation of several figures. Their contributions are acknowledged in the appropriate sections of the book. I am very grateful for assistance provided by Dr Rod Westhorpe, retired anaesthetist and formerly Honorary Curator of the Geoffrey Kaye Museum of Anaesthetic History, Melbourne, Australia, in my efforts to track down ownership of Figure 8.8. I am also grateful to Dr Westhorpe for giving me permission to use the image of the Kimpton Brown Flask used in Figure 8.9. I am grateful to Colonel Mike Stewart for allowing me to read his paper 'War Wound: The prevention of Infection in Battlefield Wounds and Fractures', which was the subject of his presentation for the Sir Gordon Gordon-Taylor Memorial Lecture at the Royal College of Surgeons of Edinburgh in 2012. I am grateful to Dr Pamela Molyneux for providing me with information relating to her late grandfather, Sir Lionel Whitby and to Neil Kerr for allowing me to use two of his late father's poems. I would also like to thank the organisations and institutes which have granted me permission to use images selected to illustrate the book. I have made strenuous efforts to establish ownership of every image I have used.

Preface

The purpose of this book is to examine important developments in the surgical management of wounded soldiers of the British Expeditionary Force in France and Flanders between 1914 and 1918. The work sets out to explain how improving treatment regimes delivered in casualty clearing stations, rather than at distant base hospitals near the French coast, resulted in much better outcomes. There were many ground-breaking developments in resuscitation, anaesthesia and surgery during the four years of conflict and the chances of surviving wounds of the limbs, skull and brain and of the chest and abdomen significantly improved as the war progressed. The work does not deal with patients who had facial wounds, since such individuals were evacuated to Great Britain where they underwent major reconstructive surgery extending over many months or years. The reader who wishes to learn more about the management of facial wounds is referred to the chapter written by John Holmes in *War Surgery 1914-18*[1] or to Dr Andrew Bamji's book on the subject.[2]

In the opening months of the Great War, medical officers were in possession of the knowledge and expertise passed on to them by their immediate predecessors of the late 19th and early 20th centuries, although unfortunately many important clinical or administrative skills acquired by men such as Sir James McGrigor, George James Guthrie and Baron Dominique Larrey during the early part of the 19th century had been forgotten. Most British military surgeons in 1914 were disciples of Joseph Lister and were schooled in the surgical practices of the Second Boer War. During this latter conflict, most wounds had been regarded as sterile. To ensure that they remained so, they were often sutured as soon as possible, and an antiseptic dressing applied to prevent harmful organisms from gaining access. Listerian principles were adopted in a similar way to deal with many casualties in 1914. Wounds were sutured and antiseptic dressings were applied in the dressing stations of field ambulances before patients were sent by hospital train to base hospitals for definitive surgery, a journey that sometimes took several days. Results were appalling and many wounded soldiers died as a result of overwhelming septic infections or from gas gangrene. It needed pioneering surgeons to challenge established doctrine and to introduce a new surgical procedure called wound excision to deal with multiple, filthy, contaminated wounds caused by high explosive shell fire or by rifle and machine gun bullet. These enterprising clinicians had to endure much opposition and hostility from those who lacked the vision to see beyond existing methods of treatment. It took some time before wound excision became

1 Scotland, T., Heys, S., *War Surgery 1914-18* (Solihull: Helion and Company, 2012).
2 Bamji, A., *Faces from the Front: Harold Gillies, the Queen's Hospital, Sidcup and the Origins of Modern Plastic Surgery* (Solihull: Helion and Company, 2017).

established as the new standard of care. Wound excision is quite simply the early radical removal of all devitalised and contaminated tissue, converting a filthy wound into a macroscopically clean one, thereby reducing the chances of overwhelming septic infection and gas gangrene and increasing the probability of survival.

For wound excision to become accepted, it required an acknowledgement that wounds sustained in the richly fertilised fields of France and Flanders were extremely filthy and were contaminated from the outset by deadly infecting organisms. Suturing such wounds in dressing stations of field ambulances ensured that these potentially lethal organisms were locked inside wounds, where conditions for their proliferation were ideal. In many cases, inappropriate immediate wound closure was a virtual death sentence and by the time definitive surgery was finally performed at base hospitals, it was far too late, since bacteria had become firmly established. Many soldiers succumbed to pyogenic (pus forming) infections caused by staphylococci, streptococci and by faecal organisms, there being no shortage of excrement on the battlefield. The presence of devitalised muscle, caused mainly by high explosives, was very common and this meant there was no oxygen in the affected tissues, giving the organisms responsible for gas gangrene the opportunity to thrive, often with deadly consequences for the patient.

In 1915, at Casualty Clearing Station Number 17 near Ypres, Geoffrey Marshall documented a mortality rate of 90 percent in patients undergoing above knee amputations for completely mangled and grossly infected lower limbs, and who were in a state of circulatory collapse at presentation. Wounds had been sustained many hours and sometimes days before surgery and the general condition of the patients was very poor. These men were suffering from the effects of shock caused by blood loss (surgical shock) to which was often added the impact of shock due to superimposed infection (septic shock). More than one hundred years previously, in the pre-anaesthetic era, Peninsular War surgeon George James Guthrie published his results for a series of 128 soldiers who had undergone very early lower limb amputations after being removed from the battlefield, quoting an operative mortality of 15 percent. His operative mortality figure for late lower limb amputations, performed after a couple of days once inflammation (infection) had become established was 58 percent, proving conclusively that early surgery was beneficial and increased the chances of survival. Had Guthrie's work been better appreciated, and had steps been taken in 1914 to emulate his practice, ensuring that definitive surgery was delivered as soon as possible after the infliction of wounds, results in the early months of the war would have been much better than they were. Lessons had to be relearned unfortunately, as is so often the case.

As time went by, ways *were* sought to deliver surgical care as soon as possible, at first in casualty clearing stations and latterly in the main dressing stations of field ambulances, when Australian Medical Services introduced Field Ambulance Resuscitation Teams after the re-establishment of mobile warfare in the spring of 1918. Early surgical intervention saved lives in two fundamental ways. The first was to stop severe bleeding and the second was to prevent sepsis, the latter being the biggest killer in patients surviving for more than a few hours, regardless of whether their wounds were in their brains, their chests and abdomens or their limbs.

Since many important advances were made in surgery during the Great War, particularly in the treatment of fractures, it would be reasonable to suppose that clinical progress made during the conflict would translate seamlessly into civilian practice afterwards by ensuring that clinicians who had learned important lessons from their wartime experience could use their hard earned skills to maintain the standards achieved and to make further progress. While this was true of surgery as it affected the brain, the chest and the abdomen, the treatment of fractures made little progress in Britain during the inter-war years, because general surgeons who had managed (or in many cases mismanaged) fractures before August 1914, ensured that they continued to look after them once the conflict was over. A powerful lobby of general surgeons led by those in the big London teaching hospitals was resentful of the success enjoyed by orthopaedic surgeons between 1914-18 and this surgical lobby fought doggedly to retain the treatment of fractures, setting orthopaedic surgery in Britain back by a quarter of a century or more. Thankfully, the efforts of a few determined individuals prevailed, and orthopaedic surgeons finally gained control of fracture treatment after a long and sometimes bitter struggle.

1

A Time to Die and a Time to Live

A Time to Die

It was 13 November 1914. The boy shivered uncontrollably as his stretcher was lifted from the hospital train and was transferred to the ambulance wagon which transported him the short distance to the general hospital in Rouen. He was barely conscious and incapable of communicating in a coherent way with the stretcher bearers who carried him to his bed. He had been wounded during heavy fighting near Ypres two days before while playing his part in defending a shallow trench against a determined attack by German forces near Polygon Wood, where Prussian Guardsmen had tried to break through his position and capture the small city of Ypres a couple of miles behind the British line. Beneath some stinking dressings, his right forefoot was badly damaged with much skin loss and he had an open fracture dislocation of his right ankle. He had suffered appalling pain every time this leg was jolted or twisted on the long journey from his shallow trench to the advanced dressing station, then onward to the casualty clearing hospital, before he was finally put onto a hospital train. Injections of morphine partly controlled his agony, for a time at least, but they made him confused and the pain always came back to sap his fading energy.

There was also a terrible problem brewing in his left thigh. A medical officer at the advanced dressing station had sutured a wound on its outer aspect midway between his knee and his hip and had wrapped an antiseptic dressing firmly round the thigh. The ward sister in the general hospital looked sadly at the boy as she removed the dressing and saw that there were many closely spaced sutures which were now straining and fit to burst. His whole thigh was horribly swollen to more than twice its normal size and was very red. Nothing had been written in his very brief record to describe the nature of the wound or if anything had been found within it before stitching it up.

The consulting surgeon standing behind the sister groaned with dismay when he saw how far gone the boy was. He had dealt with many similar cases resulting from the fierce fighting which had been going on around Ypres since mid-October. So many young men had arrived at his base hospital in a similar state. It had taken them far too long to get there. For many it was too late, and they had died as a result of overwhelming septic infections or of gas gangrene.

"Good God Almighty!" the surgeon exclaimed, looking at the boy's left thigh. "What kind of idiot stitches up filthy contaminated wounds like this and then chucks poor boys onto a train, expecting me to sort out their mess? Are supposedly intelligent surgeons still stuck in the days of the Boer War, believing that wounds should be sutured to prevent infection getting in? Don't they realise that everything has changed? In this war we are dealing with filthy contaminated wounds sustained in heavily manured fields. Wounds aren't caused by the supposedly 'humane bullets' of the Boer War.[1] They are caused by exploding shells which rip through human tissue, destroying everything in their path. You never got wounds like this in the Boer War."

While the consultant was busy working himself into a rage at the incompetence of others, one of his juniors inserted a rubber catheter through the boy's anus into his rectum and connected it by a length of rubber tubing to a bottle of isotonic saline in order to replace much needed fluid. Saline is readily absorbed through the rectal mucosa into the circulation, although unfortunately once there, it escapes just as quickly. For good measure, the young medical officer put a hollow needle into the skin fold below the boy's right arm pit and connected it to a bottle of normal saline to run the solution into the subcutaneous tissue, in the hope that it too would be absorbed and improve the boy's condition. In 1915, this method of treatment was discredited by a physician called Geoffrey Marshall, who was working as an anaesthetist in a casualty clearing station near Ypres. Medical officers in 1914 had little idea of the consequences of severe blood loss and how to deal with them and the next four years would turn out to be a painful and difficult learning curve. For the time being, however, the measures the young doctor had taken were the only ones available.

The boy's systolic blood pressure was below 80 and his pulse, barely palpable, was around 140/minute. The surgeon shook his head as he palpated the boy's left thigh. It was very tense and felt as tight as a drum. He looked at the right leg. The foot was obviously dead, as were the muscles visible in the wound extending from his ankle to the mid-calf. He palpated upwards towards the knee and to the lower thigh, where he stopped in his tracks. He could feel crepitus, a fine crackling beneath his gently examining fingers. He knew full well that this meant gas gangrene. Caused by the organism Clostridium Perfringens, gas gangrene is associated with the formation of bubbles of gas in the tissues as the infection spreads rapidly along muscle fibres, releasing a deadly toxin and producing further muscle destruction as it gallops inexorably onwards. The only treatment which just might save the boy's life would be a high thigh amputation, but the surgeon knew from bitter experience that the outlook was practically hopeless. Nevertheless, he felt duty bound to give it a try. He could have given the boy some more morphine and left him to die. It wouldn't have taken long, but he was only nineteen after all, and some poor mother's son.

Minutes later, the surgeon was scrubbed in theatre with his assistant, waiting impatiently for the anaesthetist to put the patient under, which he did with ether dripped onto an open mask. The surgeon began. He decided to deal with the left thigh first. He had to move fast. He removed the sutures and plunged his hand into the wound. Immediately, a river of pus poured from the wound and gushed over his protective apron onto the floor. The stench of putrefaction was terrible. He extended the incision from hip to knee immediately, saying to his young assistant 'Always make your incision twice as big as you think you'll need to, then you won't have to enlarge it much'. Recently arrived in France and unaccustomed to such sights and smells, his junior colleague promptly fainted. An observant orderly caught him before he hit the back of his head on the floor, and after ascertaining that he was alright, scrubbed up to assist

1 Most wounds inflicted by the Boers were caused by bullets fired from long range which were believed to be less traumatic to the tissues.

the surgeon, who by then had removed all necrotic tissue and a large fragment of shell casing from the thigh wound and had irrigated it with saline. Now he was calling for the antiseptic EUSOL (Edinburgh University Solution of Lime) in the hope that the disinfectant would kill the bacteria which had colonised the wound. Likely infecting organisms were staphylococci, judging by the smell of the pus, although they could be streptococci or faecal organisms. There was always plenty of shit on the battlefield. The surgeon hated using antiseptics. He felt they were of little use. The best way to deal with contaminated wounds was to prevent severe sepsis such as this by completely excising all dead and contaminated tissue as soon as possible after the infliction of wounds before bacteria had a chance to become established.

Following this, he turned his attention to the right leg and performed a high thigh amputation in the hope of getting clear of the rapidly advancing gangrene. The stumps of muscles close to the hip joint looked alright. He very loosely apposed the skin edges with a couple of loosely tied sutures and the procedure was finished. The entire operation from beginning to end had taken him less than three quarters of an hour. The young anaesthetist had already stopped dripping ether onto the mask and was hoping for the best. He had never intended to spend his life putting patients to sleep. In civilian life before the war he was training to become a physician, but there were very few trained anaesthetists in 1914.

The boy never regained consciousness. He died during the night with the night sister in attendance. She wrote a kindly letter to the boy's mother, explaining what had happened to her only son and that the surgeon had done his best. The surgeon meanwhile was outside, ostensibly getting some fresh air but all the while puffing vigorously on a pretty foul cigar. He was careful not to let anyone see the tears of frustration and anguish running down his cheek caused by yet another avoidable death. He pledged to himself that he would make every effort do something to put a stop to this dreadful sort of thing happening in future.

A Time to Live

It was 4 July 1918. The young soldier was content. He felt no pain and was barely aware of the stretcher bearers as they carried him towards the dressing station. He thought fleetingly that he must have been in a battle, but that was of no concern to him now. He was imagining himself back home in Australia on the farm with his widowed mother and two younger brothers. "What will they be doing now, I wonder?" He sighed repeatedly, gasping for air but unable to get enough oxygen into his lungs. He felt dizzy and had an overwhelming feeling of fatigue. He decided there was no point in fighting it, so he would take a nap for a few minutes and drifted imperceptibly into unconsciousness.

He awoke with a start as the stretcher bearers put down their load with a bump at the shelter close to the entrance of the dressing station. One of the stretcher bearers looked at his watch. It was just after 0600. The Battle of Hamel had begun less than three hours ago at 0310. The other attendant walked quickly through the entrance into the receiving room where two trained orderlies were assessing the wounded who had now just begun to arrive. He approached them and said he had an urgent case, a young lad who had been badly wounded in both legs. They brought him quickly into the receiving room. The dressing station orderly looked at the boy who was very pale with beads of perspiration on his white and clammy forehead. The boot on his right foot had been blown off and the mid-foot and fore-foot were reduced to pulp. Only his devitalised big toe was recognisable, hanging on by a strand of tendon. The bones of his dislocated ankle joint were visible, as was his shattered lower tibia, impregnated with bits of shrapnel, grass, earth and something that looked suspiciously like a piece of someone else's skull. The leg was bleeding profusely from damaged blood vessels around mid-calf.

The khaki trousers covering his left thigh had a large rent in them and blood had seeped through onto the stretcher beneath and was now dripping onto the floor, creating an expanding crimson puddle. "Quick," cried the orderly, "we need to get this one through to the operating theatre and let the surgeon see him. Otherwise we'll lose him." They grabbed the stretcher and rushed into the operating theatre, which was within a designated section of the treatment room at the heart of the dressing station. It was laid out with an array of instruments for performing surgical procedures and nitrous oxide and oxygen cylinders for administering general anaesthetics.

The young soldier woke from his dream-like state. He was aware of his trousers being cut using a pair of scissors and someone was removing his tunic to expose his chest and arms. He made some clumsy movements to help but was so weak that he was unable to make any useful contribution before drifting into unconsciousness again. There were two medical officers standing over him. One was skilled in resuscitation and in administering anaesthetics, while the other was an experienced surgeon, capable of making important decisions very quickly and able to perform urgent operative procedures. They were members of a newly established Field Ambulance Resuscitation Team which Australian Medical Services had developed in response to the restoration of mobile warfare in 1918. Their aim was to deliver limb and life-saving surgery in their medical headquarters at the main dressing station (MDS) at Les Alençons near Amiens. There was an ambulance wagon standing outside and at their disposal in case they were required further forward at an advanced dressing station even closer to the front line. Four orderlies trained in general resuscitation were part of the team and they had all the equipment necessary to perform their various tasks. An orderly applied a very substantial and firm dressing to the boy's shattered right leg to temporarily stop the bleeding by direct pressure.

One of the medical officers who was the surgeon checked the boy's pulse and blood pressure. The pulse was 140/minute and was so weak that it was barely palpable. The systolic blood pressure was 80 mm. Hg and he was clearly in a state of shock due to blood loss. Examination of his chest, abdomen and pelvis revealed no abnormality and there was no evidence of any head injury. The boy's only wounds were those already found, so that was something at least. The surgeon decided on the course of action he must take to save the boy's life. He would have to take off the boy's right leg, hopefully getting away with a below knee amputation and he would have to excise the wound on his left thigh.

Whilst the first medical officer was making his assessment, the other found a good vein in front of the boy's elbow and inserted a metal cannula into the vessel. He attached the cannula to a litre bottle of saline via a decent length of sterile rubber tubing and ran the saline into the boy's arm quite quickly till the bottle was empty. He knew from experience that any beneficial rise in blood pressure would be transient, because saline escapes very quickly from the tiniest blood vessels, called capillaries, into the interstitial tissues between the body's cells, pushed out by hydrostatic pressure. Next he ran in sodium bicarbonate to counteract the effect of acidosis caused by a build up of lactic acid in the tissues which would further compromise the state of their shocked patient. Then he reached for a bottle of Gum Arabica in saline to act as a blood volume expander, because it remains within the circulation rather than escaping into the surrounding tissues like saline.[2] What the boy needed most, however, was blood to replace the considerable amount he had lost. The medical officer went over to a wooden icebox standing in the corner and removed one of several bottles of preserved blood which were inside it.[3] He looked at the blood, which was in two definite layers. The bottom layer was dark red and consisted of the red blood cells which had settled. The top layer was straw coloured supernatant fluid. After taking it from the ice box, he had to first remove the supernatant by siphoning it off, before replacing it with 2.5 percent gelatine and saline solution to make it up to a litre. After preparing the blood he connected it to the patient and began the transfusion.

Had the opportunity arisen, he would have preferred transfusing fresh blood from a lightly wounded donor, but this required a supply of suitable donors and it took time to do the necessary tests to establish their blood groups. He would also have had to do a blood test on the badly wounded boy to make sure his group was compatible with the proposed donor otherwise a serious transfusion reaction or even death might result. Since their patient was one of the first casualties to arrive, and there were therefore no potential fresh blood donors, his only option was to use preserved blood.

The boy's pulse became stronger and his blood pressure began to rise. He regained consciousness, was less pale and was better perfused. It was now safe to operate. After reassuring the boy that all would be well, the medical officer administering the anaesthetic held a mask to the boy's face and gave him a mixture of nitrous oxide and oxygen. Other anaesthetic drugs were available, but for very severely wounded soldiers who had lost a lot of blood and were in surgical shock, nitrous oxide and oxygen were the safest agents to use. Recovery from nitrous oxide/oxygen anaesthesia was rapid, which meant that the wounded soldiers could be evacuated from the MDS very soon after surgery, making room for other casualties in need of urgent help. Use of other agents such as ether or chloroform in such circumstances was fraught with difficulty, delay and danger.

The surgeon scrubbed up to make a start with one of the orderlies assisting him. They wore aprons and sterile gowns over their uniforms and used surgical gloves, although many surgeons at the time still operated in their bare hands. The firm padding was removed from the right leg and blood immediately welled up from the wound. 'It's no use," he said, "I can't see a bloody thing. You'll need to put a tourniquet on." He elevated the leg and an orderly applied a tourniquet around the mid-thigh, noting the time. Now able to see, the surgeon disinfected the skin with 3% solution of picric acid in spirit before fashioning skin flaps and began performing a below knee amputation, resecting all the damaged muscle in

2 Gum Arabica is an inert complex high molecular weight polymer of polysaccharides (carbohydrate with sugar molecules bound together) and glycoproteins (protein with carbohydrate chains bound to the molecules), which was shown by scientific experiment in 1916, and by clinical application in 1917, to remain in the circulation and assist combat shock.

3 An American doctor in the US Army, Oswald Hope Robertson, had discovered that blood taken from a donor and mixed with dextrose to provide nutrition for the oxygen carrying red blood cells and with sodium citrate to stop the blood clotting, could be preserved for up to 26 days provided it was kept cold. Robertson used donors with Group IV blood, which we now call Group O. This is the universal donor group, which means that Group IV or O can be safely transfused into any patient, regardless of that patient's own blood group, because no antibodies will form and there will be no transfusion reaction. In the heat of battle, this was very important because it meant that no time-consuming blood test was required to ascertain the blood group of the recipient.

the calf as well as removing the ankle and foot. He found the posterior tibial artery and vein, which had holes in the side of them and had been the source of most of the bleeding. He tied them off to secure haemostasis. He used a saw to transect the tibia around twelve centimetres below the knee joint and cut though the fibula at the same level with bone cutters. He was very pleased to note that the remaining muscle stumps below the knee looked healthy, although he wouldn't know for sure until he took the tourniquet off. His principal concern had been that a below knee amputation might not be enough. It had been an easy decision to amputate. Much good work had been done to show that the sooner a mangled limb was taken off, the better it was for the patient. The clinical condition of the victim usually improved significantly straight away following its removal. The tricky bit was to decide at what level to amputate. It was clear from the outset that the lower part of the leg was unsalvageable, but he was a bit doubtful about the viability of the calf muscles. 'Right boys, you can take the tourniquet off now', he said, putting a pad of swabs over the stump till he was sure he had controlled the bleeding. He whistled softly to himself, which was the way he coped with the incredible stress he was under. Every surgeon has a way of dealing with these occasions to avoid letting others detect his or her anxiety. Then, ever so slowly, he removed the pad. "Thank Christ, the bleeding's stopped", he said. He checked one final time that all dead muscle had been resected, now that the tourniquet was off. Everything looked fine. The muscle stumps were nice and pink with little bleeding vessels appearing all over their cut surfaces and the skin too was pink. "Thank Christ" he said again. The surgeon was now confident he would get away with a below knee amputation which was much better for the boy than an amputation through the thigh. Rehabilitation is much faster for a below knee as opposed to an above knee amputation. He very loosely apposed the muscle and skin flaps, making sure the two or three sutures he used were not tight. There must be no build-up of pressure within the stump. Finally, he applied a padded dressing. While doing this amputation, he had just performed wound excision, which is the removal of *all* devitalised and contaminated tissue. In this instance, wound excision had necessitated the removal of a dead ankle and foot. Without doubt, wound excision was the single most important operation to be developed during the Great War. Early wound excision greatly reduced the probability of major infections caused by pus forming organisms and by the organisms responsible for gas gangrene. The procedure was pioneered by two surgeons, Henry Gray, a Scot from Aberdeen and Edward Milligan, an Australian from Melbourne, back in 1914 and early 1915.

Next the surgeon directed his attention to the left thigh, where there was a ragged hole in the skin on the lateral (outer) side of the thigh with soil and debris around its margins. He excised the skin edges of the penetrating wound before extending it by making an incision for several inches upwards towards the hip and another of equal distance downwards towards the knee. He systematically removed huge chunks of dead muscle from the lateral compartment of the thigh until all that was left was healthy bleeding tissue. At the bottom of the wound, lying adjacent to the femur but fortunately not damaging it, was a piece of shell casing, with several fragments of the boy's uniform lying close by. The surgeon removed the foreign bodies and washed the thigh out with two litres of saline before doing a final check to see if everything looked healthy. He was confident he had performed a complete wound excision. He might have closed the wound primarily but decided it would be safer to leave it open for the time being before applying a dressing. The wound would have to be looked at in a casualty clearing station in a couple of days, and if everything was fine, closed formally by delayed primary closure. The same applied to the amputation stump on the other side.

The operation was over. The anaesthetist gave the patient an injection of omnopon to help combat post-operative pain, and switched off the nitrous oxide, keeping the oxygen going till the boy had wakened up. The patient looked up at the members of the team who had saved his life, although he was not aware of it at the time. He didn't even realise that he had lost his right leg. At least he would get home to Australia to his mother and his brothers. Many less fortunate than he would not. "Thanks," he said, as they wheeled him out of the treatment room. "No worries cobber," said the surgeon.

In this chapter I have described two clinical scenarios, one from 1914 and the other from 1918, to illustrate how two patients with similar wounds had very different outcomes. Both cases are made up, but they could just as easily have been factual, since I based their clinical presentations on the types of cases seen and on existing knowledge and expertise at the time.

The surgeon referred to in the 1914 case is modelled on the character of Henry Gray, referred to above. Gray spent three and a half years in France, at first in charge of a group of base hospitals in Rouen, and then from 1917, he was Consulting Surgeon to the British Third Army. Gray was a fiery and volatile character, who was very forceful and did not suffer fools gladly, especially when they happened to be surgical establishment figures from London. This unfortunately led him to make many enemies amongst his peers. At the same time, he was loved and respected very much by young surgeons working in casualty clearing stations because he was very supportive of them, helping them with very difficult cases. He was certainly one of the best surgeons to serve his country in France during the four years of conflict. I will return to Henry Gray in later chapters to explain his many contributions in full. He certainly went on to fulfil his pledge to do his very best to stop patients arriving in base hospitals in a moribund state as a result of overwhelming sepsis caused by dreadful initial management and totally unacceptable delay.[4]

By 1918, Australian Medical Services had developed Field Ambulance Resuscitation Teams in response to the restoration of mobile warfare. A Resuscitation Team was first used at the Battle of Hamel on 4 July 1918 and the person most responsible for its development was Dr Alan Holmes à Court, a Major in the 4th Australian Field Ambulance. Holmes à Court would have been one of the two medical officers in the case presentation. He had particular expertise in blood transfusion and anaesthesia. The Field Ambulance Resuscitation Team proved to be so successful that very soon all five Australian Divisions had similar teams to deal with urgent cases. Australians had developed a standardised advanced dressing station which could be assembled and dismantled quickly and could be carried in three lorries to where it was needed. When there was an infantry advance, what had been the main dressing station (MDS) could leapfrog over the original advanced dressing station (ADS) to become the new ADS. In this way, the ADS always remained in close contact with the battle front. The Field Ambulance Resuscitation Teams were based in the MDS to deal with patients requiring resuscitation, arrest of bleeding from otherwise salvable limbs and emergency amputations in limbs doomed from the outset.

4 Scotland, T., Boyer, A., *Henry Gray, Surgeon of the Great War: Saving Lives in a Theatre of Destruction*, (Edinburgh: Capercaillie, 2015).

Chapter 2 deals with individuals who made landmark discoveries during the 19th Century, or displayed outstanding administrative skills, or made important advances in the practice of medicine and surgery, and whose contributions greatly influenced how medical services were organised and delivered at the outbreak of the Great War in 1914. It aims to provide the reader with an appreciation of the starting point from which so many developments took place during the four years of conflict and which by 1918 had completely transformed the treatment of wounded soldiers.

2

Key developments in the 19th century and their impact on management of the wounded in 1914

In proper execution of their duties, medical officers are frequently under fire and during the late war the cases of wounded medical officers were numerous. Some had been killed and not a few lost limbs in sieges or battles. Yet it has ignorantly been advanced by some military men that the medical officers have no business in exposed situations and in this professed opinion they would deny the medical officer a pension for the loss of a limb. Yet it is well known that the cases are numerous wherein the lives of officers and soldiers have been saved by the zealous medical officers of their regiments being at hand to suppress haemorrhage. In alleviating pain, it is no small advantage to have the surgeon at hand to extract cloth, splinters etc. Circumstances may subsequently prevent this being done till a long period afterwards, when the state of inflammation has been considerably advanced and when their extraction must necessarily be attended with infinitely more pain; whereas, by promptness, life or limb might have been saved, especially the former, as at an early period, amputation would have been successful.[1]

The above observations on the speed with which war wounds are treated were made by Sir James McGrigor, who was Sir Arthur Wellesley's Chief Medical Officer in the Peninsular War between December 1811 and June 1814. Wellesley became the Duke of Wellington following the exile of Napoleon Bonaparte on Elba in 1814. McGrigor's remarks could have been equally applicable to the First World War between 1914 and 1918 and to every conflict before and since. The aim of this chapter is to make the reader aware of very important advances which were made in medicine and surgery during the 19th century and to demonstrate how these advances influenced, or in some cases, failed to influence military surgical practice in 1914 at the outbreak of the Great War. There were many individuals who made outstanding contributions to medical science during the 19th century. They may have had particular administrative skills, or shown great clinical expertise, or made a discovery which changed the face of medicine forever. Whatever they achieved helped to provide personnel of the Royal Army Corps in 1914 with the scientific background and clinical expertise to do the best they could when they were confronted by dreadful wounds, the likes of which had never been seen before.

1 McGrigor, Mary (ed.), *Sir James McGrigor, The Scalpel and the Sword; the Autobiography of the Father of Army Medicine,* (Dalkeith: Scottish Cultural Press, 2000), pp. 229-230.

Volume II of the *Official History of Australian Medical Services of the war of 1914-18* was published in 1940.[2] Its author was military historian Arthur Graham Butler, who served with distinction as a medical officer with the Australian Imperial Force at Gallipoli in 1915, then on the Western Front at Arras and Ypres in 1917. By 1918, the Director of Medical Services, AIF, was Major General Sir Neville Howse, VC, whom Butler regarded as the most capable medical officer of his day. In the Official History, Butler makes a direct comparison between Howse and his two most outstanding counterparts from the early 19th century, James McGrigor and Baron Dominique Larrey. Here is what Butler had to say about them:

> It may be doubted whether, since Baron Larrey directed medical affairs for Napoleon and Sir James McGrigor for Wellington, any head of a medical service has gained so completely the confidence of the military command, or exercised so great a personal influence in military affairs as did Surgeon- General Howse within the scope of the A.I.F. And it is a matter of more than passing interest to observe that, in each instance, the same causes operated to bring this about, namely, the combination of great professional and administrative ability with qualities of more directly military significance- personal courage and battle-sense, and flair as a soldier and 'man of affairs' for understanding and dealing with the problems not only of campaigns but also of the home front.[3]

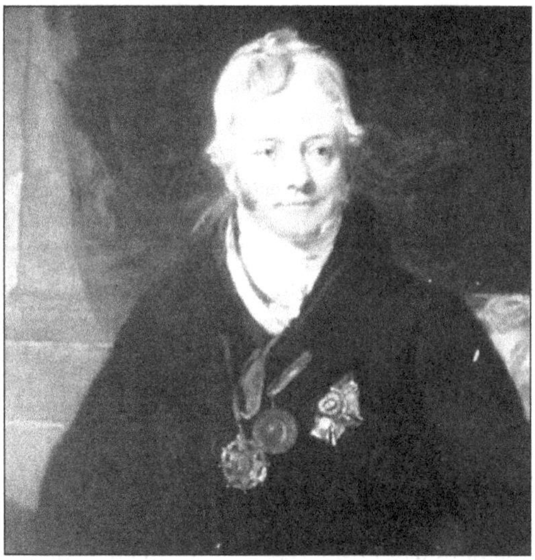

Figure 2.1 Portrait of Sir James McGrigor (1771-1858) by Andrew Geddes. (Courtesy of Aberdeen Medico-Chirurgical Society)

James McGrigor was born in the small village of Cromdale in the north east of Scotland. His father was a wealthy merchant in Aberdeen, where the young McGrigor grew up and attended Aberdeen Grammar School. He went to Marischal College, part of the University of Aberdeen, from where he graduated Master of Arts before enrolling to study medicine. He spent three years working at Aberdeen Royal Infirmary before going to Edinburgh for one year, where he studied under the great anatomist Monro Secundus, the second of three generations bearing the name Monro. McGrigor joined the army in 1794 as a regimental surgeon with the Connaught Rangers. He had an eventful early career with postings in Flanders and the West Indies where his outstanding ability was noted. There followed a series of rapid promotions, culminating in December 1811 with his appointment as Chief Medical Officer to Sir Arthur Wellesley (later the Duke of Wellington) in the latter stages of the Peninsular War campaign. The Peninsular War (1807–14)

2 Butler, Arthur G., *Official History of the Australian Army Medical Services in the war of 1914–1918 Volume II – The Western Front*, (Canberra: Australian War Memorial, 1940).

3 Butler, *Official History*, Vol. II, p. 803.

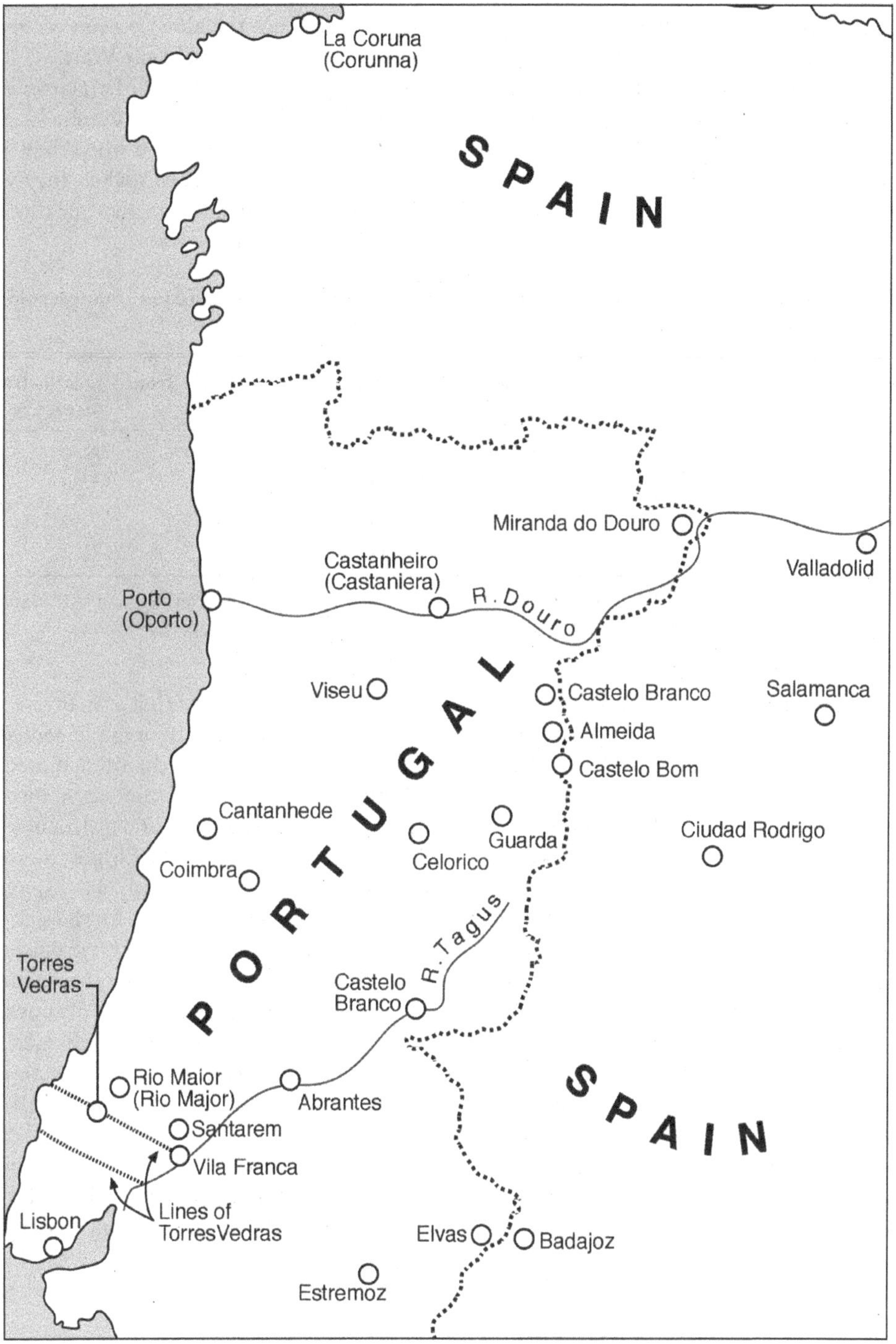

Figure 2.2 Map of Spain and Portugal showing important locations for Peninsular War. (With thanks to Gordon Stables, Department of Medical Illustration, University of Aberdeen)

was a military conflict between Napoleon Bonaparte's empire and the allied powers of Spain, Britain and Portugal, for control of the Iberian Peninsula during the Napoleonic Wars.

McGrigor's organisational and administrative skills were outstanding and he enjoyed the complete confidence of Wellesley. As a medical officer, he had two principal duties. He was responsible for the wellbeing of the men, who were his patients, treating them when they were sick or wounded and helping them avoid catching potentially lethal diseases when they were healthy. Many of the ailments which affected soldiers frequently resulted in their deaths and four times as many soldiers died from disease as succumbed to wounds.[4]

Table 2.1 Figures summarising deaths from disease and deaths from enemy action amongst soldiers admitted to regimental and general hospitals in 1812, 1813 and 1814

Year	Total treated	Total deaths	Deaths from wounds	Deaths from wounds %	Deaths from disease	Deaths from disease %
1812	176,180	7,193	944	13.1	6,249	86.9
1813	123,019	6,866	1564	22.8	5,302	77.2
1814	53,073	2,909	845	29.0	2,064	71.0
Total	352,272	16,968	3,353	19.8	13,615	80.2

McGrigor, James, Sketch of the Medical History of the British Armies in the Peninsula of Spain and Portugal during the late campaigns, *Medico Chirurgical Transactions*, 6 (1815), pp.482-486.

McGrigor also had a responsibility to his commanding officer, to ensure that as many men as possible were available to fight, thus enabling Wellesley to wage war. McGrigor implemented all the measures about to be described to fulfil his dual responsibilities. He redistributed medical personnel more effectively. When he arrived in Portugal, there were far too many medical officers 'working' at base hospitals in Lisbon, spending time with their wives and girlfriends and too few enduring the hardships of looking after soldiers at the battle front. McGrigor improved the distribution of various supplies which had been stockpiled very inefficiently. He expanded regimental hospital systems closer to the front, providing more rapid treatment for the sick and wounded and avoiding energy sapping journeys to more distant base hospitals. He established a regulation at Coimbra (Figure 2.2) soon after he arrived in Portugal, segregating the sick from the wounded and subsequently applied it to all other hospitals. He opened a series of convalescent hospitals after observing that many soldiers suffering from diseases were discharged too soon back to cold and overcrowded barracks, only to suffer fatal relapses. Soldiers were now to spend three weeks in convalescent units where they had a greater chance of making a full recovery, and where medical officers could keep a close eye on them and look out for any recurrence of symptoms. McGrigor reduced hospital overcrowding and had wooden huts transported from Britain to accommodate the sick and wounded, who were also supplied with bunk beds to replace the straw on which they had lain previously. This reduced the incidence of typhus

4 McGrigor, James, "Sketch of the Medical History of the British Armies in the Peninsula of Spain and Portugal during the late campaigns , Medico Chirurgical Transactions 6 (1815), pp. 482-486.

fever and of hospital gangrene. The latter was contagious and could spread very rapidly from the wound of one patient to that of a neighbour in the adjacent bed. McGrigor observed:

> I may say of the whole of our hospitals in the Peninsula as well as of this station (Celorico) that at all times the utmost cleanliness of the wards and bedding and especially of the persons and linen of the patients have now been rigidly enforced. We regard cleanliness and ventilation not only as means of cure and of comfort but as essentially requisite to prevent contagion.[5]

Hospital gangrene

Hospital gangrene was a very serious contagious wound infection, and descriptions of it suggest that it was probably caused by a virulent streptococcus, although McGrigor was ignorant of the existence of bacteria, which only became recognised in 1865 with the work of Louis Pasteur. John Bell (1763-1820) was a prominent Edinburgh-trained surgeon who described the typical course of the disease. A patient with a wound would at first make satisfactory progress and then, after a few days, everything would go wrong. The wound would break down and form a deep ulcer which had its origin in small beginnings.[6] Bell described what happened during the development of this progressive, ulcerating lesion as follows:

> The sore inflames, then come vomiting, diarrhoea and a distinct fever, and the disease seizes plainly in the wound part. In the first day, the wound swells, the skin retracts, wastes, has a dark erysipelatous redness verging to black, the cellular membrane is melted down into a foetid mucus, and the fascia is exposed but, in the second stage, the fascia and skin unable to bear the inflammation, and deprived of mutual support, become black, foetid, soft and fall into perfect gangrene.[7]

Bell continued:

> If the patient is to die, the gangrene proceeds; the skin first sloughs off; then the fascia which dive between the muscles to enclose, protect and nourish them are next affected; the muscles are divided from each other more and more. In many you could have laid your hand edge-ways betwixt the several muscles of the thigh. Then the vomiting, diarrhoea, and nervous systems increase, the pain is dreadful; they are exhausted in the course of a week and die.[8]

Bell's description is of a condition we recognise today as necrotising fasciitis, which is most commonly seen when it occurs as a complication of intravenous drug abuse using contaminated, dirty needles. There is extensive and rapidly spreading infection within the skin and subcutaneous

5 McGrigor, Mary, *The Scalpel and the Sword*, p. 218.
6 Bell, John, *The Principles of Surgery in Two Volumes*, (Edinburgh: For T. Cadell & N. Davies; T.N. Longman & O. Rees & others, 1801), pp.107-109.
7 Bell, *The Principles of Surgery* in Two Volumes, pp. 107-109.
8 Bell, *The Principles of Surgery in Two Volumes*, pp. 107-109.

planes, which quickly involves the deep fascia, and sub-fascial plane, before running unchecked through muscle planes, culminating in the death of the body tissues it affects. Septicaemia, circulatory collapse and death may occur. When it produces this aggressive clinical picture, the organism is referred to in lay terms as "a flesh-eating bug", a descriptive yet fitting term. This must have been similar to how hospital gangrene presented in the 19th century.

One hundred years later, Sir Anthony Bowlby, Senior Consulting Surgeon to the British Expeditionary Force during the Great War had never seen hospital gangrene when he declared: "True hospital gangrene, or sloughing phagadaena, I have neither seen nor heard of in any hospital in France."[9]

While Bowlby never saw hospital gangrene typical of that of the 19th century, he most certainly did see cases suffering from another major infection known as gas gangrene, a completely separate entity caused by the organism Clostridium Perfringens, which only grows in dead tissue where there is no oxygen. The infection causes further massive tissue destruction as it spreads rapidly along tissue planes, producing toxins as it does so which frequently cause death. Gas gangrene was a major problem during the Great War and is discussed in Chapter 4.

Epidemics of hospital gangrene were all too common during the Peninsular War in overcrowded wards. There was a serious outbreak of hospital gangrene in February 1813 at Ciudad Rodrigo in Spain, but in 1814 following the Battle of Toulouse there were no recorded cases of the disease. This was attributable to greatly improved facilities provided by James McGrigor.

Contagion, which is the transmission of disease from one person to another by direct contact between those persons or by things belonging to them, often played a part in the transmission of diseases, although their causes remained obscure, being attributed in varying degree to intemperance, exposure to excesses in temperature, and miasma, which was foul smelling marsh vapour from putrefying organic matter. McGrigor thought that typhus fever was contagious, but it is not. Typhus is a louse borne disease, prevalent in squalid, overcrowded conditions, and caused by a micro-organism called Rickettsia Prowazekii. A Brazilian doctor called Henrique da Rocha Lima isolated the micro-organism responsible for typhus fever in 1916. He named it after his colleague Stanislaus von Prowazekii, who had died of typhus in Hamburg in1915 where both men had been carrying out research at a prison hospital to investigate the cause of the disease. While McGrigor was ignorant of its cause, he reduced the incidence of typhus and saved lives by reducing overcrowding.

McGrigor's skills were tested to the limit when Wellesley's army was forced to retreat from Spain into Portugal after the Battle of Salamanca in July 1812, rather than risk being cut off by numerically superior French forces. During a prolonged and arduous withdrawal, the sick rate rose from a baseline 25% ration strength in June 1812 to 37% ration strength in October of that year. By using all his skills, McGrigor restored the army to health over the winter months and by April 1813 the sick rate was down to 20%. This made many men available to fight and thus enabled Wellesley to take the initiative in the spring of 1813.

Previous documentation of battle and non-battle casualties was poor and McGrigor rectified this. He was a meticulous collector of statistics and was able to meet with Wellesley every day to give him a precise account of the army's fighting strength.

9 Bowlby, A., The work of the clearing hospitals during the past six weeks, *British Medical Journal*, 2:2816 (19 December 1914), pp. 1053-1054.

A comparison can readily be drawn between the impact made by measures introduced by McGrigor in the Peninsular War during the winter of 1812-1813 and efforts made by medical personnel of the five British Armies in 1918 to minimise wastage from disease at a time when men were in precariously short supply. Australian Medical Services used every means at their disposal to minimise such losses, enabling their infantry to attack very effectively between August and October 1918. This explains why Butler refers to McGrigor in such glowing terms in the Official History of Australian Medical Services.

When he became Director General of Army Medical Services in 1815, McGrigor insisted that every medical officer, wherever he might be in the Empire, should complete regular returns for sickness and disease for the troops under his care. These returns were sent initially to the Principal Medical Officer of the colony before being sent onwards to the Director General in Britain. McGrigor declared:

> Perhaps it may be thought that I have descended to a degree of minuteness: however, I conceive, that, from the facts stated, important and useful deductions may be made. I think it a matter of regret that such journals are not more frequently kept; with a little industry on the part of the profession they might always be so. Had such records been always faithfully kept, many practical points would not, as they now are, be involved in doubt and uncertainty. We should not now be so ignorant of some diseases, of the countries where we have so often made campaigns, or of which we have so long been in possession. Humble as the labours may seem, and confined as the abilities of an individual may be, were he only faithfully to relate observations made with care, to compare them with those of his contemporaries, and by them to correct the opinions of his predecessors, he would perform no mean service to his art.[10]

McGrigor's diligence was rewarded in 1838, when two statisticians called Henry Marshall and Alexander Tulloch used the data collected to publish a groundbreaking work, *Statistical report on the mortality and invaliding among the troops in the West Indies,* published in 1838.[11] The West Indies was one of the most dangerous places to be posted and soldiers could fall victim to many diseases including dysentery, typhus and yellow fever, or yellow jack as it was known. Marshall and Tulloch disproved the erroneous notions of temperature variations and miasma as causative factors of disease and did so from statistics they gathered and interpreted. Their work represents an early example of evidence based medicine. Unfortunately, while they successfully disproved existing concepts of causes of disease, it would be many years before the agents responsible would be identified. The greatest single cause of mortality in the West Indies was yellow fever. In 1881, a Cuban doctor by the name of Carlos Finlay (who was actually of French and Scottish descent) showed that yellow fever is carried by mosquitoes. We now know that it is caused by a virus, which is transmitted by the bite of female mosquitoes (the yellow fever mosquito, Aedes Aegypti and other species). It is found in tropical and subtropical areas in South America and Africa.

10 McGrigor, James, *Medical Sketches of the Expedition from India to Egypt* (London: John Murray, Fleet Street, 1804), pp. 56-57.

11 Marshall, H., *Statistical report on the sickness, mortality, and invaliding among the troops in the West Indies,* (London: W. Clowes and Sons, 1838).

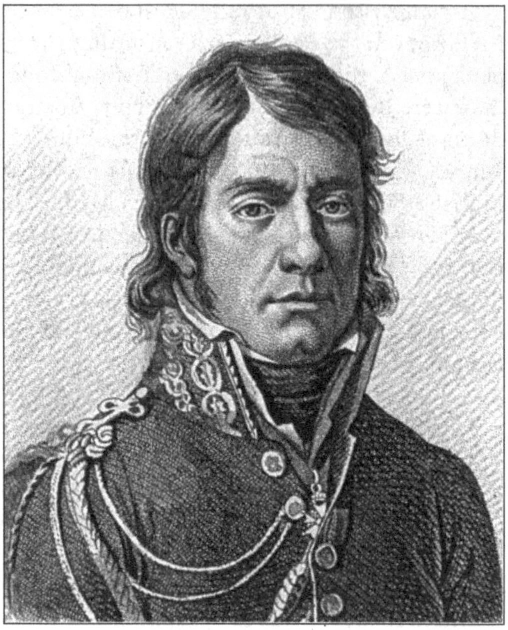
Figure 2.3 Baron Dominique Larrey (1766-1842). (Courtesy Wellcome Library, London)

Dominique Larrey was senior surgeon to Emperor Napoleon Bonaparte and was appointed Chief Surgeon of the Imperial Guard in 1814. He was born in Beaudéan, a small village in the Pyrenees, the son of a shoemaker. After his father died, he was raised by his uncle Alexis, who was chief surgeon in Toulouse. He served an apprenticeship with his uncle for six years, and then went to Paris to serve under Pierre-Joseph Desault, chief surgeon at the Hôtel-Dieu de Paris. He went on to serve first in the navy and then in the army. He became Surgeon-in-Chief to the Napoleonic armies in 1797. Larrey showed outstanding organisational skills and was also a very capable surgeon. British surgeon George James Guthrie (see below) admired his work very much and referred frequently to Larrey's operative ability in his writings.[12] During Napoleon's Italian campaign in 1797, Larrey was impressed by the speed at which supply wagons of the 'flying artillery' made their way around the battlefield and he thought that a flying ambulance or 'ambulance volante' could be designed to evacuate wounded soldiers quickly from the battlefield. Larrey's flying ambulance consisted of three divisions under the command of the chief surgeon. Each division had 113 men who performed their allotted tasks to assist in the rapid removal of the wounded from the battlefield. Each division had twelve light and four heavy carriages, or wagons, in which to transport the wounded. Larrey observed:

> With these ambulances, the most rapid movement of the advanced guard can be followed up, and when necessary, they can be separated into a great many divisions, every officer of the medical staff being mounted, and having at command a carriage, a mounted overseer, and everything necessary for affording the earliest assistance on the field of battle.[13]

Larrey's 'ambulance volante' certainly resulted in more rapid evacuation and treatment of wounded soldiers who might otherwise have lain on the battlefield for many hours. Larrey's ambulance became a template for subsequent ambulance designs in the 19th century. For example, during the American Civil War (1861-5), Dr Jonathan Letterman, Medical Director of the Union Army of the Potomac, developed a field ambulance as part of a strategy to deal

12 Guthrie, George James, *A Treatise on Gunshot Wounds: On Inflammation, Erysipelas, And Mortification, On Injuries of Nerves* (London: Burgess and Hill, 1827).
13 Larrey, D.J., *Memoirs of Military Surgery of Campaigns of the French Army Vol. I, Translated by R.W. Hall* (Baltimore: J. Cushing, 1814), pp.23-24.

with large numbers of casualties. His ambulance bore similarities to that of Larrey. Letterman declared:

> It will be perceived that the ambulance system, with that of supplies and of field hospitals, were ordered as essential parts of that new organisation from which, I earnestly hoped, the wounded and sick would receive more careful attendance and more skillful treatment.[14]

Letterman's anbulance system was put severely to the test at the Battle of Gettysburg between 1and 3 July 1863. The Medical Director of one corps wrote:

> It is with extreme satisfaction that I can assure you that it enabled me to remove the wounded from the field, shelter, feed them, and dress their wounds within six hours after the battle, and to have every capital operation performed within twenty four hours after the wound was received.[15]

After the battle was over, Letterman reflected:

> The Ambulance Corps performed its duty well. Before daylight on the morning of the 4th July, all wounded within our lines(numbering on those two days about twelve thousand) were removed to the hospitals.[16]

Once again, it is easy to draw direct comparisons between the rapid removal of casualties from the field of battle by Larrey and Letterman during the Napoleonic Wars and American Civil War respectively,and the evacuation of wounded on the Western Front between 1914 and 1918, where experience soon showed that delay in instigating definitive treatment frequently led to life threatening complications, while early intervention was beneficial and saved lives (Chapter 4). Indeed, as will be explained in Chapter 8, by July 1918 the five Australian divisions making up the Australian Corps introduced Field Ambulance Resuscitation Teams, with the very clear aim of treating soldiers as soon as possible after they had been wounded. The Official Historian of Australian Medical Services must certainly have had Larrey in mind when he described the activities of the Australian Field Ambulance Resuscitation Teams.

George James Guthrie was the most experienced and competent surgeon in Wellesley's Peninsular Army. He was a brave and innovative clinician who made very important contributions to military surgery. He was descended from a Scottish family from Forfarshire. His father was a London chiropodist who worked in Lower James Street, Golden Square. Young Guthrie became a hospital assistant at York Military Hospital when he was 15 and a member of the Royal College of Surgeons of England when he was 16. He joined the army and gained surgical experience in North America before going to the Peninsula in 1808. There were no anaesthetics to relieve pain, so surgery had to be rapid, decisive and involved the limbs predominantly. Abdominal procedures and chest operations were never seriously considered. Guthrie debunked

14 Letterman, J., *Medical Recollections of the Army of the Potomac*, (New York: D. Appleton and Company, 1866), pp.22-23.
15 Letterman, *Medical Recollections*, p. 157.
16 Letterman, *Medical Recollections*, p. 158.

the myth that amputations should only be performed after inflammation (infection with pus formation) had taken place, a management regime introduced by surgeon John Hunter (1728-1793) in the late 18th Century. Guthrie proved conclusively, in a series of amputations performed between 21 June and 24 December 1813 that patients who underwent early surgery had a much lower operative mortality than those whose surgery was delayed.

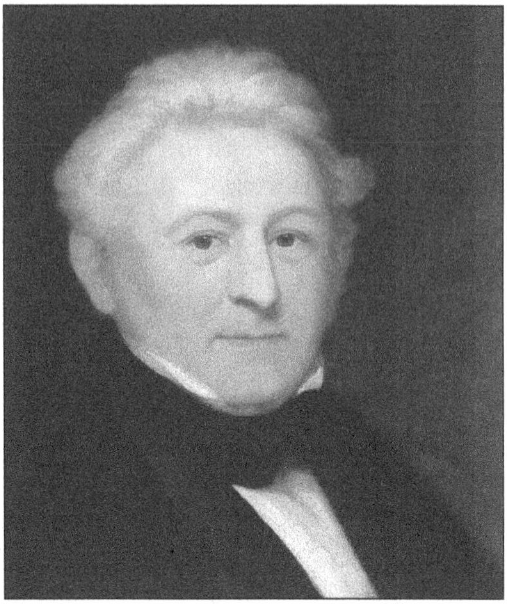

Figure 2.4 George James Guthrie (1785-1856), oil painting by Henry Room. (Courtesy Royal College of Surgeons of England)

Table 2.2 demonstrates very clearly that if definitive surgery was performed early, before infection became established, patients stood a much greater chance of surviving the operation. The reader may care to review the two case histories outlined in Chapter 1, where it should become clear that the policy in 1914 of delaying definitive surgery till wounded soldiers reached base hospitals near the French coast took far too long and cost many lives, because by then wounds were grossly infected. It would be 1915 before measures began to be put in place to undertake limb and life-saving surgery closer to the battle front at casualty clearing stations, which could be reached much more quickly before infecting organisms had become firmly established.

One particularly serious lower limb wound was the compound gunshot fracture of the femur (thigh bone), which was a source of very high mortality throughout the 19th century and for the first two years of the Great War (Chapter 7). One of Guthrie's colleagues, an Irish surgeon called John Hennen wrote:

Table 2.2 Figures comparing results of early and delayed amputations

	Total	Died	Deaths %
Delayed Amputations in hospital stations between 21st June and 24th December 1813			
Upper Extremity	296	116	39
Lower Extremity	255	149	58
Total number of operations	551	266	48
Early amputations in field between 21 June and 24 December 1813			
Upper Extremity	163	5	3
Lower Extremity	128	19	14.8
Total number of operations	291	24	8.2

Guthrie, G. J., *A Treatise on Gunshot Wounds: On Inflammation, Erysipelas, and Mortification, On Injuries of Nerves,* (London: Burgess and Hill, 1827), p. 228.

> The estimate of the mortality occasioned by compound fractures of the thigh from gunshot is most melancholy. In the French army, Baron Percy has calculated that scarcely two in ten recover. In the English army in the Peninsula, Mr. Guthrie found, that, on a review of his cases, not more than one-sixth recovered, so as to have useful limbs; two thirds of the whole died, whether amputation was performed or not; and the limbs of the remaining sixth were not only useless, but a constant source of uneasiness to them for the remainder of their lives. Not a single case has done well where amputation was deferred, and even where it has been performed, two out of three have died. [17]

It would be in April/May 1917 at the Battle of Arras when Henry Gray from Aberdeen (Chapter 1) successfully reduced the mortality of compound gunshot fractures of the femur from 80% to less than 20%, finally improving the results of a wound which had vexed military surgeons throughout the 19th century and for the first two and a half years of the Great War.

Guthrie was the first surgeon to appreciate that a bleeding artery must be tied off at both ends of the divided vessel. This is required because there is an extensive network of very small vessels which supply blood to the artery beyond the transacted vessel which then 'back bleeds'. This seems obvious now and must have been employed thousands of times in war surgery since Guthrie's discovery, but it was ground breaking work then. Guthrie declared:

> My paper in the New Medical and Physical Journal, demonstrated the necessity for performing the operation at the wounded part of the vessel, and not at a distance. It showed, what is not yet well understood by many, that in no case (and this is without exception) should one ligature above the wound be depended upon, but that another should be applied below.[18]

Amputations were undertaken frequently and were probably the first thing to come into a surgeon's mind when confronted by serious wounds of the arm or leg. Without any effective measures to eliminate pain during surgery, there must have been a natural desire on the part of both surgeon and patient to get the operation over with as quickly as possible. Having said that, Guthrie preserved limbs where at all possible, even when very serious wounds had been sustained. For example, a musket ball injury to the upper humerus adjacent to the shoulder joint was a relatively common wound and resulted in a smashed humeral head. In such a case, Guthrie opted for a limb sparing excision of the humeral head, which left the patient with a "flail" arm lacking stability, but which nevertheless retained a functioning hand and therefore was very much better than an amputation.

Guthrie had a confrontation with Scottish civilian surgeon Charles Bell, who went to Brussels after the Battle of Waterloo in June 1815 looking for a bit of excitement by offering his services to treat the wounded. After returning to London, Bell was clearly feeling confident in his ability and dared to criticise the method employed by one of Guthrie's staff in performing excision of the humeral head at York Hospital. Clearly riled by Bell's tactless and ill-advised comments about the operation, Guthrie stated:

17 Hennen, John, *Principles of Military Surgery 3rd Edition*, (London: John Wilson, 1829).
18 Guthrie, *A Treatise on Gunshot Wounds*, p. 228.

> If Mr Charles Bell had been thoroughly acquainted with the subject upon which he was writing, he would not have hazarded the criticism he has done. Mr Charles Bell has charged the medical officers of York Hospital with having confused notions on the subject of this operation, and with negligence of the anatomy of the parts. I now appeal to the profession to decide with whom the confusion of ideas, and the negligence, really exists[19]

Guthrie wrote these words in 1827, twelve years after the Battle of Waterloo. Bell must really have upset him! Guthrie documented that Larrey had performed the operation of excision of the head of humerus ten times and Larrey had written:

> I have had the good fortune, in ten cases, to prevent the unfortunate result (amputation) by extracting either the head of the humerus or its fragments without delay. This operation should be performed as soon as possible, as it prevents irritation, inflammation, abscesses, sinuses, and excessive caries of the humerus that would require amputation of the arm [20]

Larrey is sending a very clear message to future generations of military surgeons which they would do well to pay heed to. Early surgical intervention before infection becomes established is both beneficial to the patient and is associated with a much better outcome.

First general anaesthetics

General anaesthesia was first used in 1846 and was a development of great importance, since surgical procedures could be performed painlessly following its introduction. The impact made by three agents, nitrous oxide, ether and chloroform will be explained, since they were the ones used most frequently subsequently during the Great War. Nitrous oxide, a gas, never realised its potential during the 19th century although it became indispensable in 1915, when it became clear that it was the only safe agent to use in many cases (Chapter 5). Its anaesthetic properties were first noted by Humphrey Davy.

Humphrey Davy was born in Penzance, Cornwall. He was apprenticed to a surgeon for a time before going to Bristol to study science. In 1798, Davy joined the Pneumatic

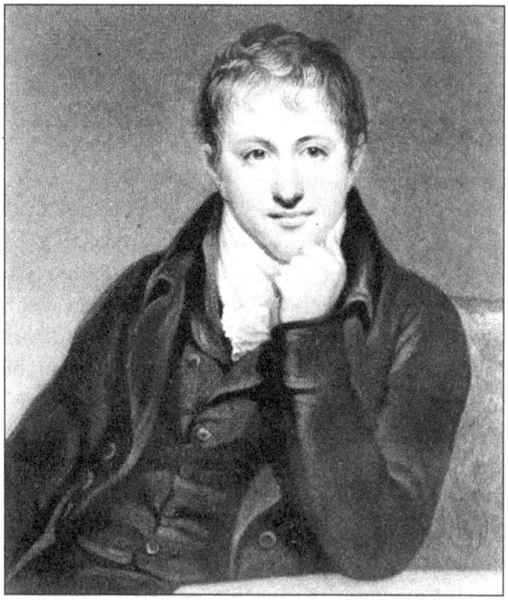

Figure 2.5 Humphrey Davy (1778-1829). (Courtesy Wellcome Library, London)

19 Guthrie, *A Treatise on Gunshot Wounds:* pp. 502-05.
20 Guthrie, *A Treatise on Gunshot Wounds*, pp. 476-77.

Institution at Bristol, which had been established to investigate the medical powers of various gases. While experimenting with nitrous oxide, he noticed that after breathing the gas he felt light headed and happy. This resulted in nitrous oxide becoming known as "laughing gas." Davy also noticed that its inhalation helped with the pain from a troublesome wisdom tooth. Instead of becoming recognised as a possible anaesthetic agent, however, nitrous oxide was taken along to parties to add to the frivolity of such occasions.

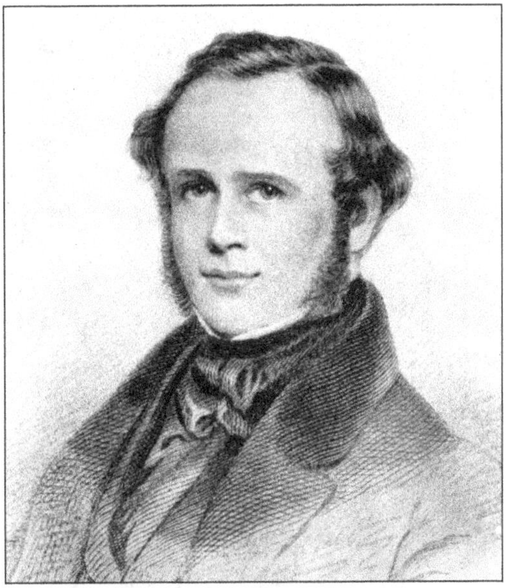

Figure 2.6 Horace Wells (1815-1848). (Courtesy Wellcome Library, London)

In 1844, realising there were potential commercial possibilities for nitrous oxide, American Gardner Quincy Colton (1814-98) gave up his studies as a medical student and began giving nitrous oxide demonstrations. At one such demonstration, a member of the audience sustained a leg injury while inhaling the gas but felt no pain. A dentist from Connecticut called Horace Wells (1815-48) was in the audience and wondered if nitrous oxide had potential for dental anaesthesia. He tried it successfully on several patients in his office but then unwisely gave a demonstration of a dental exaction in front of medical students at the Massachusetts General Hospital which ended in disaster when the patient cried out and the demonstration ended in disarray. Wells never got another chance, although the patient subsequently revealed that he had felt no pain.

At a subsequent demonstration in Paris in 1867, Colton administered nitrous oxide while a dentist successfully extracted a tooth. Always the entrepreneur, Colton realised he really should concentrate on using the gas for tooth extractions and it wasn't long before compressed nitrous oxide became available in liquid form in cylinders for dental work.

During the Franco-Prussian War (1870-71), clinicians in Germany showed interest in nitrous oxide, while in Britain an editorial in the British Journal of Dental Science suggested that the military should use the war to evaluate the gas but there is no evidence that this ever happened.[21] The 19th century was a missed opportunity, and nitrous oxide only came into its own during the Great War. A 'quick whiff of nitrous oxide and oxygen', while not sufficient for a healthy individual, would allow a speedy amputation or arrest of haemorrhage in the limb of a badly wounded soldier suffering from surgical shock who might succumb using any other agent (Chapter 5).[22]

21 Gray, T. Cecil, Mitchiner Memorial Lecture 'Another Side of Mars', *Journal of the Royal Army Medical Corps*, 130 (1984), pp.3-11.

22 Robertson, A., in Scotland, T., & Heys, S., Wars *Pestilence and the Surgeon's Blade, The Evolution of British Military Medicine and Surgery During the 19th century*, (Solihull: Helion and Co., 2013).

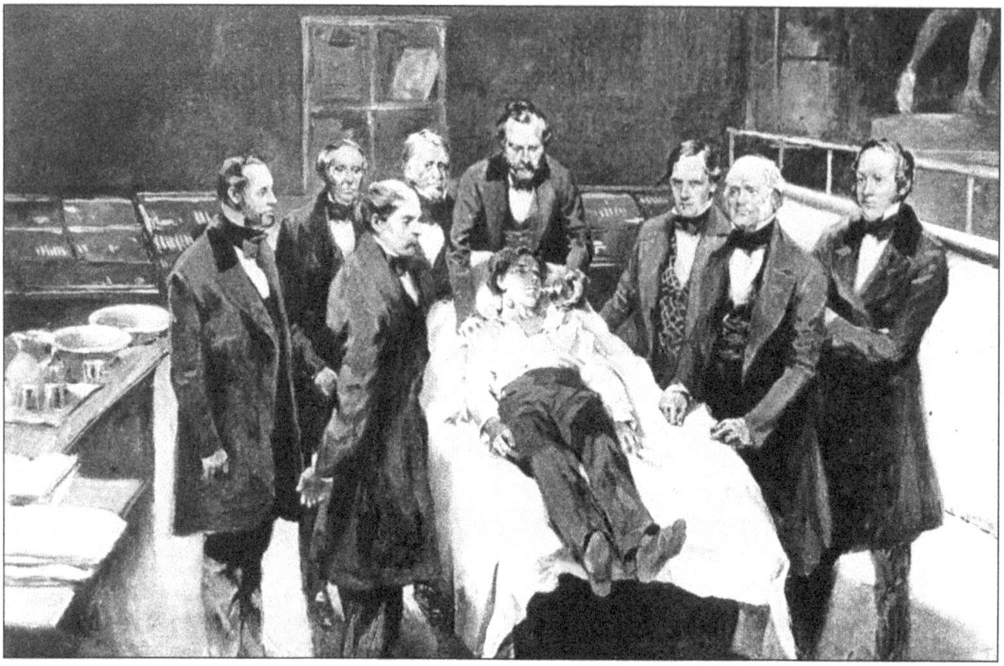

Figure 2.7 First demonstration of surgical anaesthesia by William Morton (1819-1868) at Massachusetts General Hospital, 16 October 1846. (Courtesy Wellcome Library, London)

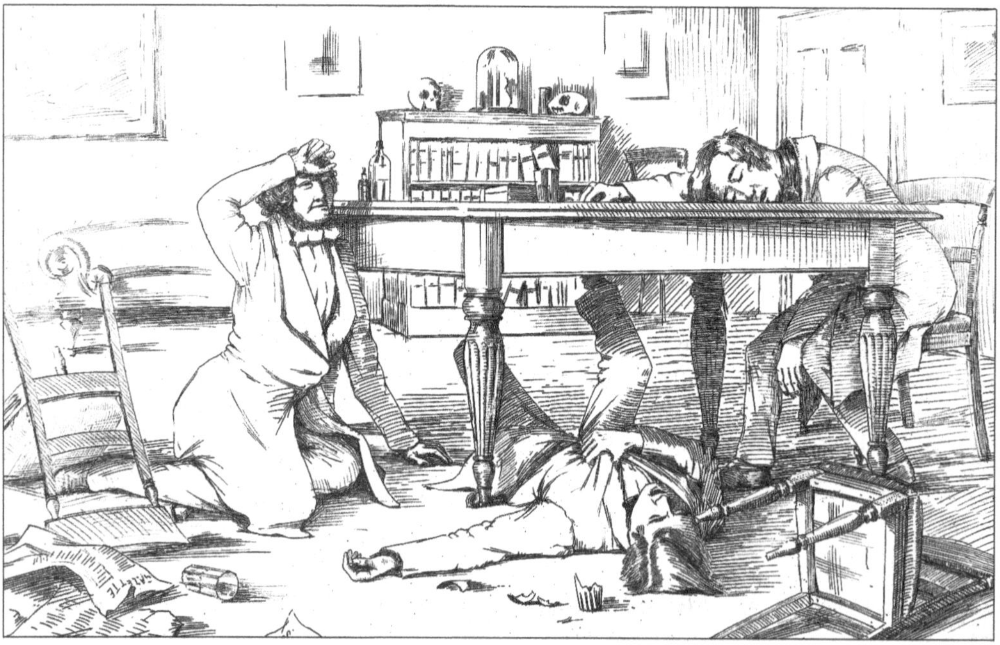

Figure 2.8 James Young Simpson (1811-1870) and two colleagues recovering from the effects of chloroform inhalation. (Courtesy Wellcome Library, London)

On 16 October 1846, at Massachusetts General Hospital, a dentist called William Morton (1819-1868), a colleague of Horace Wells, used ether to anaesthetise a young man with a tumour in his neck, while Chief-of-Surgery Dr John Collins Warren removed the tumour. Surgery changed forever and it wasn't long before news about this momentous event spread far and wide. Ether was soon used for treating wounded soldiers. The Mexican War had been terminated by treaty on 15 June 1846, but frequent skirmishes continued for many years. Morton wrote to the Surgeon Generals of the United States Army and Navy, promoting the use of ether anaesthesia. He offered to sell them ether and the equipment to administer it at wholesale prices. Both men declined, but surgeons in both Services ignored Morton's patent and used it anyway.[23]

James Young Simpson was born in Bathgate near Edinburgh. His father was a baker. When Simpson was 14, he went to the University of Edinburgh to study arts before embarking on a career in medicine, graduating at the age of 18. He was not permitted to take up his profession till he was 20 and spent the next two years working as assistant to the professor of pathology. He was determined to pursue a career in obstetrics and became Professor of Midwifery in 1839. Simpson began using ether in 1847 to relieve the pain associated with childbirth. Unfortunately, ether has a pungent aroma, irritates the patient's lungs, and is highly flammable, a major disadvantage for doctors delivering babies in patients' homes where candle light offered the only illumination. Simpson began experimenting with various agents, trying to find something better. On the evening of 4 November 1847, he and two friends inhaled chloroform, and after a brief euphoric phase, they all passed out, becoming the first humans to experience its anaesthetic properties.

Chloroform soon became very popular. It was pleasantly sweet smelling, was inflammable and produced anaesthesia quickly with nothing more than a pocket handkerchief and a small bottle of the agent for administration. Simpson publicised his discovery widely with a pamphlet and gained Royal approval from Queen Victoria who received one of Simpson's pamphlets from her friend, the Duchess of Sutherland.

Because of its ease of administration, chloroform was used much more than ether during the Crimean War (1853-56), fought between the Russian Empire and a strategic alliance comprising the British Empire, France, the Ottoman Empire and Sardinia. This was a war characterised by medical mismanagement. Conditions in hospitals in Scutari near Constantinople where the sick and wounded were treated were appalling and soldiers were extremely malnourished. Some suffered from scurvy, a disease associated with Vitamin C deficiency and caused by a diet deficient in fresh fruit and vegetables. Signs of scurvy were observed approximately three months after men left for the Crimea. The disease was associated with poor wound healing since Vitamin C is important in the formation of collagen, a key component of connective tissue, and one which is essential for healing. Things were so bad, that a Sanitary Commission Committee travelled to Scutari in 1855. The members of the committee found that wards and corridors were poorly ventilated and drains from toilets were blocked. Wards were filthy, overcrowded, damp and unhygienic. Recommendations were made and implemented. Nutrition of soldiers was improved, and the incidence, morbidity and mortality of diseases reduced, thanks to the better health of soldiers. Overcrowding was addressed with extra beds and better accommodation.[24]

23 Gray, T. Cecil, Mitchiner Memorial Lecture.

24 Scotland, T., & Heys, S., *Wars, Pestilence and the Surgeon's Blade: The Evolution of British Military Medicine and Surgery During the 19th century*, (Solihull: Helion and Co, 2013), pp. 233-34.

The French Surgeon-in-Chief reported that chloroform had been given 25,000 times, apparently without mishap. The British experience was the complete opposite, chloroform being associated with a high mortality. This led John Hall, Principal Medical Officer to recommend that the smart of the knife was a powerful stimulant and it was better to hear a man bawl lustily than to see him sink silently into the grave.[25]

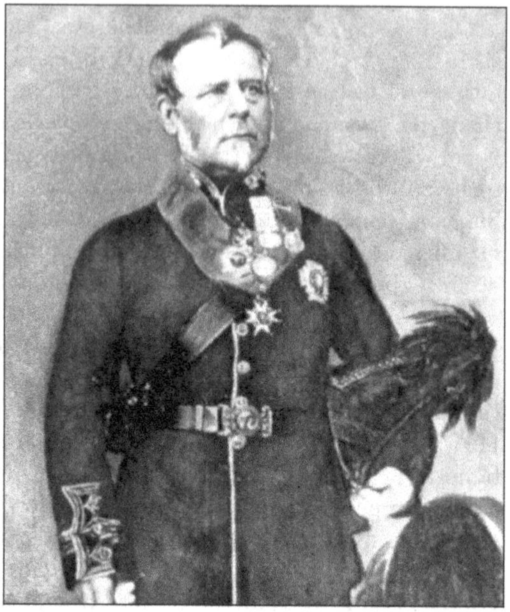

Figure 2.9 Sir John Hall (1795-1866). He was Inspector-General of Hospitals in the Crimea and was opposed to the use of anaesthetics. See text. (Courtesy Wellcome Library, London)

On 10 July 1856, Dr A. Mouat, Deputy Inspector General stood up at the meeting of the Military Medical and Surgical Society and declared:

> The subject of the administration of chloroform in the well-known shock or depression following severe gunshot injuries is a fit and proper one for discussion in this Society. The profession at home naturally looks to the medical officers of the army to contribute their mite of practical experience towards the settlement of this important and disputed question; but I much fear they will be somewhat disappointed in the results and conclusions arrived at. Great and grave doubts are beginning to arise in the minds of some unprejudiced surgeons and thinking observers at home and abroad as to the indiscriminate use of this powerful anaesthetic, so tempting to the sufferer, yet at times so fraught with danger ....[26]

The American Civil War (1861-65) began five years later. When Abraham Lincoln was elected the 16th President of the United States in 1860 as the first Republican president on a platform pledging to keep slavery out of the territories, seven slave states in the Deep South seceded and formed a new nation, the Confederate States of America. The incoming Lincoln administration and most of the Northern people refused to recognize the legitimacy of secession. They feared that it would discredit democracy and create a fatal precedent that would eventually fragment the no-longer United States into several small, squabbling countries. The American Civil War was a very bloody conflict which resulted in the death of approximately 700,000 men. Chloroform remained the frontline anaesthetic agent used by both northern and southern states because it was so easy to administer, while ether was the favoured anaesthetic in base hospitals in the north.

25 Gray, T. Cecil, Mitchiner Memorial Lecture.
26 Mouat, A., Observations on some points connected with the use of chloroform in military practice, *The Lancet* (1856), ii, pp.78-81.

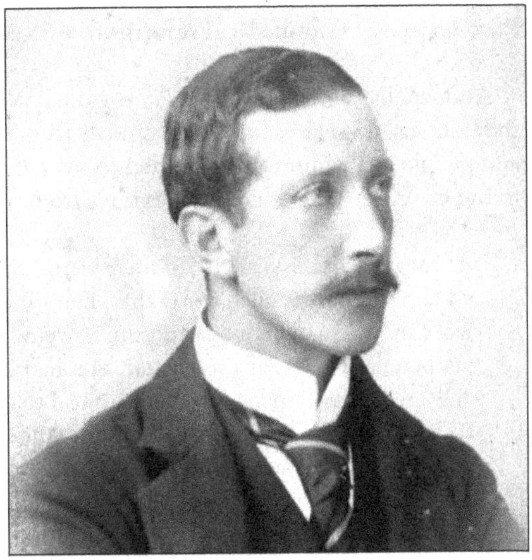

Figure 2.10 Alfred Goodman Levy (1866-1954). (Courtesy Wellcome Library, London)

In the Franco-Prussian War, a conflict between the Second French Empire of Napoleon III and the German states of the North German Confederation led by the Kingdom of Prussia, chloroform remained the anaesthetic of choice. In the Boer War (1899-1902), fought between the British Empire and the two independent Boer Republics of Afrikaans-speaking Dutch settlers in the independent Transvaal and Orange Free State, there was no need to look beyond chloroform. The Surgeon General reported: "The proper anaesthetic for the field and the only one desirable in hot climates is chloroform."[27]

Thus chloroform was clearly the anaesthetic of choice in military surgery throughout the 19th century despite a growing body of evidence that it's use was not without danger. Between 1864 and 1901, no fewer than seven chloroform committees investigated its potential hazards, but it was not until 1911 that Dr Alfred Goodman Levy demonstrated beyond reasonable doubt that strong stimulation under light chloroform anaesthesia caused ventricular fibrillation, a fatal cardiac arrhythmia. Whether this was the primary cause of all chloroform deaths will never be established, but chloroform was potentially dangerous.

Although the first use of general anaesthesia in surgery in 1846 for anything other than tooth extraction was a cause for much celebration, it never reached its full clinical and scientific potential and in the latter part of the 19th century, other scientific and surgical breakthroughs grabbed the limelight. It was felt that anaesthesia had gone as far as it ever would. After all, a hanky impregnated with chloroform and held over the nose and mouth of a patient was all that was required to administer a general anaesthetic and there was nothing difficult about it. Writing in "War Surgery 1914-18", Robertson pointed out that the teaching of anaesthesia was not on the curriculum of most medical schools. It wasn't thought to be necessary. In 1909, a bill proposing that all general anaesthetics should be administered by a medical practitioner failed to get through parliament. In 1912, the GMC finally accepted that anaesthesia should be the last of 16 subjects on the undergraduate curriculum of all medical schools. Two years later came the Great War and with it, unsurprisingly, a distinct shortage of trained anaesthetists.[28]

27 Metcalfe, N.H., "Military Influence upon the development of anaesthesia from the American Civil War (1861-1865) to the outbreak of the First World War", *Anaesthesia*, 60:12, (2005), pp. 1213-17.

28 Robertson, A. in Scotland, T., Heys, S., *War Surgery 1914-18*, (Solihull: Helion and Company 2012), p. 89.

Post-Crimean War medical reforms in preventive medicine and their impact up to 1914

A journalist writing for *The Times* called William Howard Russell (1820-1907) travelled to the Crimea and sent back regular reports from the front line. He was the first war correspondent and people in Britain were horrified to read about the appalling conditions endured by soldiers in the Crimean War. Here is an extract from one of his reports:

> At the close of the year (1855) there were 3,500 sick in the British Camp before Sebastopol, and it was not too much to say that their illness had, for the most part, been caused by hard work in bad weather or by exposure to wet without any adequate protection. Think of a tent pitched, as it were, at the bottom of a marsh, into which some twelve or fourteen miserable creatures, drenched to the skin, had to creep for shelter after twelve hours of vigil in a trench like a canal, huddled together without any change of clothing and lying packed up as close as they could be stowed in saturated blankets. But why were they in tents? Where were the huts that had been sent out to them? The huts were on board ships in the harbour of Balaclava. Some of the huts were floating about the beach; others had been landed, and now and then I met a wretched pony, knee deep in mud, struggling on beneath the weight of two thin deal planks, a small portion of one of these huts, which were probably converted into firewood after lying for some time in the camp, or turned into stabling for officers' horses.[29]

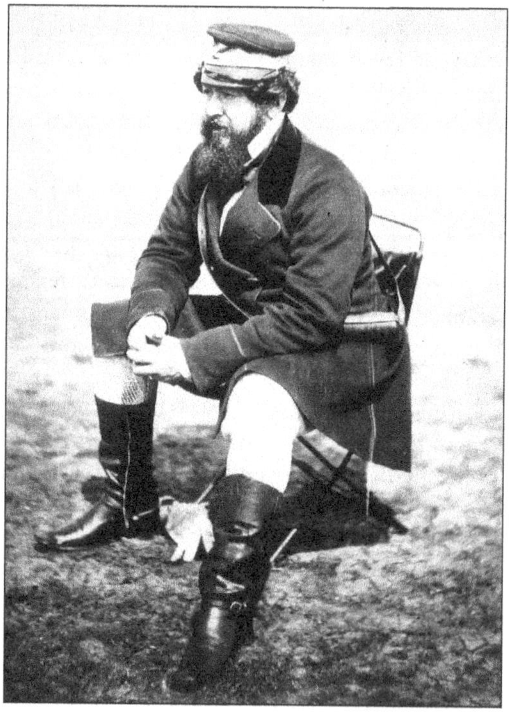

Figure 2.11 William Howard Russell (1820-1907). (Wikimedia Commons)

Following the Crimean debacle and the terrible resulting publicity, a Sanitary Commission with four sub-committees was set up in 1857 to improve the health and well-being of soldiers. The Medical Department was reorganised, a barrack and hospital improvement scheme was established, a new Department of Medical Statistics provided accurate information on the health of soldiers and an Army Medical School aimed at promoting education and research was opened at Netley in 1860 with Chairs in Surgery, Medicine, Hygiene and Pathology. The various measures introduced by the four sub-committees of the Sanitary Commission all helped to improve matters in the second part of the 19th century as Table 2.3 sets out to demonstrate.

29 Hudson, Roger (Editor), *William Russell, Special Correspondent of the Times*, (London: The Folio Society, 1995), p. 44.

Table 2.3 Mean annual mortalities for 1860-1898 and for 1817-1820

Location	Mean Annual Mortality 1817-21	Mean Annual Mortality per 1,000 for each decade			
		1860-69	1870-79	1880-89	1890-98
U.K.	17	9.95	12.67	6.40	9.03
W. Indies	185	5.58	10.99	14.94	9.56
S. Africa	12	13.16	39.12	37.96	7.38
Ceylon	111	13.03	14.90	14.34	9.66
China		52.04	14.14	9.82	11.03
India	85	25.46	19.25	16.36	16.42
Egypt				26.72	13.22
W. Africa	362				45.13

Data column 2: From Chaplin, A., The rate of mortality in the British Army 100 years ago, *Proceedings of the Royal Society of Medicine*, 1916; 9 (section History of Medicine); pp.89-99. Remainder of data from: Rosenbaum, S., More than a century of Army medical statistics, *Journal of the Royal Society of Medicine* 83 (1990) pp. 456-463.

It must be pointed out, however, that despite figures showing a steady improvement, there were still more deaths caused by disease than from enemy action in all wars fought by the British during the 19th century. In the Second Boer War (1899-1902), for example, twice as many soldiers died from disease as were killed or died from wounds. Most deaths were caused by typhoid fever, a waterborne infection acquired by drinking contaminated water or by eating food prepared in it. Better hygiene would have prevented many deaths. Almroth Wright, who was Professor of Pathology at the Army Medical School at the time, had developed a vaccine effective against typhoid fever which was available for use during the Boer War but fears about the safety of the vaccine meant that it failed to gain approval for use. Wright was so disgusted that he resigned from his position. At the outbreak of war in 1914, typhoid vaccination was still not compulsory although the Secretary of State for War, Lord Kitchener, encouraged all men to be inoculated against the disease before being despatched to the front.

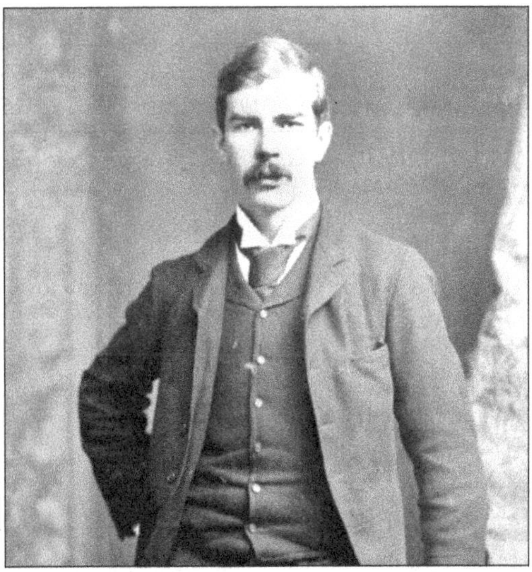

Figure 2.12 Sir Almroth Wright (1861-1947). (Wikimedia Commons)

One very important measure introduced after the Crimean War, which was aimed at improving the health of soldiers, was the appointment of a sanitary officer, whose duty was to advise the commanding officer on matters relating to hygiene and avoidance of disease, such as procurement of clean drinking water and safe disposal of human excreta. The first ever sanitary officer to be appointed was Staff Surgeon Rutherford during the Second China War in 1857.[30] Unfortunately, not all commanding officers were prepared to listen, and the advice given by sanitary officers was frequently ignored. General Viscount Wolsely (1833-1913) was Commander-in-Chief of the British Army from 1895 to 1900, having served in Burma, the Crimean War, the Indian Mutiny and the Sudan. He felt there was no need for a sanitary officer in the field, declaring:

> As long as this fad continues, my recommendation is to leave the sanitary officer at the base, where he may find some useful occupation as a member of the sanitary board. In the numerous campaigns where I have served with a sanitary officer, I can conscientiously state I have never known him to make any useful suggestion, whereas I have known him to make many silly ones.[31]

It is to the everlasting shame of senior officers that there were so many unnecessary deaths from disease during the Second Boer War, despite the formation of the Royal Army Medical Corps in 1898. Senior officers were frequently slow to accept advice from medical officers, who were regarded as neither officers nor gentlemen. James McGrigor's close association with the Duke of Wellington stands out in stark contrast to the general perception of medical officers throughout the remainder of the 19th century. Following the appointment of Sir Alfred Keogh as Director General of Army Medical Services in 1904, things finally changed for the better and preventive medicine became recognised as being of utmost importance and the overwhelming majority of fatalities on the Western Front between 1914-18 were the result of enemy action as Table 2.4 clearly shows.

Table 2.4 Deaths from disease and deaths from enemy action for Boer War and for Western Front, 1914-18

War	Killed in action or died of wounds	Deaths from disease
Boer War	7,999 (36%)	14,048 (64%)
Great War Western Front 1914-18	677,515 (95.5%)	32,098 (4.5%)

Mitchell, T.J., Smith, G.M., *History of the Great War Medical Services Casualties and Medical Statistics*, (London: His Majesty's Stationery Office, 1931).

The evolution of the evacuation pathway for wounded soldiers from post-Crimea to the Great War

Sir Thomas Longmore was appointed Professor of Surgery at the Army Medical School in 1860, and his contributions were noteworthy. Longmore was born in London, the son of a Royal Navy surgeon. He served with distinction in the Crimea and was promoted Deputy Inspector

30 Cantlie, N., *A History of the Army Medical Department, Vol. 2,* (Edinburgh: Churchill Livingston, 1974), p. 250.
31 Cantlie, *A History of the Army Medical Department, Vol. 2,* p. 286.

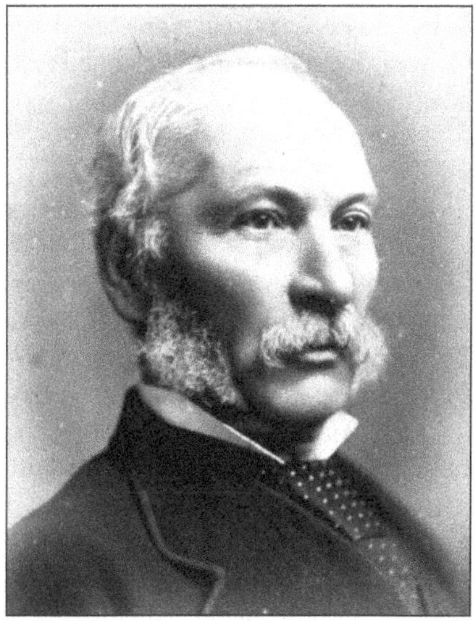

Figure 2.13 Sir Thomas Longmore (1816-1895). (Courtesy Wellcome Library, London)

General of Hospitals in 1858. During his tenure at Netley, Longmore published a much-acclaimed book dealing with gunshot wounds and their treatment which became *the* standard reference.[32] He was involved in the modernisation of an evacuation pathway for wounded soldiers, and to this end was a most influential member of a committee chaired by the then Director General of Army Medical Services, Sir William Muir. The proposed pathway put into effect was as follows. A regimental medical officer had 16 regimental stretcher bearers who brought the wounded to the regimental aid post. A stretcher bearer company then transported the wounded to a field hospital in ambulance wagons. Field hospitals were mobile bell-tented units with 200 beds and divided into three or four sections capable of independent activity. There were four field hospitals per division. The personnel in field hospitals treated soldiers with minor wounds, while more seriously wounded men were taken to larger stationary hospitals (in marquees) on the lines of communication. There were 13 stationary hospitals of 200 beds for each army corps. General hospitals at the base had 500 beds and a hospital ship often functioned as an additional base hospital. Following some administrative problems in the Second Boer War (1899-1902), the field hospitals and bearer companies combined in 1905 to form single functional units called field ambulances. Some lessons were learned from the Russo-Japanese War of 1904-05, a conflict brought about by the rival imperial ambitions of Russia and Japan towards Manchuria and Korea. The Russo-Japanese War resulted in a great many casualties. It has been estimated that the Japanese sustained 227,000 killed, wounded and missing, and the Russians between 190,000 and 270,000.[33] If, as was very likely, there were similar numbers of casualties in a European conflict, then existing medical facilities would be inadequate. The regimental medical units and field ambulances represented the entire medical organisation in front of the lines of communication and would be insufficient for the rapid collection and evacuation of large numbers of wounded. Field ambulances would become congested and bogged down so that another layer was required behind them to which casualties could be moved quickly prior to evacuation to hospitals on lines of communication. These new units were named clearing hospitals. The role of the regimental medical services and field ambulances was to collect the wounded and transfer them to the clearing hospitals, which received the wounded and then transferred them onward by hospital trains to stationary hospitals on lines of communication and to general hospitals at the base for definitive treatment prior to them being sent them back to Britain. This was the pathway used by the BEF in 1914.

32 Longmore, Thomas, *Gunshot Injuries: Their History, Characteristic Features, Complications and General Treatment*, (London: Longmans Green and Co., 1877).

33 Steinberg, John, *The Russo-Japanese War in Global Perspective, World War Zero, Vol. 2,* (Brill Academic Publishers, 2007), p. 196.

In 1864 Longmore represented the British Government at the International Congress in Geneva, when the International Treaty, which became known as the Geneva Convention, was adopted.

The Geneva Convention and Internaional Red Cross

The Geneva Convention and International Red Cross owe their origin to a Swiss businessman called Henry Dunant (1828-1910), who was an observer at the Battle of Solferino on 24 June 1859. Fought between an Austrian army of 175,000 men and an allied force of 150,000 French, Piedmontese and Sardinians, the battle took place a few miles to the south of Lake Garda in Italy. Austria lost the battle with 13,317 killed and wounded and 9,220 missing. Allied losses were 14,415 killed and wounded, with 2,776 missing. Solferino was a catastrophe of medical mismanagement where men died unattended in appalling conditions. Dunant personally intervened to help when he could and from his experience at Solferino he nurtured the hope and belief that the treatment of wounded soldiers could and should be significantly improved. Dunant proposed a permanent relief agency for humanitarian aid in time of war and a government treaty recognising the neutrality of the agency and allowing it to provide aid in a war zone. The former, was the International Red Cross, and the latter the Geneva Convention. The rules of the Geneva Convention apply only in times of armed conflict and seek to protect people who are not in or are no longer taking part in hostilities. These include the sick and wounded of armed forces in the field, wounded, sick, and shipwrecked members of armed forces at sea, prisoners of war, and civilians. The Convention also guarantees neutrality to medical staff, to ambulances and to field hospitals. The rules of the Geneva Convention first applied during the Prussian War against Denmark in 1864, and then the Austro-Prussian War in 1866.[34] The aim of the International Movement of the Red Cross is to protect human life and health, to ensure respect for all human beings, and to prevent and alleviate human suffering, without any discrimination based on nationality, race, sex, religious beliefs, class or political opinions. Dunant's firm conviction that this must be so became the starting point for the International Red Cross and he used some of his personal fortune to help.

Discovery of bacteria and antiseptic surgery: Louis Pasteur (1822-1895) and Joseph Lister (1843-1910)

The names of Louis Pasteur and Joseph Lister are indelibly linked. Louis Pasteur was a French biologist, who at the age of 32 became Dean of the Faculty of Science at Lille University. When engaged in research to find out why beer turned sour, he identified thousands of micro-organisms when he looked at samples of sour beer under the microscope. He deduced they were the cause of beer turning sour rather than the result. He also studied sour milk and sour wine and drew the same conclusions. In 1865, he was asked to investigate his first disease called "pébrine"

34 Cooter, R.M., Harrison, M., Sturdy, S., *War, Medicine and Modernity,* (Stroud, Gloucestershire: Sutton Publishing Limited, 1998), p. 25.

which affected the silk worm industry. Larvae of the silkworm affected by pébrine are unable to spin thread. If adult moths are affected, they transmit the disease to their larvae and the larvae die. Pasteur established a bacterial cause for the disease and became convinced that bacteria were also responsible for causing disease in humans. This was the germ theory of disease which would change medicine forever.

Joseph Lister, Professor of Surgery at the University of Glasgow, was inspired by Pasteur's work and remarked:

> When it had been shown by the researches of Pasteur that the septic property of the atmosphere depended not on the oxygen or any gaseous constituent, but on minute organisms suspended in it, which owed their energy to their vitality, it occurred to me that decomposition in the injured part might be avoided without excluding the air, by applying as a dressing some material capable of destroying the life of the floating particles.[35]

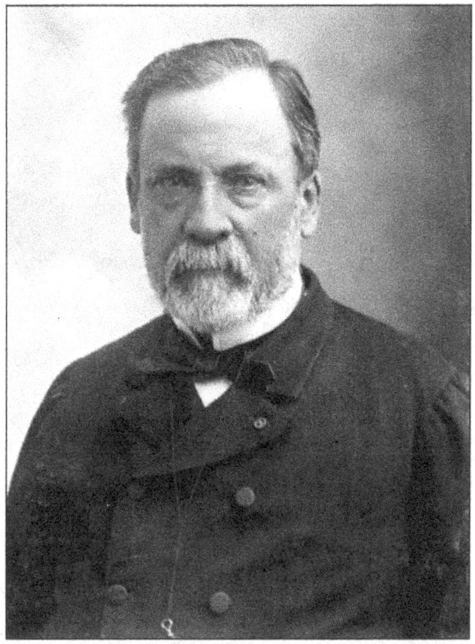

Figure 2.14 Louis Pasteur (1822-1895). (Courtesy Wellcome Library, London)

Lister began applying carbolic acid (phenol) dressings to wounds to prevent organisms gaining access. In August 1867, he applied a piece of lint which had been soaked in carbolic acid to the injured leg of an eleven-year-old boy who had been admitted to Glasgow Royal Infirmary. His young patient had sustained a compound fracture of his tibia and fibula as a result of an accident where his leg had been run over by the wheel of a cart. Until then, such an injury would almost certainly have resulted in a major infection. After four days, Lister renewed the pad and discovered to his delight that the wound looked clean. After five weeks he was amazed to discover that the boy's fractured bones had united. Lister

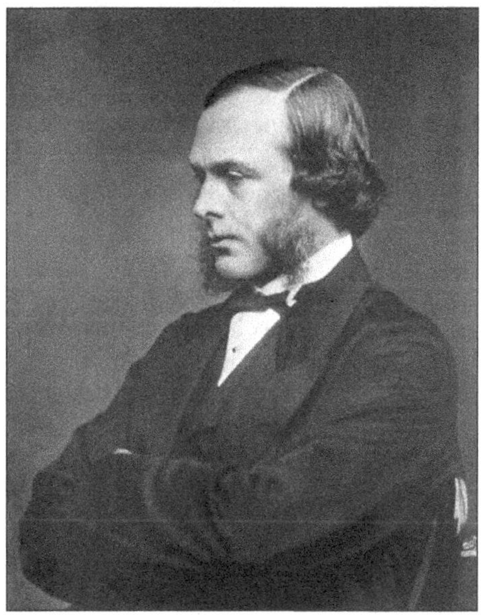

Figure 2.15 Joseph Lister (1827-1912). (Courtesy Wellcome Library, London)

35 Lister, J., On the antiseptic principle in the practice of surgery, *British Medical Journal*, 2: 351 (21 September 1867), pp.246-248.

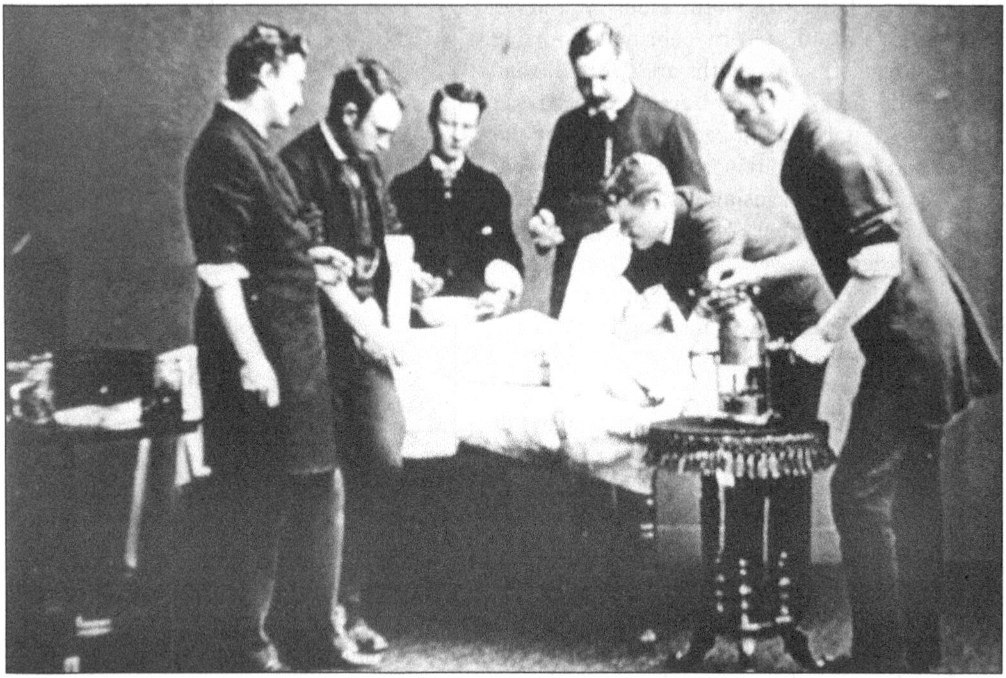

Figure 2.16 Sir Alexander Ogston (1844-1929), standing far left, demonstrating antiseptic surgery at Aberdeen Royal Infirmary; the surgical wound and instruments are sprayed with carbolic acid mist. (Courtesy Aberdeen Medico-Chirurgical Society)

published his findings in the Lancet in a series of articles, and in the British Medical Journal on 21 September 1867.[36]

Carbolic acid is derived from creosote, which had been discovered by Friedlieb Runge, a prominent German analytical chemist. Creosote was used by Runge to protect wood from rotting and to treat railway sleepers to prevent decomposition. Runge did not understand that it was bacterial action which brought about the decomposition and disintegration of the wood. Lister tested the results of spraying instruments, surgical incisions and dressings with a fine carbolic acid mist and found that wounds healed better. Surgeons still operated wearing blood-caked outdoor clothes and relied entirely on the carbolic acid to kill any bacteria.

Antiseptic surgery soon became widely used in civilian practice and Sir Alexander Ogston (1844-1929), Regius Professor of Surgery at the University of Aberdeen (Figure 2.16), introduced antiseptic surgery to Aberdeen Royal Infirmary. Ogston discovered the existence of the staphylococcus aureus in 1880, the micro-organism which was and still is the commonest cause of surgical wound infection.

The North German Federation led by the Prussians were quick to embrace antiseptic surgery during the Franco-Prussian War (1870-71), the first time it was used militarily. Robert Koch (1843-1910), who was an arch rival of Louis Pasteur, served as a surgeon during that conflict.

36 Lister, *British Medical Journal*, 1867, pp.246-48.

Koch made many microbiological discoveries after the Franco-Prussian War and while Pasteur concentrated on developing vaccines to treat individual patients by immunising them against specific diseases, Koch favoured public health measures to control infectious diseases in entire populations. The two men hated each other, partly because of personal animosity and partly because they were on opposite sides during the Franco-Prussian War which Prussia won and humiliated France. Koch identified the anthrax bacillus in 1877, mycobacterium tuberculosis in 1882 and vibrio cholerae, the cause of cholera in 1883.

Aseptic Surgery

Aseptic surgery is defined as surgery performed under sterilised conditions to prevent the introduction of infectious microorganisms. It was a natural progression from Lister's antiseptic surgery, which depended on carbolic acid killing bacteria which landed on a wound from surgeons wearing their normal outdoor clothes and operating with contaminated instruments. If surgeons wore gowns which had been sterilised and if the surgical instruments they used were likewise sterilised, then bacteria would have much less chance of gaining access to the wound. In 1885, Ernst von Bergmann, who was Professor of Surgery at the Universities of Berlin and Wurzburg, successfully sterilized surgical instruments and wound dressings by steam. Bergmann's method used steam under pressure and was the basis for modern sterilization procedures using autoclaves. Aseptic surgery soon gained acceptance in the latter years of the 19th century and surgeons became accustomed to operating in a clean environment.

In 1892 on Pasteur's 70th birthday, a Jubilee Celebration was held in Paris to mark his outstanding contributions to science. Pasteur, who had suffered a stroke, shuffled slowly onto the stage at the Sorbonne on the arm of the French President, in front of a distinguished audience from all over the world. As he made his entry to rapturous applause, he was greeted from the floor by Lord Lister.

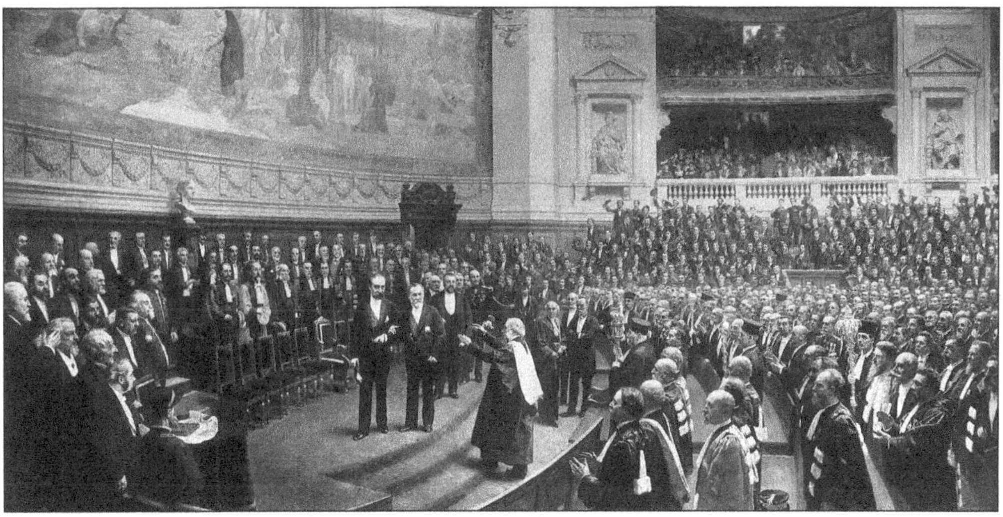

Figure 2.17 Lord Lister hails Louis Pasteur at the Sorbonne, Paris, on the occasion of Pasteur's Jubilee Celebration, 27 December 1892. (Courtesy Wellcome Library, London)

An era of antiseptic surgery in warfare

Whilst the North German Federation had been quick to embrace antiseptic surgery during the Franco-Prussian War, it would be in Egypt in 1882 before British military surgeons used antiseptic surgery in warfare. By the time of conflict in the Sudan in 1885, it was being used regularly.[37] During the Second Boer War (1899-1902), Listerian principles of wound antisepsis dominated surgical thinking and practice. The aim of surgical treatment of wounds was to operate on patients before infecting organisms gained access and to achieve healing without suppuration (pus formation). The general management of wounds in the Boer War became a blueprint for treatment during the Great War. The Boer War, however, was fought in the dry grasslands of the Transvaal and Orange Free State, while the First World War on the Western Front was fought in richly manured fields of Northern France and Flanders where the soil was teeming with deadly bacteria. Most wounds in the Boer War were inflicted by small-bore lead rifle bullets with a copper or steel jacket, giving them a higher muzzle velocity than older and slower soft lead bullets. When non-vital structures were hit by these new bullets fired by Boer marksmen from long range, less tissue damage resulted and this led to the Hague Convention of 1899 banning the use of soft deforming bullets for the 'sake of humanity'. The prospect of being shot by a humane bullet is not one the reader should find particularly reassuring, given that during the Boer War the ratio of killed to wounded on the battlefield, the uncorrected lethality, was 0.28 for officers and 0.32 for soldiers, an approximate ratio of one killed for three wounded.[38]

William Flack Stevenson (1844-1922) was Professor of Military Surgery at the Army Medical School from 1892 to 1895. He held the position of Surgeon General from 1899 to 1900, whilst Principal Medical Officer on Lines of Communication in South Africa. He authored the monograph *Wounds in War* which was published in 1904.[39] The methods used to treat wounds in the Second Boer War were destined to be the methods employed in August 1914. Some of Stevenson's observations were as follows:

> A certain amount of suppuration occurred in gunshot wounds in South Africa, but it was of a singularly mild and localised character and was followed in comparatively few cases by general infection: cases of septicaemia, no doubt, were seen, but the percentage of these was low. One medical officer, who saw over 2,000 cases of gunshot in a general hospital, expressed his belief that 80 per cent of them healed by first intention and that only a few of the other 20 per cent showed signs of septic infection. Messrs. Bowlby and Wallace remark in this connection that 'although a good many bad cases of suppuration occurred, pyaemia only rarely appeared, and then only in isolated cases, and never assumed the epidemic form'.[40]

37 Scotland, T., & Heys, S., *Wars, Pestilence and the Surgeon's Blade: The Evolution of British Military Medicine and Surgery During the 19th century*, (Solihull: Helion and Co., 2013), p. 310.

38 Parker, P.J., Commentary in Stevenson, W.F., Surgical Experiences from the Boer War, *Journal Royal Army Medical Corps*, Vol 1, No.2, (1903), pp. 89-95.

39 Stevenson, W.F., *Wounds in War, the mechanism of their production and treatment,* (London: Longman Green and Co, 1904).

40 Stevenson, *Wounds in War*, p. 152.

It is noteworthy that Messrs. Bowlby and Wallace mentioned in the above quotation by Stevenson, became senior surgeons during the Great War. Bowlby eventually became Surgical Advisor for the entire British area, while Cuthbert Wallace became Consulting Surgeon to the British First Army. Much more will be said about them in subsequent chapters.

Some surgeons attributed the lack of suppuration in South Africa to climate, sunshine and dry, pure air. The soil lacked the lethal organisms to be found subsequently in the richly fertilised fields of France and Flanders Others thought that the wounds inflicted by small-bore bullets were less traumatic to the tissues and were indeed more 'humane'. Stevenson disagreed with these views, claiming that better surgery and the use of antiseptics were responsible for the good results. He declared that unless antiseptic cleansing of the wound and of the skin around was possible from the first, suppuration was sure to occur. Stevenson was in fact saying that the wounds inflicted were clean and bacteriologically sterile and became infected subsequently. Only the rapid application of an antiseptic agent to occlude the wound would prevent harmful organisms from gaining entry and causing infection. If wounds did become infected due to delay in application of a suitable dressing, then antiseptics would solve the problem. In fact, Lister's antiseptic surgical regime was the solution to every military surgical wound problem:

> In the treatment of suppurating wounds, irrigation, drainage, and dry absorbent dressings frequently renewed are the means to be relied on. The best procedure is to wash the wound to its deepest recesses with an 8 per cent, solution of chloride of zinc, having previously scraped away the granulations with a Volkmann's spoon, and then thoroughly irrigate it with a 1-20 carbolic solution, these irritating germicide solutions being subsequently removed by irrigating with boiled water; provision for complete drainage should then be made, and the dressings applied. During the first few days these wounds should be dressed twice a day after the same plan, only omitting the zinc solution. By these means they will be brought into a healthy condition, and the suppuration will gradually decrease. MacCormac pointed out that the difficulty in this treatment consists in the complete disinfection of the wound in its more inaccessible parts and in its efficient drainage. When this could be done, the wounds, without exception, became aseptic after four or five dressings. Mr. Watson Cheyne has recommended that the surfaces of septic wounds should be lightly painted with pure carbolic acid, and I have latterly had good results from this method. [41]

Stevenson continued:

> If Lord Lister had done nothing more for surgery than teaching the surgeon the necessity and importance of avoiding contamination of the wound he treats, and pointing out that the means of doing this was to asepticise his hands and instruments before applying them to open wounds, he had done well for the science of surgery; he had, indeed, done more for the general treatment of wounds than any of the great men who had been his predecessors had achieved. But he has done much more than this: he has revolutionised the whole science of surgery and made modern surgery possible. Yet, while we may stand amazed at the advances surgery has made of late years under his teaching, we probably hardly suspect

41 Stevenson, *Wounds in War*, p. 153.

> the possibilities of the future. In no branch of surgery, abdominal and brain surgery not excepted, has antiseptic treatment brought forth more marvellous changes for the better than in the treatment of wounds in war.[42]

Stevenson may well have been partly correct in his assertion that better surgery and Lister's antiseptics contributed to improved outcomes during the Second Boer War with fewer infections and low incidence of suppuration. For the time being, military surgery was up to the mark, and was dealing well with the wounded. Then twelve years later came the Great War and everything changed as Chapter 4 clearly illustrates.

Summary of surgical progress in the 19th century: A blueprint for the Great War

During the first half of the 19th century, surgeons like Guthrie and Larrey operated without anaesthetic agents and dealt mainly with wounds of limbs, because arms and legs were readily accessible. A tourniquet could be used to control bleeding, or direct pressure exerted over a vessel if the wound was too proximal (far up the limb) for its application. Guthrie and Larrey were exceedingly skilful surgeons and operated with great speed and precision. They could perform amputations in a few minutes, but they also gained experience in limb preserving operations. Musket ball injuries involving the humeral head adjacent to the shoulder joint could be dealt with by excising the humeral head, leaving the patient with a flail arm, but with a functioning hand. This was infinitely better than performing an ablative procedure. Both Larrey and Guthrie showed that early surgical intervention was associated with much better outcomes. Guthrie proved conclusively that patients undergoing early amputation had a much lower operative mortality than those subjected to late surgery, when wounds were inflamed due to infection. John Hunter's management of major limb wounds requiring amputation had been to delay the procedure until there was inflammation. Hunter (1728-93) was the most distinguished surgeon of the 18th Century and the Hunterian Museum in the Royal College of Surgeons of England preserves his name and collection of anatomical specimens. Inflammation was regarded by Hunter as a normal part of the healing process. Guthrie was very bold to contradict such an established figure as John Hunter just as pioneering surgeons would be in 1914 to disagree with those who persisted with Listerian principles of wound management (Chapter 4). Compound gunshot fractures involving the femur were especially troublesome throughout the 19th century and primary amputation was Guthrie's treatment of choice. During the Second Boer War, limb surgery still dominated military operating lists and fractures of the femur carried a mortality of greater than 50 percent, when patients with inadequately splinted compound fractures were subjected to a 600-mile rail journey to distant base hospitals.[43] If there was no alternative to patients making this long journey, then primary amputation, while not strictly necessary from a clinical standpoint, gave patients a greater chance of survival. During the opening months of the Great War, there was a school of thought that the only way of saving the lives of a few

42 Stevenson, *Wounds in War*, pp. 113-14.
43 Parker, P.J., Commentary in Stevenson, W.F., Surgical Experiences from the Boer War, *Journal Royal Army Medical Corps*, Vol 1., No.2, (1903), pp. 89-95.

patients with compound fractures of the femur was to perform immediate amputation (Chapter 7).

Wounds of the chest and abdomen were never seriously considered for surgery for most of the 19th century. Before there were anaesthetic agents, it would have taken too long and inflicted far too much pain to make such procedures bearable for both patients and surgeons alike. Furthermore, surgeons lacked the necessary skills to perform operations on the chest and abdomen. The discovery of ether and chloroform meant that patients could be rendered unconscious and surgery could be performed without inflicting pain. However, although it was employed extensively during the Crimean War, general anaesthesia made little difference to the types of procedure undertaken. Chest and abdominal wounds remained off limits to the surgeon. While it was a great advance to be able to perform surgery painlessly, anaesthesia was not without significant risk and some prominent members of the medical profession were very reluctant to use it. During the Second Boer War, a handful of enterprising clinicians attempted to perform abdominal procedures. One such surgeon was Frederick Treves, who would later remove the appendix of King Edward VII.

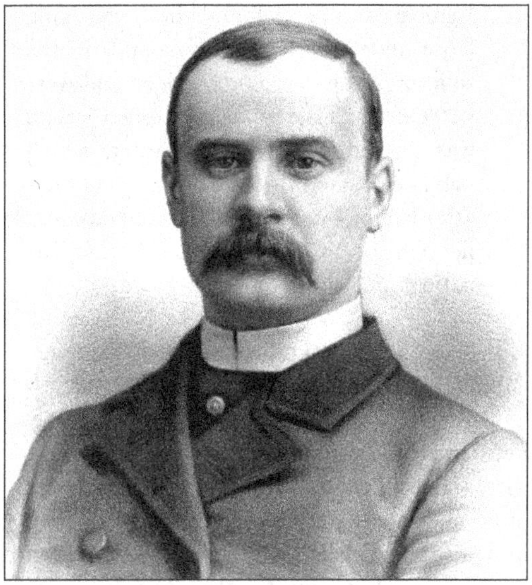

Figure 2.18 Frederick Treves (1853-1923). (Courtesy Wellcome Library, London)

Treves' description of a case that resulted in the death of a patient was a follows:

> A man was knocked down by a Mauser in the engagement of Monday, February 5th. I witnessed the engagement and saw the rifle fire and shell fire to which the men were exposed. He was hit at long range, and fell about I p.m. He was brought into hospital on a stretcher, having been carried by hand all the way. He came in at 5.30 p.m., having had to wait until the infantry and field artillery had retired. I saw him at once. He was blanched and somewhat collapsed. His pulse was small. He answered all questions promptly. He had had an injection of morphine when picked up and had vomited twice. There was still much pain, but the abdomen was quite flat. There was evidence of considerable peritoneal haemorrhage. The wound was a Mauser wound, and was over the left tenth rib in the mid-axillary line. There was no point of exit, but a well-marked ecchymosis (bruising) of the right parietes (muscles of abdominal wall) at the tip of the right twelfth rib suggested the position of the bullet. The case seemed favourable for operation, and I carried out a laparotomy by median incision at once. The following condition was found: fracture of the 10th rib, lacerated hole in the spleen, enormous quantity of blood in the peritoneal cavity and evidently from the spleen, a linear rent in the upper jejunum one inch long, four holes (entry and exit) in the jejunum at its very commencement, a hole in the lower part of the right lobe of the liver. All the five wounds in the bowel were carefully sutured, the smaller holes requiring in addition to a continuous suture of the mucous membrane – from 3 to 6

> Lembert sutures. I found the bullet lying loose under the liver. The wounds in the solid organs had ceased to bleed and were not touched. The whole peritoneal cavity was flushed out with hot water, which had been passed through a Berkefeld filter after having been boiled. The operation of necessity occupied a considerable time. The patient died shortly after.[44]

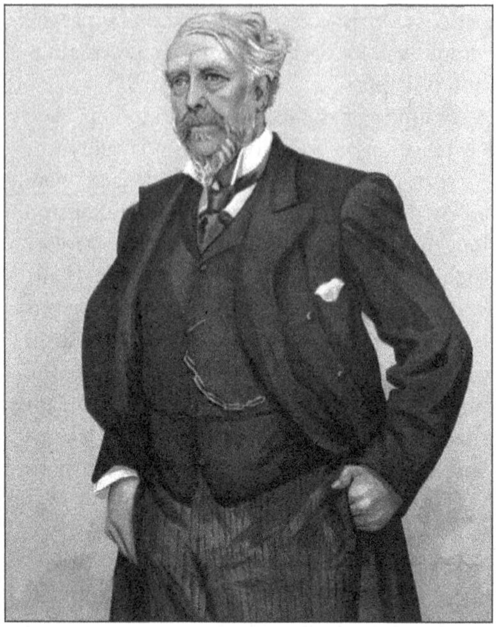

Figure 2.19 Sir William MacCormac (1836-1901). (Courtesy Wellcome Library, London)

This case is rather typical of abdominal operations performed during the Boer War, death being the usual outcome. This was partly due to lack of surgical experience and expertise and partly attributable to poor pre-and post-operative care. Whatever the reason, it prompted Sir William MacCormac, Consulting Surgeon to the British Army to proclaim: "In this war, a man wounded in the abdomen dies if operated upon and remains alive if he is left in peace."[45] His strongly expressed view was without scientific evidence but persisted to the time of the Great War when patients with penetrating abdominal wounds were treated conservatively in the opening months of the conflict with disastrous consequences.

The first real progress in the management of penetrating abdominal wounds came three years later during the Russo-Japanese War, when a female surgeon called Vera Gedroits, working in a Red Cross train, carried out early laparotomies on patients with penetrating abdominal wounds. The Russians had many Red Cross trains situated close to the front line which were equipped with operating facilities and beds for 200 or 300 patients. Each train had at least three trained doctors, 10 nursing sisters from the Red Cross Society and 40 hospital assistants. Surgical teams operated on large numbers of casualties, many with life-threatening abdominal wounds. Early surgery was the key to success. Any delay in treatment was associated with a poor prognosis. Gedroits presented the results of her work to the Russian Society of Military Doctors and her treatment regimes, for perforating abdominal wounds were accepted as the new standard of care by Russian surgeons. Her results were far better than those of any other surgeons. This was probably because she made every effort to operate within three hours of wounding and because she was a very skilful surgeon.

Gedroits never achieved recognition outside Russia. This may have been because she was a woman. Perhaps it was because nobody in the west knew about her work. There were no on-line

44 Treves, F., The War in South Africa after Spion Kop, *British Medical Journal,* 1: 2045, (10 March 1900), pp. 599-607.

45 Bennett, J.D., Abdominal surgery in war-the early story, *Journal of the Royal Society of Medicine*; 84: 9, (1991), pp.554-557.

literature searches in 1905. Perhaps it was because she was Russian, and all things Russian were viewed with suspicion. Britain had formed an alliance with Japan in 1902 to guard against Russian expansion around the Pacific coast and to bring an end to 'splendid isolation' in the wake of much criticism of Britain's conduct during the Second Boer War, when Boer women and children were interned in concentration camps. This British invention was used in an attempt to persuade Boer men to lay down their arms if they wanted to see their families again. Whatever the reason, this vital surgical principle was never acted upon by western surgeons and had to be 'rediscovered' and eventually applied during the Great War.[46]

Neuro-surgical procedures gained in popularity during the Boer War, particularly on patients with depressed skull fractures who did not necessarily display any signs of underlying brain damage. Surgeons frequently operated on patients with such wounds, believing it was essential to elevate depressed fragments of bone to relieve pressure on the underlying brain. In fact, given that wounds in South Africa were relatively uncontaminated compared with those sustained in France and Flanders during the Great War, many of these patients would probably have done perfectly well without such invasive surgery, so it is little wonder that results were perceived as good.

46 Bennet, J.D., Princess Vera Gedroits: military surgeon, poet and author, *British Medical Journal,* No. 305: 6868 (19 December 1992), pp. 1532-34.

3

Overview of military events and medical organisations, 1914-1918

This chapter sets out to provide an overview of British Medical Services in France and Flanders between August 1914 and November 1918 and to explain how these services evolved in response to important military engagements which took place during the four years of the Great War.

Following Britain's declaration of war against Germany on 4 August 1914, a small British Expeditionary Force sailed to France from the south coast of England under cover of darkness on the nights of 12 and 13 August 1914. It consisted of two infantry corps and one cavalry division. I and II Corps, each with approximately 30,000 men, were commanded by Lieutenant-Generals Sir Douglas Haig and Sir Horace Smith Dorrien respectively and the Cavalry Division of 10,000 men was commanded by Major-General Sir Edmund Allenby.

Personnel of the Royal Army Medical Corps made preparations to activate their plan to deal with the wounded. An evacuation pathway had been devised during the latter part of the 19th century and was modified by lessons learned during the Second Boer War and by observations made during the Russo-Japanese War.

Each infantry battalion of approximately 1,000 officers and men had a regimental medical officer (RMO) who was responsible for treating the sick and wounded. The RMO had sixteen regimental stretcher bearers tasked with retrieving the wounded and transporting them to the regimental aid post (RAP), where they were given first aid before personnel of a field ambulance took over their care. Field ambulances were formed as single functional units in 1905 by amalgamating the stretcher bearer companies and field hospitals employed during the Boer War (Chapter 2). Each field ambulance had 10 officers and 224 men, who worked in either a tent division or a stretcher bearer division, serving a brigade of approximately 4,000 infantrymen. Each ambulance was subdivided into three identical sections, lettered A, B or C, which were potentially capable of independent action. Three field ambulances were allocated to an infantry division of 3 brigades, each of which had four battalions. The tent divisions of the ambulances were responsible for establishing a divisional advanced dressing station (ADS) approximately 2 miles behind the front line and a main dressing station (MDS) a further 2 miles to the rear. The ADS and MDS were treatment facilities for the wounded although major surgery was rarely performed in these facilities, particularly during the early years of the conflict. Cavalry field ambulances were arranged differently, each ambulance having only two sections. Between July and November 1918, Field Ambulance Resuscitation Teams were employed by personnel of the five Australian Divisions to perform limb and life-saving surgery at main dressing stations and occasionally at advanced dressing stations (Chapter 8).

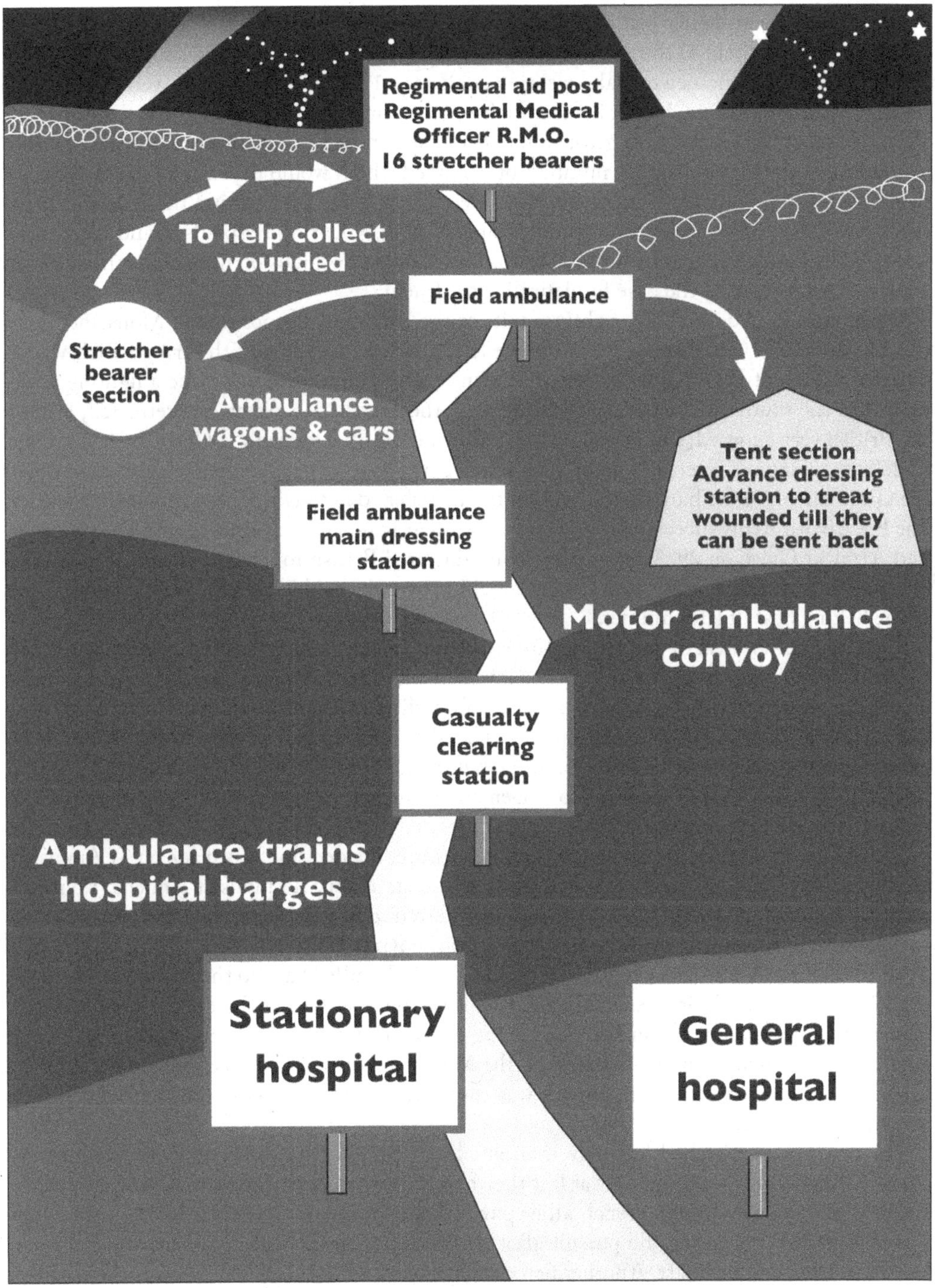

Figure 3.1 Evacuation Pathway for the wounded. (With thanks to Gordon Stables, Department of Medical Illustration, University of Aberdeen.)

The ambulance stretcher bearer divisions were responsible for collecting the wounded from RAPs and taking them to the ADS or MDS. From there, patients were transported to casualty clearing hospitals (renamed casualty clearing stations in 1915) if their wounds were of sufficient severity. As explained in Chapter 2, clearing hospitals came into being after the Russo-Japanese War, a conflict associated with great numbers of casualties. Fearing that a European conflict would be associated with similar numbers of wounded which would overwhelm the facilities in field ambulances, casualty clearing hospitals were introduced close behind the MDS to allow rapid evacuation of wounded from the dressing stations. Clearing hospitals would receive the wounded and transfer them by hospital trains to stationary hospitals on lines of communication and general hospitals at the base for definitive treatment.

On Sunday 23 August 1914, fighting units of the BEF took up position at Mons and along the Mons–Condé Canal in Belgium on the left flank of the French 5th Army which was at Charleroi. Men of II Corps fought the Germans before being forced to make a fighting withdrawal to the south on the Sunday evening after the French 5th Army had retreated, leaving the British very exposed. On 26 August at le Cateau, Smith-Dorrien's II Corps turned around to deliver a stinging reverse to von Kluck's 1st Army, in a manoeuvre designed to slow down the Germans who were hard on the heels of the British and not giving them a moment's respite. The French 5th Army successfully performed a similar manoeuvre against von Bulow's German 2nd Army at Guise on 29 August, permitting the tired British to have a rest day, and tend to blistered feet, which ached after constant marching over the cobbled streets of Northern France in the baking heat of late summer.

The rapid withdrawal of the BEF from Mons and Le Cateau made life particularly difficult for the field ambulances of II Corps, since it was involved in very heavy fighting. Further problems were created when the clearing hospitals providing the vital link between the field army units and the lines of communication were forced to withdraw. Clearing hospitals had been gathering at St Quentin prior to distribution, but the rapid German advance made this position untenable and they were transferred to Rouen on 26 August. St Quentin had been the principal point to which evacuation of the wounded was directed, but it had to be abandoned on the night of 27 August. As a result of sustained German pressure, the decision was made on 31 August to establish a new line of communication. General and stationary hospitals at Amiens, Rouen, le Havre and Boulogne were closed down and transferred to St Nazaire on the Atlantic coast and to Nantes, 40 miles upstream from St Nazaire on the River Loire.

With the French 5th Army to its eastern side, the BEF pulled back to the River Marne, fewer than 30 miles east of Paris. General Joffre, who was Commander-in-Chief of the French forces, launched a major counter-offensive against the Germans between 6 and 9 September, in what later became known as the First Battle of The Marne. It was a decisive action and brought the German advance to a standstill. Now it was the Germans' turn to withdraw, with the French and British in pursuit.

The British had marched for more than one hundred and fifty miles under severe pressure since the Battle of Mons, and now at last they had an opportunity to attack. Re-invigorated by the prospect, they and their French allies pursued the Germans across the River Aisne. They had anticipated continuing the pursuit after the crossing, but instead the Germans dug in on the north bank and held fast. Another fierce engagement, which became known as the Battle of the Aisne was fought between 12 and 15 September 1914. Each side then tried to outflank the other, in a series of manoeuvres which to the north became known as the 'race to the sea'. Each

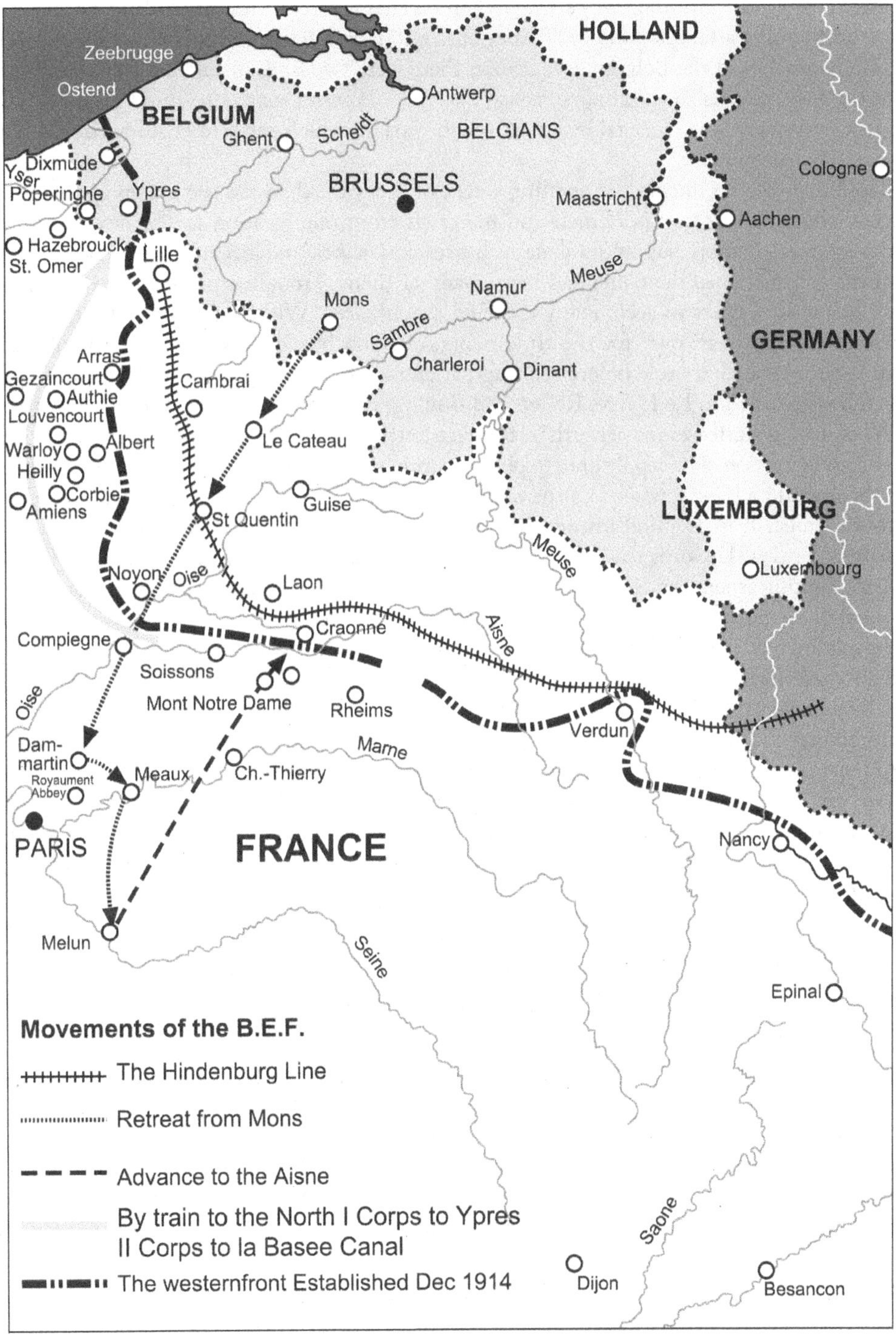

Figure 3.2 Map of Western Front showing key locations, including those of some casualty clearing stations. (With thanks to Gordon Stables, Kirsten Reilly and Lewis Taylor)

side tried to gain an advantage by getting in behind enemy forces, and then 'rolling up their line'. These outflanking attempts were only brought to a standstill when the opposing armies reached the sandy beaches of the Belgian coast. Soon there were two lines of soldiers facing each other from the Swiss border to the channel coast, and the Western Front came into being. A conflict of great movement was replaced by static trench warfare which came to characterise the Great War until spring 1918.

Rapid manoeuvres during the opening weeks of the war exhausted the horses of field ambulances, which had to transport men and materials from one location to the next. Motorised transport was in short supply and many horses lost shoes and became lame, because such frequent and sustained demands had been made of them. Troublesome delays were common, there being no farriers to accompany the field ambulances. With the danger of an imminent German breakthrough over for the time being, clearing hospitals were finally distributed to fulfil their intermediary role before sending patients on to the stationary and general hospitals which had returned to Le Havre, Rouen and Boulogne during the second half of September.

When troops started to move north in the 'race to the sea', the BEF was transported by train in the general direction of its supply lines to play its part in the unfolding conflict. II Corps went north to fight around La Bassée, while I Corps went further north and arrived at the Belgian city of Ypres by mid-October 1914. Reinforcements arrived as quickly as possible to replace growing numbers of casualties. British III Corps reached France in time for the Battle of The Aisne, and IV Corps in time for fighting around Ypres in October and November 1914, where the character of the fighting changed dramatically. The Belgian Army to the North blocked access to the coastal plain in what became known as the Battle of The Yser, an engagement it only won by opening the dyke sluices and flooding the flat coastal plain from the coast to Dixmuide, thus securing the northern flank of the allied line for the duration of the war. Fighting round Ypres offered the Germans a final opportunity to break through and end fighting in the West by inflicting a defeat on their hated enemy, the French, and by knocking the 'contemptible' little British Army out of the war. This was to be no outflanking manoeuvre. This was to be a hammer blow to punch a hole through the heart of the allied defences. Only after defeating the British and the French, could they turn their full attention against the Russian Armies on the Eastern Front. The British had to call on all their experience to prevent a catastrophic breakthrough. As a result of their efforts and those of French and Belgian forces, the allies came to hold a roughly semi-circular area of ground with a four to five-mile radius bulging out from Ypres against the higher and more advantageous German positions. Thus was born the infamous Ypres Salient. The Germans looked down on the positions held by the allies, where defenders could be fired at from the front, from the sides, and even from the rear.

During the fighting around la Bassée and Ypres in October and November 1914, clearing hospitals were moved to St Omer, Hazebrouck, Bethune, Bailleul, Ypres and Poperinghe. Ambulance trains ran daily to the Flanders front, taking great numbers of casualties to the stationary and general hospitals for definitive management of their wounds. In December 1914, Sir Anthony Bowlby, Senior Consulting Surgeon to the British Expeditionary Force, published a paper in the British Medical Journal outlining the recommended treatment for different wounds at the clearing hospitals during the opening months of the war.[1] For example, simple

1 Bowlby, A., The work of the 'clearing hospitals' during the past six weeks, *British Medical Journal*, 2:2816 (19 December 1914), pp. 1053-54.

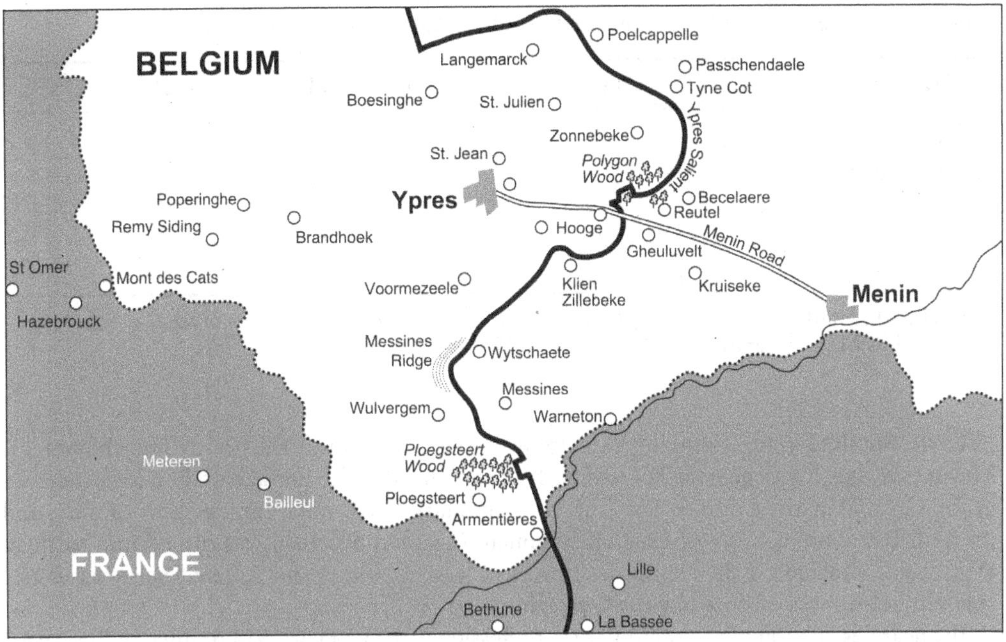

Figure 3.3 Map of Ypres Salient showing key locations, including those of casualty clearing stations. (With thanks to Gordon Stables, Kirsten Reilly and Lewis Taylor)

flesh wounds needed an antiseptic dressing, while fractured forearm bones required an antiseptic dressing and splintage. A fractured femur needed the wound washed out with an antiseptic solution before applying an antiseptic dressing and a splint for the fracture. Patients with chest wounds were not dealt with surgically and abdominal wounds were managed the same way as in the Boer War and were not as a rule dealt with operatively. Those patients considered to be in need of surgery were transferred to base hospitals for definitive management.

Bowlby's observations are most illuminating because the management of wounds soon changed completely. Dreadful problems were identified in those patients arriving at base hospitals and many lives were lost needlessly as a result of overwhelming pyogenic (pus forming) infections and from gas gangrene. These deaths were caused by appalling delays in delivering effective wound treatment. This is illustrated by the first case history in Chapter 1 and will be discussed further in Chapter 4.

Opposing forces spent four years killing and maiming each other in the confined area of the Ypres Salient. There were three major battles around Ypres, but even when nothing of importance happened, men were killed or wounded in the Salient on a daily basis. The heavy fighting around Ypres in the closing weeks of 1914 became known as the First Battle of Ypres and resulted in the formation of the Ypres Salient. British battle casualty losses between August and December 1914 are shown in Table 3.1

It has been estimated that by the end of 1914 only 1 officer and 30 other ranks remained of each battalion of 1,000 strong which went to France in August 1914. The loss of these men was a severe blow, because they were a highly trained force of hardened professionals. In that sense they were irreplaceable, and it would be a long time before their successors acquired a matching level of ability.

Table 3.1 Battle casualties BEF, France and Flanders, August to December 1914.

Battle casualties	Officers	Other Ranks	Total
Killed	1,008	11,971	13,009
Died of wounds	228	3,429	3,657
Missing	253	6,343	6,596
Prisoners of war	530	19,385	19,915
Wounded and survived	1,877	53,812	55,689

Mitchell, T.J., Smith, G.M., *History of the Great War Medical Services Casualties and Medical Statistics*, (London: His Majesty's Stationery Office 1931), p.122.

To the South of Ypres, swinging away from the city and towards the nearby French border is Messines Ridge. It was here on 31 October 1914 that the first Territorial battalion to be involved in the Great War went into action. The Expeditionary Force was running short of men, and the 14th Battalion, County of London Regiment (London Scottish) was rushed into battle at Wytschaete situated on the central part of the Messines Ridge and suffered heavy casualties before the ridge was captured by the Germans.

The near destruction of the small British professional army in late 1914 resulted in Territorial divisions being sent to the Western Front. The Territorial Force was originally created to guard Britain's shores, but casualties in France and Belgium in 1914 were so heavy, that the Territorials were invited to sign up for overseas service. When the British took over more of the front line from their French allies in 1915, Territorial troops went to France in increasing numbers, partly as single battalions to reinforce depleted divisions already in France and partly as divisions to participate in the British offensives of 1915. Soon there were six Territorial divisions in France, the 46th (North Midland), 47th (London), 48th (South Midland), 49th (West Riding), 50th (Northumbrian), and 51st (Highland). By then, there were two British Armies, which had been formed on Christmas Day 1914. The First Army in northern France was under the command of Lieutenant-General Sir Douglas Haig and the Second Army at Ypres under Lieutenant-General Sir Horace Smith-Dorrien.

On 22 April 1915, the British Second Army had to defend the Ypres Salient against the first German chlorine gas attack. This marked the start of the Second Battle of Ypres which lasted until 25 May. Chlorine was discharged from gas cylinders late in the afternoon of 22 April between the villages of Poelcappelle and Langemarck a few miles from Ypres. This resulted in the complete collapse of the northern segment of the Ypres Salient when French Colonial troops occupying the trenches around Langemarck fled, leaving a huge gap in the front line. Fortunately, the Germans had not made preparations to fully exploit the advantage gained, and men of the Canadian 1st Division, who had recently arrived in the Ypres Salient, deployed rapidly and saved the day. The Salient contracted to a tight defensive position round Ypres, making it easier to defend.

Casualty clearing hospitals were renamed casualty clearing stations in 1915 and they began to take on vital surgical roles. Many urgent operations were performed there before patients were sent by train to distant base hospitals. This change in management followed the recognition that early definitive surgery was essential in many cases to save limbs and lives. Casualty clearing stations for the Second Battle of Ypres were at Poperinghe (3 and 50), Bailleul (2 and 8), Hazebrouck (10 and South Midland) and Mont Des Cats (North Midland).[2]

The personnel at a casualty clearing station comprised 8 officers and 77 other ranks. One medical officer had dental qualifications. Nursing sisters were introduced in 1915, at first five and then seven. Casualty clearing stations were usually out of range of shell fire, at a minimum of 10,000 yards from the front line and could be reached relatively quickly by motor ambulance wagon convoys from advanced dressing stations. They were often constructed from prefabricated wooden huts and were near a railway line. Each had accommodation for 800-1,200 wounded and were staffed by personnel who were experienced in the treatment of soldiers with limb and life-threatening wounds. Each casualty clearing station normally had two surgical teams during "quiet" spells, each consisting of a surgeon, anaesthetist, theatre sister and an operating theatre orderly. When reinforcements were required during a battle, surgical teams were sent from tent sections of field ambulances, from other clearing stations in quiet sectors and from base hospitals. While casualty clearing stations performed the vital role of limb and life-saving surgery, this was not their sole function. Many clearing stations also dealt with soldiers who had minor wounds. This was important because it kept the lightly wounded in the forward area and returned them to the front line quickly. There was also a group of patients who needed surgery, but whose condition was not so severe that they could not wait till they reached base hospitals for treatment. After careful assessment, such patients were put directly onto ambulance trains and sent down the line to the base.

While the British Second Army defended the Ypres Salient in April and May 1915, the First Army conducted offensives between March and September in Northern France at Neuve Chapelle, Aubers Ridge, Festubert, and Loos at the insistence of their French allies who wanted British support while the French attacked the Germans further south.

The first of Kitchener's volunteer divisions arrived on the Western Front in 1915 and played a major part in the fighting over the next three years. Lord Kitchener, Secretary of State for War, harboured a prejudice against the Territorial Army and had little faith in these 'part time soldiers'. Kitchener was one of the few who did not believe that the war would be 'over by Christmas'. Realising that it would be a long and costly conflict, he began to recruit volunteers. Posters appeared with Kitchener's stern face and pointing finger, challenging men to join up. Men flocked in their thousands to enlist. Two of the first resulting volunteer (service) divisions were the 9th and 15th Scottish Divisions. They were in the field by mid-1915, in time to take part on the first day of the Battle of Loos on 25 September 1915. Loos can justifiably be described as 'a very Scottish battle', because in addition to the 9th and 15th Divisions, there were Scottish battalions in the three regular participating divisions on the first day of the battle. Loos was partly fought over ground which was industrialised with many slag heaps (crassiers) from coal mines and partly over flat and featureless open country with no natural cover. Because of a severe shortage of artillery pieces and ordnance, reliance was placed on chlorine gas to compensate for these deficiencies. The strategy failed miserably. The wind, such as it was, was blowing in the wrong direction over much of the battlefield and men frequently became victims of their own gas.

2 Macpherson, W.G., *History of The Great War based on official documents Medical Services General History Vol. II,* (London: MacMillan, 1923), p.396.

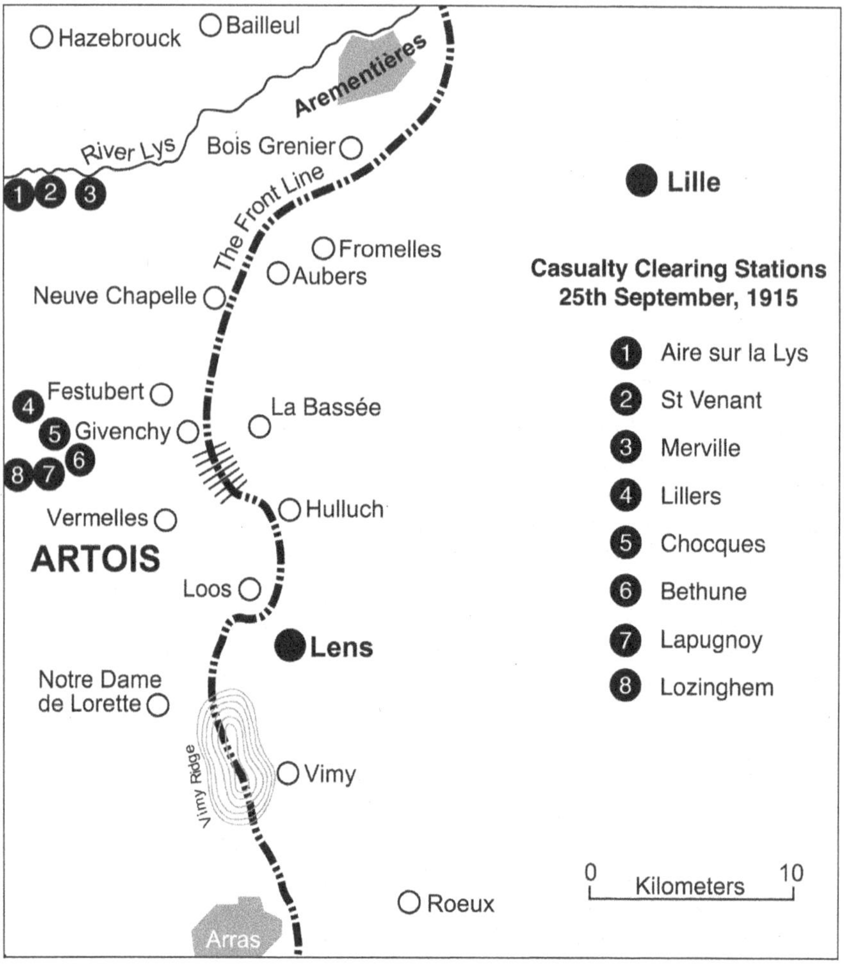

Figure 3.4 Map of Northern France showing key locations of battles and casualty clearing stations. (With thanks to Gordon Stables, Kirsten Reilly and Lewis Taylor)

Casualty clearing stations for the First Army were located at Merville (CCS 7, 1st/2nd London, Lahore), St Venant (Lucknow), Lillers (6, 9, 2nd/1st W. Riding)), Chocques (No 1and detachment of No 1 Canadian) and Aire (No 22, No 1 Canadian), Lapugnoy (No 18), Lozinghem (No 23) [3]

The battles fought in northern France in 1915 provided the British Medical Services with the opportunity to prepare for premeditated attacks and to gain much needed experience in performing urgent surgical operations in casualty clearing stations. By 1915 it had become clear that penetrating wounds of the abdomen did very badly without surgery and steps were taken to rectify this.

3 Macpherson, *History of The Great War, Vol II,* p.452.

During the Battle of Loos, advanced operating centres were established to deal with abdominal wounds and patients were taken to two centres at Bac St. Maur and Noeux-les-Mines as quickly as possible. Surgeons from casualty clearing stations staffed these facilities (Chapter 7). The Medical Research Committee (MRC) began codifying medical records which resulted in greater accuracy of documentation. Battle casualties for 1915 are shown in Table 3.2.

Table 3.2 Battle casualties BEF, France and Flanders, 1915

Battle casualties	Officers	Other Ranks	Total
Killed	3,032	45,572	48,604
Died of wounds	745	14,159	14,904
Missing	412	15,523	15,935
Prisoners of war	390	8,231	8,621
Wounded and survived	7,434	217,529	224,963

Mitchell, T.J., Smith, G.M., History of the Great War Medical Services Casualties and Medical Statistics (London: His Majesty's Stationery Office 1931), p.136.

By July 1916, there were three more British Armies in France as a result of ever-increasing numbers of men being posted to the Western Front. A Third Army was formed in France in July 1915. Initially, it was commanded by Lieutenant-General Sir Charles Monro and was deployed astride the River Somme. Lieutenant-General Rawlinson then briefly held command when Monro went elsewhere. A Canadian Corps containing three divisions (soon there would be four) was formed. Australian and New Zealand Forces (Anzacs) arrived in France in early 1916, so that with many more troops at his disposal, General Sir Douglas Haig, who had taken over command of British Forces from Field Marshall Sir John French in December 1915, was able to further expand his armies. Rawlinson was given command of the newly formed Fourth Army on 5 February 1916, while Lieutenant-General Sir Edmund Allenby took over the command of the Third Army from Rawlinson. A Reserve Army under Lieutenant-General Sir Hubert Gough, which first fought at the Battle of the Somme in July 1916, was renamed the Fifth Army in October 1916.

Saturday 1 July 1916, the first day of the Battle of the Somme, was the worst day in British military history with more than 57,000 casualties, 20,000 of whom were either killed or died from their wounds. Casualty clearing stations for seriously wounded were located at Corbie (5, 21), Vecquemont (34, 45), Heilly (36, 38), Puchevillers (3, 44), Beauval (No 4) and Gézaincourt (No 29). Casualty clearing stations at Heilly, Vequemont and Gézaincourt also dealt with lightly wounded. So numerous were the casualties on 1 July that during the night of 1/2 July, congestion in the casualty clearing stations was acute. There were insufficient ambulance trains to evacuate the wounded and casualties arrived in the clearing stations from field ambulances more quickly than anticipated. The favourable weather and increased capacity of a narrow-gauge railway between Acheux and Gézaincourt added to the rapidity with which CCSs filled. Furthermore, unexpectedly large numbers of lightly wounded arrived at Vequemont, Heilly and Gézaincourt. During the first 24 hours of the battle, 863 officers and 22,826 men were admitted to the field ambulances of Fourth Army alone and of these, 797 officers and 13,603 other ranks were transferred to casualty clearing stations. Everything became bogged down and casualties were also evacuated by road and by barge to help relieve the congestion till more ambulance trains were provided. Steps were taken to avoid any repetition of this very unsatisfactory state of affairs.[4]

Generally speaking from a medical standpoint, 1916 was notable for arrangements made to collect casualties from a very large force fighting a series of battles and advancing very slowly. Improvements in collection and evacuation were introduced. The number of regimental stretcher bearers was doubled from 16 to 32 and more accommodation and better shelter was provided in RAPs and ADSs. Casualty clearing stations were formed into groups of two or three, employing a system of admitting 150-300 casualties in rotation, which facilitated evacuation and treatment.[5] Additional surgical teams were supplied during battles. It has already been noted that abdominal wounds required urgent life-saving surgery and advanced operating centres to deal with such cases were opened at Authie, Warloy and Heilly.[6] Crisis expansion of base hospital accommodation was required to accommodate the unprecedented numbers of wounded, so that many existing hospitals were enlarged and new ones were opened.[7] To keep pace with ever increasing numbers of casualties over the following two years, stationary and general hospitals continued to expand for the remainder of the war. Stationary hospitals were originally designed to be positioned on the line of communication, providing a link between the casualty clearing station and general hospital at the base. Given the static nature of warfare, there was no need for this distinction and stationary hospitals fulfilled exactly the same role as general hospitals. The only difference was one of size, stationary hospitals being smaller. Figure 3.5 depicts the number of beds available in different centres by 1918.

Table 3.3 shows the casualties for 1916. The majority were from the Battle of the Somme which lasted for four and a half months.

Table 3.3 BEF Battle Casualties, France and Flanders 1916

Battle casualties	Officers	Other Ranks	Total
Killed	6,506	100,905	107,411
Died of wounds	1,814	35,065	36,879
Missing	878	27,281	28,159
Prisoners of war	750	14,766	15,516
Wounded and survived	20,345	443,352	463,697

Mitchell, T.J., Smith, G.M., History of the Great War Medical Services Casualties and Medical Statistics (London: His Majesty's Stationery Office 1931), p. 149.

While Kitchener's New Army Divisions fought on the Somme in 1916, volunteer numbers had diminished during 1915 as a result of ever-growing casualty lists. Men had to be found to

4 Macpherson, W.G., *History of The Great War based on official documents Medical Services General History Vol. III*, (London: His Majesty's Stationery Office, 1924), pp. 37-47.
5 Mitchell, T.J., Smith, G.M., *History of the Great War Medical Services Casualties and Medical Statistics*, (London: His Majesty's Stationery Office, 1931), p. 147.
6 Macpherson, *History of The Great War, Vol. III*, pp. 37-38.
7 Macpherson, *History of the Great War, Vol II*, p. 69.

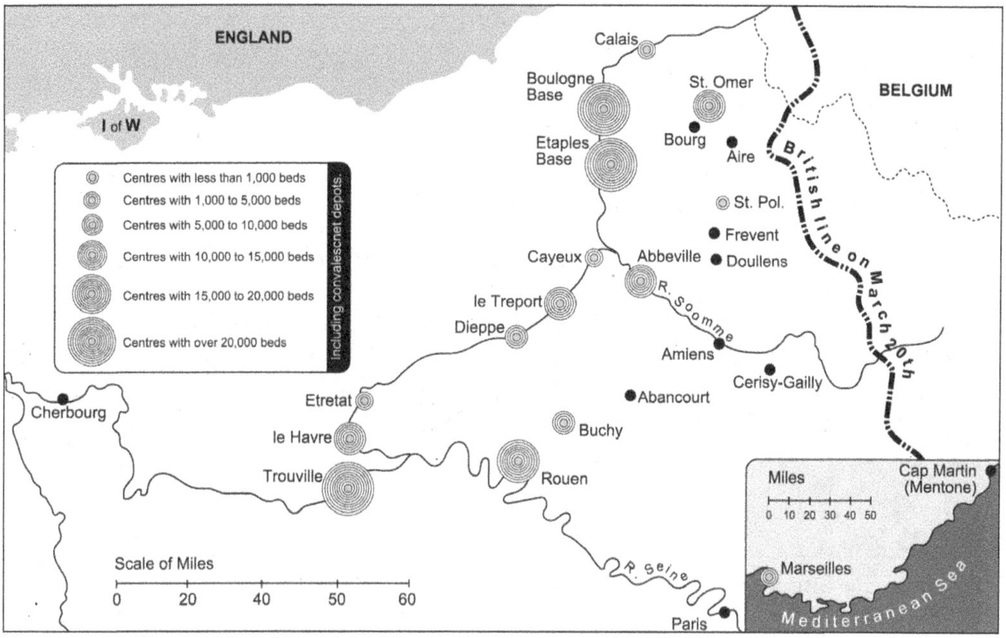

Figure 3.5 Map showing hospital centres in France, from MacPherson, WG, *History of the Great War based on official documents, Medical Services, General History* (London: HMSO, 1921-24), p. 138. (With thanks to Gordon Stables, Department of Medical Illustration, University of Aberdeen)

maintain battalion strength and by late 1915, all men between the ages of 15 and 65 years who were not already in the forces had to register and notify the authorities which trade they were in. In October 1915 Lord Derby was appointed to the position of Director of Recruiting. He encouraged all those between the ages of 18 and 40 to either enlist or to attest with an obligation to enlist if called upon. The carrot to encourage enlistment, if it can be called that, was the assurance of a war pension in the event of being killed or wounded. Unsurprisingly, this did not have the desired result and consequently conscription was introduced with the Military Services Act in January 1916.

Many young conscripts first saw action in 1917, when the four principal battles were the Battle of Arras, in April and May 1917, the Battle of Messines on 7 June, the Third Battle of Ypres between 31 July and 10 November 1917 and the Battle of Cambrai between 20 November and 7 December. Arras was fought to support an abortive attempt by General Nivelle, Commander-in-Chief of the French Armies, to break through German defensive positions on the Chemin des Dames. Losses at Arras were approximately 158,660, of whom 29,505 were killed. Messines was a successful preliminary action to remove the Germans from Messines Ridge before beginning the Third Battle of Ypres on 31 July 1917. The strategic aim of Third Ypres was to break out from the Ypres Salient and capture the Belgian ports of Ostend and Zeebrugge, thereby denying their use to the Germans as U-boat bases. The offensive became completely bogged down in the mud and ended on 10 November 1917 at the ruined village of Passchendaele, where men fought and died in the most appalling conditions. The Third Battle of Ypres involved Australian, New Zealand and Canadian Divisions as well as British and South African Forces.

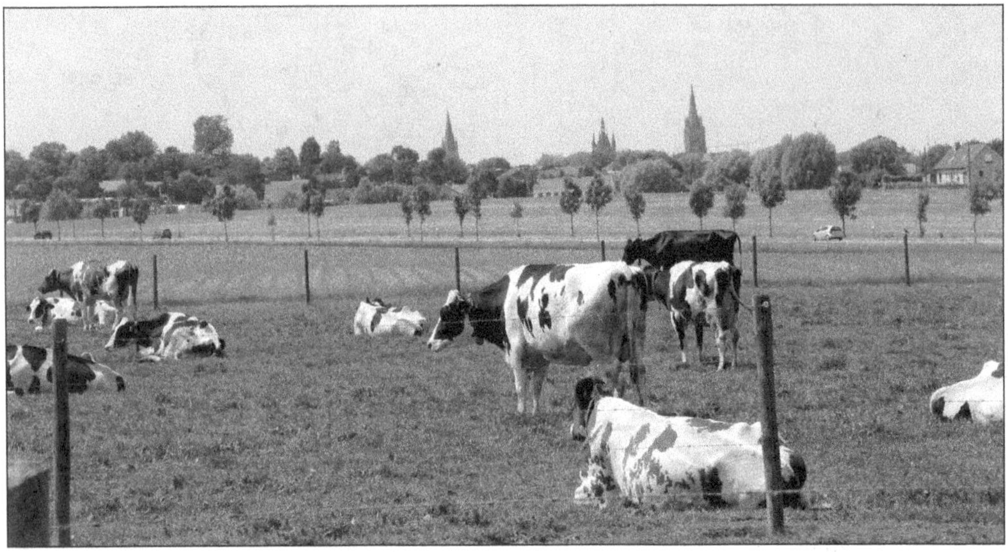

Figure 3.6 The City of Ypres is surrounded by rich agricultural land today, just as it was at the start of the Great War in 1914. Lethal organisms occurring naturally in the soil were responsible for colonising wounds with potentially devastating consequences. (With thanks to Dr Derek King)

More than a quarter of a million British and Commonwealth soldiers died in the confined area of the Ypres Salient during four years of the Great War. The bodies of a great many of those who died were never found and lie buried forever beneath the richly fertilised fields of Flanders. Those same fertilised fields were partly responsible for the deaths of many soldiers whose wounds became colonised by the lethal organisms which cause gas gangrene and tetanus, and which occur naturally in the soil.

During the Third Battle of Ypres, casualty clearing stations were arranged in groups of 3 or 4, each group sharing particular areas of expertise. There had been many important advances made in the surgical management of different types of wound and this was reflected in the organisation of medical services.

Casualty clearing stations (CCSs) 32, 44 and Australian 3rd at Brandhoek were closest to the front line and therefore reached most quickly. They dealt with chest wounds, penetrating abdominal wounds and compound fractures of the femur. There were four CCSs at Remy Siding, British 10 and 17 and Canadian 2 and 3. They were the largest clearing stations on the Western Front and dealt with all types of cases including penetrating chest and abdominal wounds and compound fractures of the femur. The three CCSs 12, 46 and 64 at Proven (Mendinghem) dealt with wounds of the skull and brain, while the two at Haringhe (Bandaghem), CCSs 62 and 63, dealt with those who were sick. Casualty figures for 1917 are shown in Table 3.4

If the allies were finding it difficult to replace losses, the Germans too were feeling the strain by 1917. They had suffered very heavy casualties in 1916, both on the Somme and at Verdun, where they had fought a prolonged battle of attrition against the French between February and December of that year. As a result, they withdrew to a prepared defensive line which shortened the length of their front by eliminating a broad-based salient. This formidable defensive position was christnened the Hindenburg Line by the British.

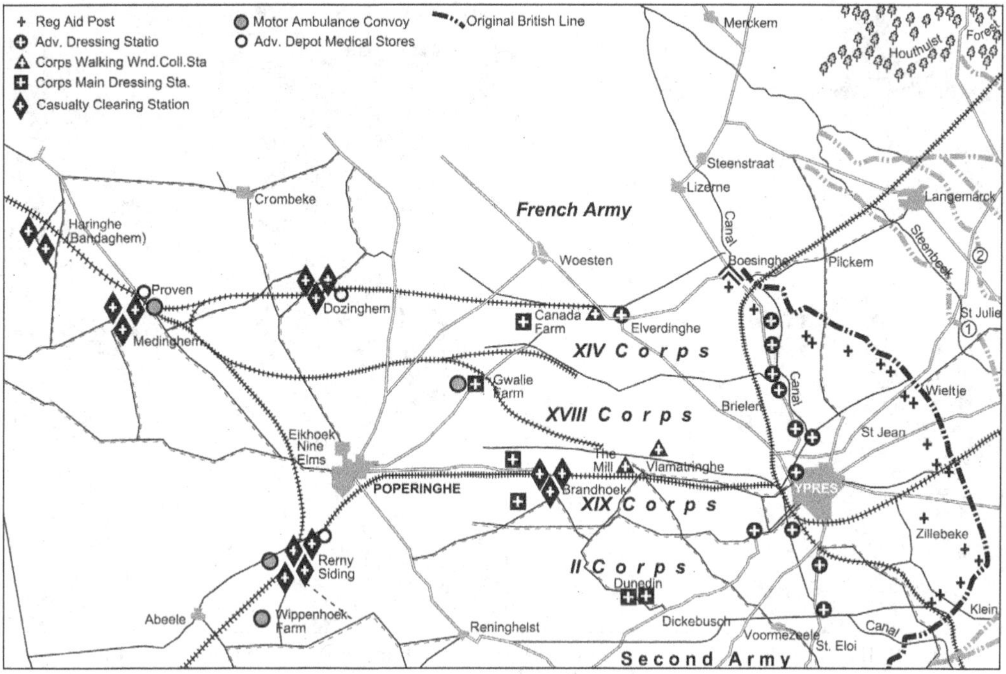

Figure 3.7 This map shows the general situation of Medical Units of 5th Army, 31 July 1917. Casualty clearing stations were in groups of 2-4 to make it easier to deal with massive numbers of casualties. (Macpherson, W.G., *History of the Great War based on official documents Medical Services General History Vol. III*, London: His Majesty's Stationery Office, 1924, p. 138)

Table 3.4 Battle casualties BEF, France and Flanders, 1917

Battle casualties	Officers	Other Ranks	Total
Killed	7,659	124,102	131,761
Died of wounds	2,627	47,205	49,832
Missing	1,405	29,162	30,567
Prisoners of war	1,229	21,998	23,227
Wounded and survived	20,835	494,027	514,862

Mitchell, T.J., Smith, G.M., *History of the Great War Medical Services Casualties and Medical Statistics*, (London: His Majesty's Stationery Office 1931), p.158.

Meanwhile in Russia on the 16 December 1917, the leaders of the Bolsheviks-Lenin, Trotsky, and Stalin sued for peace with the central powers, and an armistice was declared. A peace treaty was signed on 29 March 1918 at Brest-Litovsk, and Russia was finally out of the war.

Massive numbers of German troops moved from what had been the Eastern Front, across to the Western Front. On 21 March 1918, a major German offensive was launched against the British Third and Fifth Armies from the Hindenburg Line in an attempt to break through and end the war (Figure 3.8). This was the *Kaiserschlacht*, the Kaiser's Battle, otherwise known as

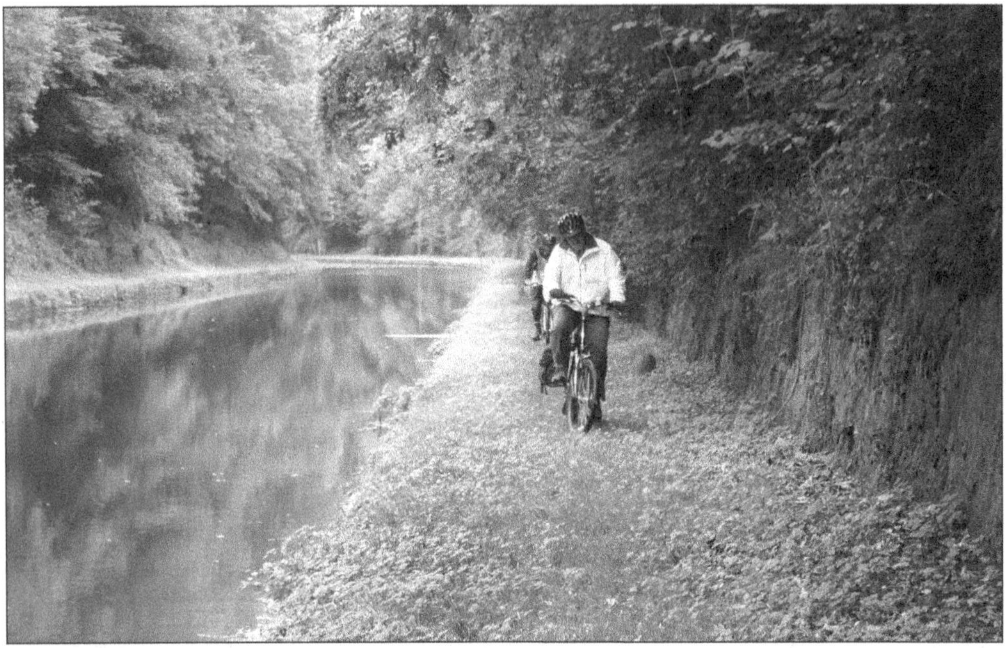

Figure 3.8 The St Quentin Canal was an integral part of the Hindenburg Line from which Ludendorf launched Operation Michael on 21 March 1918. It was from here that mobile warfare on the Western Front was re-introduced after more than three years of static trench warfare. (Author photograph)

Operation Michael. German *stormtruppen* overwhelmed Forward Zone positions of the Fifth Army and made deep inroads into the Battle Zone. Operation Michael failed in its objective to break through, but the British Fifth Army was pushed back 37 miles to Villers-Bretonneux before the German advance was finally halted. There were four further German offensives, one against the British Second Army, attacking through Armentières and over Messines Ridge towards Ypres and the railway junction of Hazebrouck, and three against the French around Rheims. While much ground was lost to the enemy, the allied lines held, and the attacks failed.

A counter-attack by French and American forces on 16 July 1918 on the Marne was a turning point. It was now the turn of the allies to attack. On 8 August 1918, the British Fourth Amy launched a major offensive at the Battle of Amiens, pushing the Germans back eight miles in a single day. German resistance stiffened by 11 August, so Field Marshall Sir Douglas Haig, who had been promoted on 1 January 1917, switched his attack to the British Third Army and the Battle of Albert commenced on 21 August. Men who had gone to war in the warm summer of 1914 would not have recognised the army of 1918. It had been transformed by sophisticated artillery, capable of locating German batteries accurately by sound ranging, and destroying them with accurate high explosive shellfire. Infantry attacks were launched behind scientifically calculated creeping barrages which were orchestrated to protect the advancing troops, who instead of going forward in waves, advanced in small groups equipped with Lewis Guns and rifle grenades to attack German positions. The British Armies had become unstoppable. The Hindenburg Line was breached on 29 September 1918, and the final advance to victory was over open ground. An armistice came into effect on 11 November 1918.

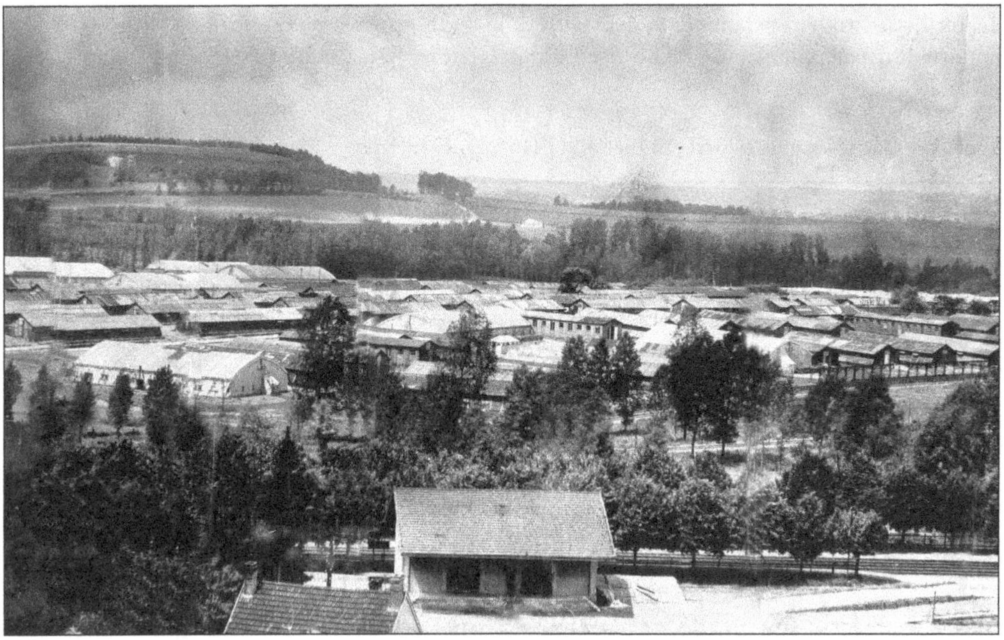

Figure 3.9 Casualty Clearing Station 37 captured by the Germans on 27 May 1918. (Courtesy Wellcome Library, London)

From a medical standpoint, events in 1918 were reminiscent of the fighting in 1914, beginning with a retreat under great pressure followed by an advance, but whereas in 1914 there was a small expeditionary force of less than 150,000 men, there were five British Armies in 1918 with a combined strength of around 2,000,000. As a result of rapid German advances in the spring of 1918, casualty clearing stations were forced to pack up and retire rapidly. They lost their stability and the important role they had fulfilled for so much of the war was suddenly curtailed. Much of the surgery undertaken in casualty clearing stations had once again to be done at the base hospitals. Between 25 and 29 March 1918, thirteen base hospitals at Étaples admitted 19,292 wounded and performed 3,698 operations, representing an operative procedure rate of 19 percent. [8]

On 27 May 1918, Casualty Clearing Station No 37 at Mont Notre Dame, including all staff and patients, was overrun and captured by the Germans before it could be evacuated. Casualty Clearing Station 48 at nearby Montigny-sur-Vesle was evacuated just in time, but 47 seriously wounded soldiers had to be left behind.[9]

The loss of these facilities and personnel made medical authorities very cautious, with the result that by July 1918, some casualty clearing stations were located further behind the lines than they otherwise might have been, and it took much longer to reach them. This had important practical implications which resulted in the formation of Field Ambulance Resuscitation

8 Whitehead, I.R., *Doctors in the Great War* (Barnsley: Leo Cooper, 1999), p. 211.
9 Macpherson, *History of The Great War Vol. III*, pp. 275-76.

Teams by Australian personnel to deal with limb and life-threatening wounds. This was a very important development and will be discussed in Chapter 8. Casualty figures for 1918 are shown in Table 3.5.

Table 3.5 Battle casualties BEF, France and Flanders, 1918

Battle casualties	Officers	Other Ranks	Total
Killed	5,111	75,365	80,476
Died of wounds	3,044	43,040	46,084
Missing	1,317	62,324	63,641
Prisoners of war	3,749	103,898	107,647
Wounded and survived	25,733	552,669	578,402

Mitchell, T.J., Smith, G.M., *History of the Great War Medical Services Casualties and Medical Statistics*, (London: His Majesty's Stationery Office 1931), p.168.

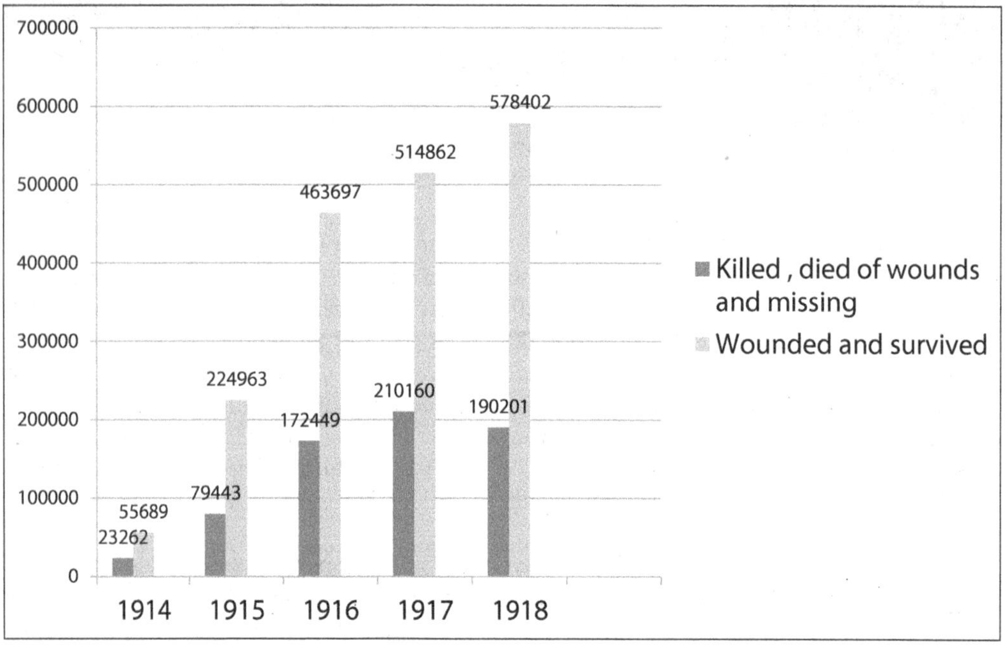

Figure 3.10 Casualty Figures showing those killed and died of wounds (dark shade), and those who survived their wounds (light shade). (From Mitchell, T.J., Smith, G.M., *History of the Great War Medical Services Casualties and Medical Statistics*, (London: His Majesty's Stationery Office 1931))

Official battle casualty figures between 1914 and 1918 are reproduced in Figure 3.10. There was a steady increase in casualties year by year throughout the war. The dark columns show the numbers of those who were killed in action, died of their wounds or were missing in action. I have assumed that all those recorded as missing were killed, although this is not entirely accurate. Some of the missing may have been taken prisoner, only to reappear at the end of the war.

Most, however, had been blown to pieces by shellfire or had sunk into the mud without trace. The light column shows those who were wounded and survived. The last year of the war had the greatest number who were wounded and survived (578,402), and there was a small drop in the number who were killed or died from wounds compared with the figures from 1917 (190,201 for 1918 and 212,160 for 1917). The ratio of killed plus died of wounds to wounded and survived is 0.32. This is a corrected lethality, since it considers those who died while under medical care. The crude figure for uncorrected lethality in the Boer War was 0.32. This represents men killed on the field of battle but takes no account of those who died subsequently from wounds sustained. During the D-Day landings in June 1944, the lethality for British soldiers was 0.39 and the cumulative figure for US troops in WW2 was 0.38. The lethality of high velocity wounds in Northern Ireland in more recent times was 0.37.[10]

10 Parker, P.J., Commentary in Stevenson, W.F., Surgical Experiences from the Boer War, *Journal Royal Army Medical Corps*, Vol. 1, No.2, (1903), pp. 83-91.

4

1914-15: Early operative disasters and a surgical breakthrough

Case history

The young corporal was struck in his right thigh by a small fragment of shell casing on the evening of 24 August 1914 during the gruelling retreat from Mons. He felt a slight stinging sensation in his thigh but nothing more. He walked back in the general direction of the retreat and was directed to the rear by a stretcher bearer pointing towards the approximate location of the advanced dressing station. The field ambulance had deployed for action that day, and while the tent division had set about establishing a dressing station, the bearer division had gone forward to collect the wounded. Unfortunately, the stretcher bearer and tent divisions had lost contact in the confusion of the retreat, so the bearer division formed an impromptu dressing station and the corporal's wound was dealt with on the morning of 25 August. He had a small puncture wound on the outer aspect of his thigh, where the fragment of shell casing had penetrated the skin and underlying muscle. The skin defect was little more than one square inch in area and the surrounding tissue looked a bit ragged but otherwise quite healthy. The medical officer who examined him provided reassurance. 'Don't worry corporal, he said. It's nothing that a couple of stitches won't put right', and he set about cleaning the wound with antiseptic solution before inserting a few sutures and applying an antiseptic dressing. 'There you go; that'll keep any harmful bugs out till you get back to base, he said, before sending the wounded man on his way. The corporal managed to find a place on one of the ambulance wagons standing nearby which soon set off in the direction of the retreat. It reached St Quentin on the morning of 27 August where the wounded were eventually transferred to an ambulance train which left for Rouen. The corporal had begun to feel unwell during the journey to St Quentin, but now his condition deteriorated dramatically. He managed to summon a nurse who looked very anxiously at his swollen thigh. He was delirious when they took him off the train at Rouen on the morning of 29 August and was completely unresponsive when he was examined in the general hospital nearby. His pulse was 180/minute and very weak. His blood pressure was unrecordable. His entire thigh was grossly swollen, and a mottled blue discolouration extended from below his knee to above his hip and over his lower abdomen. There were huge blisters filled with black altered blood overlying the pelvic bones and hip. The skin looked very tense as though about to burst and the entire limb looked dead. The examining medical officer palpated the wounded man's limb and noted a fine crackling sensation deep within the tissues over the length of his thigh, which was a sign of multiple tiny gas bubbles, confirming the diagnosis of gas gangrene. The young corporal was beyond all help and died a few minutes later. What could and should have been a simple wound to treat effectively had resulted in his untimely death.

At the outbreak of the Great War in 1914, personnel of the Royal Army Medical Corps had put in place what they thought was a suitable regime for dealing with the wounded. Their policy was based on the Listerian principle of antisepsis (Chapter 2) and had evolved from experience gained during the Second Boer War, when most freshly inflicted wounds were regarded as clean and free from bacteria and had to be kept sterile by applying antiseptic dressings to prevent infecting micro-organisms from gaining entry. In 1914, occlusive antiseptic dressings were applied as soon as possible after the infliction of wounds and were kept firmly in place until patients underwent definitive treatment at base hospitals on or near the French coast. George James Guthrie and Dominique Larrey in the early 1800's would have regarded this plan with grave concern, since they had both demonstrated the importance of early surgery to avoid the poor results associated with delayed treatment at hospitals many miles from the front. Be that as it may, it was believed in 1914 that wound infections would not become a significant problem provided the antiseptic policy was adhered to. William Flack Stevenson (1844-1922), Surgeon General during the Boer War and Principal Medical Officer to Lord Roberts from 1899 to 1900, who was also recalled to duty during the Great War, was very clear on this matter: "Unless antiseptic cleansing of the wound and of the skin around it is possible from the first, suppuration is certain to occur."[1]

Since nothing had happened in the intervening twelve years since the Boer War to persuade clinicians to change this policy, occlusive antiseptic dressings were applied to wounds in field ambulances and clearing hospitals, where many wounds were also sutured to make certain that no infecting organisms could gain access before definitive surgery was undertaken:

> The experience of the South African War and with surprisingly moderate variation of the Russo-Japanese, led to the belief that, in a large proportion of wounds, superficial or very casual chemical antisepsis with immediate suture was not only permissible but desirable.[2]

There were so many casualties, however, and medical facilities became so congested, that journeys by hospital train to base hospitals were frequently delayed and could take days. This is stated clearly in the Official History of the Australian Army Medical Services:

> In the field ambulances during the first five or six months of the war, and later in the first clearing hospitals, wounds were superficially disinfected and sutured. The time between first aid at the front and effective operation at the Base was commonly several days.[3]

1 Stevenson, W.F., Surgical Experiences from the Boer War, *Journal Royal Army Medical Corps*, Vol. 1, No. 2, (1903), pp. 91-95.

2 Butler, A.G., *Official History of the Australian Army Medical Services, 1914–1918 Vol. II – The Western Front* (Canberra: Australian War Memorial, 1940), pp. 311-2.

3 Butler, *Official History*, p. 312.

Pyogenic (pus forming) infections

It soon became obvious to medical personnel at base hospitals that they had a disaster without precedence on their hands. Many of the wounded soldiers being unloaded from hospital trains were in an appalling clinical state and were suffering from overwhelming infections caused by a variety of organisms. Nothing on this scale had been seen in the Boer War. Some patients were delirious with high fevers and had enormously swollen limbs which were acutely painful to the slightest touch and were red and hard and were clearly the sites of major deep infections caused by pus forming organisms, mostly staphylococci or streptococci. Matters were made much worse if wounds had been stitched up in field ambulances, as was often the case. Unable to escape, pus forming deep within the wound caused a massive build-up of pressure resulting in terrible pain. If the patient survived long enough to reach the operating theatre, as soon as any procedure began and a knife was plunged into the depth of the indurated suppurating mass, pints of foul-smelling pus would gush out like magma from an erupting volcano.

Base hospital personnel on the French coast found themselves having to deal with overwhelming septic infections, which were out with the experience of even their most senior surgeons, who only had antiseptic surgical principles to fall back on. A statement in the Official Australian Medical History of the Great War sums up the position in the early months of the war:

> The results were appalling. During the first six months of the conflict the mortality and morbidity from "septic" infection dealt to the surgical profession in every nation concerned a staggering blow, from which it recovered only through tedious and painful apprenticeship.[4]

The tedious and painful apprenticeship involved finding solutions to the limb and life- threatening problems posed by bacteria in the Great War. It was now apparent that while Lister's antiseptic methods had been enough for the surgical problems encountered in the Boer War, they were completely inadequate to deal with the overwhelming infections encountered in 1914. Furthermore, surgeons themselves were inadequately prepared at the outbreak of the Great War. Most did not have the faintest idea how to deal with sepsis of this magnitude because they had never seen anything remotely like it before. They had learned their surgery in civilian practice and were accustomed to working with clean wounds using aseptic surgical techniques, developed in the latter years of the 19th century. Modern war surgery was totally different, and they had to learn it from scratch. Their lack of experience and expertise in dealing with filthy contaminated wounds exposed their patients to great risk and danger. The following paragraphs sum this up well:

> Unfortunately, the medical profession entered the war in 1914 with an interesting and very remarkable handicap. Well up in the methods of ensuring asepsis in surgical wounds, for the most part it knew little of 'septic' wounds. In the early stages of the war the more fulminant forms of wound infection fell like the scourge of an unexpected pestilence on a race of surgeons grown complacent in the atmosphere of prophylactic asepsis, with whose toilsome

4 Butler, *Official History*, p. 312.

> and tedious evolution they were acquainted chiefly by tradition and Listerian Orations. For the best part of a year, indeed, at the beginning of the Great War, the treatment of wounds in the field was vitiated by neglect of the fact that the infection was contained within the wound itself so that for the most part, paints of iodine or of picric alcohol were as whiting to a sepulchre, and repeated "dressings" of little more use than were the antics and the offerings of the priests of Baal. [5]

It is very important to appreciate that wounds sustained in the fields of France and Flanders during the Great War were never sterile. They were grossly contaminated by bacteria from the very outset. It was pointless covering them with antiseptic dressings and it was positively dangerous to suture them at dressing stations of field ambulances. Many wounded soldiers who underwent early wound closure in this way were being handed a death sentence:

> All wounds should be regarded as infective or septic. Sutures should consequently not be used as a rule ... Aseptic' surgery is out of place in septic wounds. No one antiseptic can be said to be superior to all others. Men left lying out for a day or two are often severely collapsed," and require saline, food, and stimulants before dressing. Strict precaution must be taken against tight bandages.[6]

Gas gangrene

Other patients reached base hospital suffering from gas gangrene which was associated with a very high mortality. Gas gangrene is a separate entity from hospital gangrene which is dealt with in Chapter 2. Its incidence varied from 5-6% of all wounds in 1915 to a little over 1% in 1918. The percentage mortality of patients suffering from gas gangrene in the BEF was 22%.[7] In 1915 there were 239,867 admissions to the medical services of whom approximately 14,392 (6%) were suffering from gas gangrene. A percentage mortality of 22% would have resulted in 3,166 deaths from the condition. Upon arrival, patients were often in a completely collapsed state, with a barely perceptible pulse and an unrecordable blood pressure. Examination of affected limbs revealed a sinister crackling sensation which could be felt beneath the examiners' fingers and was indicative of gas formation within the tissues. The infection had usually developed as a local gangrene with gas formation and intense toxaemia, before spreading rapidly, through the action of chemical toxins, from the zone of traumatic necrosis in the wound-most commonly in muscle but often in haematoma or other devitalised tissue, along muscle fibres causing further muscle destruction. Gas bubbles were produced as the infection advanced unchecked and the release of powerful toxins soon resulted in multiple organ failure and death. Gas gangrene is caused by the organism Clostridium Perfringens, which only thrives in the absence of oxygen, and is termed

5 Butler, *Official History*, pp. 311-2. Baal was the name of the supreme god worshiped in ancient Canaan and Phoenicia. The practice of Baal worship became widespread in Israel during the reign of Ahab. Baal was a fertility god who was believed to enable the earth to produce crops and people to produce children. Different regions worshiped Baal in different ways, and Baal proved to be a highly adaptable god.

6 Butler, *Official History*, p.316.

7 Butler, *Official History*, p. 310.

anaerobic. The infection was common in very contaminated and neglected wounds, especially if the wounds had been previously sutured in field ambulances, or if the circulation to the limb was compromised, or if the wound contained much dead muscle. Wounds of the thigh and buttock were particularly susceptible to developing gas gangrene. Fragments of clothing carrying the deadly organisms, picked up from the soil and driven into the depths of the wound predisposed to the infection, which was usually well established within a few hours of the receipt of the wound and certainly long before the victims reached base hospitals. Haemorrhage, circulatory collapse and prolonged fatigue were potent contributory factors.

Since Clostridium Perfringens is an anaerobic organism and only grows in the absence of oxygen, the only possible way to save patients suffering from gas gangrene was to resect all the devitalised soft tissues, leaving only healthy bleeding tissues which were well oxygenated. In practice this frequently meant performing an amputation. Even then, the mortality was very high due to the systemic effects caused by the toxins released by the infecting organisms.

Septic shock

From the description of the wounded corporal at the start of this chapter, it is clear that patients presenting with gas gangrene were often in a state of circulatory collapse. Some may have suffered initially from wound shock due to massive blood loss (Chapter 6), which predisposed to the development of gas gangrene, since body tissues in the damaged area would have been deficient in oxygen due to poor perfusion of blood, enabling the deadly organisms to proliferate. Others may have sustained less serious wounds and their circulatory collapse was entirely attributable to further muscle destruction and toxins released as the infection spread. This is known as septic shock.

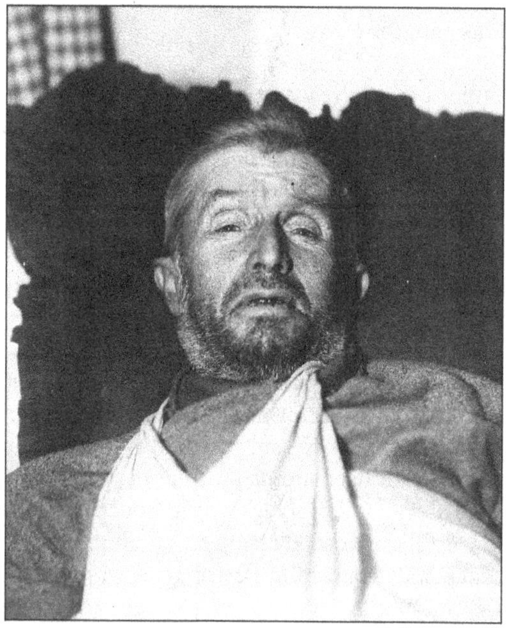

Figure 4.1 This man is suffering from tetanus; spasm of the muscles of facial expression gives rise to the appearance of a rather strange smile. In extreme acute cases, patients may have a 'risus sardonicus' in which the teeth are bared as though the patient is grinning at a funny joke. (Courtesy Wellcome Library, London)

Tetanus

Some patients arrived at base hospitals suffering from tetanus or 'lock jaw'. Tetanus is caused by the organism Clostridium Tetani which like Clostridium Perfringens is anaerobic, occurs naturally in fertilised fields and enters the body at the time of wounding. The richly manured fields of France and Flanders were a source of both Clostridium Tetani and Clostridium Perfringens. Patients with tetanus suffer from intense muscle spasms due to a potent neuro-toxin, which is a toxin affecting nerves. One of the manifestations of tetanus involves the nerves supplying the muscles of facial expression. Affected individuals often bear their teeth, as though smiling, and this is known as a 'risus sardonicus'. The percentage mortality of patients showing the full clinical picture of tetanus in 1914 was in excess of 80 percent.[8]

Why wounds were different in the Great War

The Great War differed from the Boer War in several important ways. The agents inflicting wounds were different and the severity of wounds in France and Flanders was significantly greater. There was a belief that bullets used in South Africa during the Boer War had somehow been more 'humane' than in previous conflicts. Those used in the Boer War were high velocity bullets made from lead with either steel or copper casing, which if fired from long range produced a clean drilled hole through non-vital tissue. At short range, they were much more destructive, but since the Boers were good snipers and engaged in guerrilla warfare, most bullets in South Africa were fired from a considerable distance, so the perception that the bullets employed were more humane than the soft lead versions used in previous conflicts came to be generally accepted. There was certainly nothing humane about the German sharp-nosed streamlined bullet introduced in 1905 which had a greatly increased muzzle velocity. Experiments performed by Franklin Main Mann in America into the ballistics of the new bullet, by Fessler in Germany at the Bavarian School of Musketry into its effect on the animal body, and by Sir Victor Horsley in London using wet modelling clay, all pointed to an extension of the "explosive 'effects on viscera and bones. Despite these observations, most British surgeons in 1914 could not see beyond the South African experience and underestimated the destructive capacity of bullets used in the Great War.

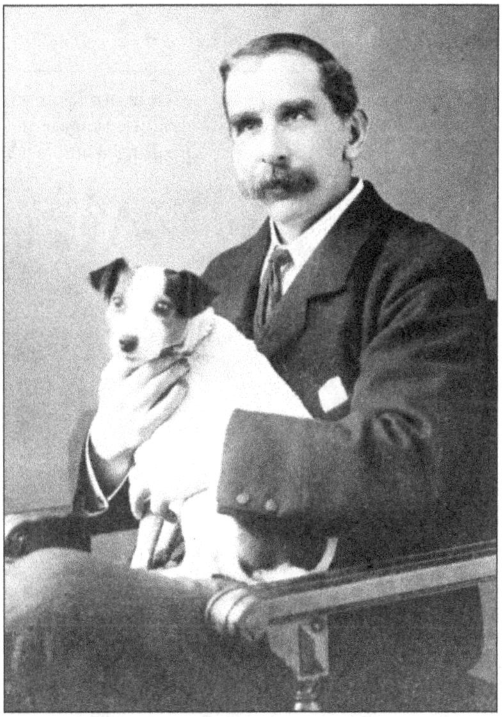

Figure 4.2 Sir Victor Horsley (1857-1916). (Courtesy Wellcome Library, London)

Sir Victor Horsley (1857-1916) was the first neurosurgeon to be appointed to the hospital in Queen Square, London, now called the National Hospital for Neurology and Neurosurgery. The Victor Horsley Department of Neurosurgery is named in

8 Hepburn, H.H., Notes on Tetanus *Canadian Medical Association Journal*, 12:5 (May 1922), pp. 312-15.

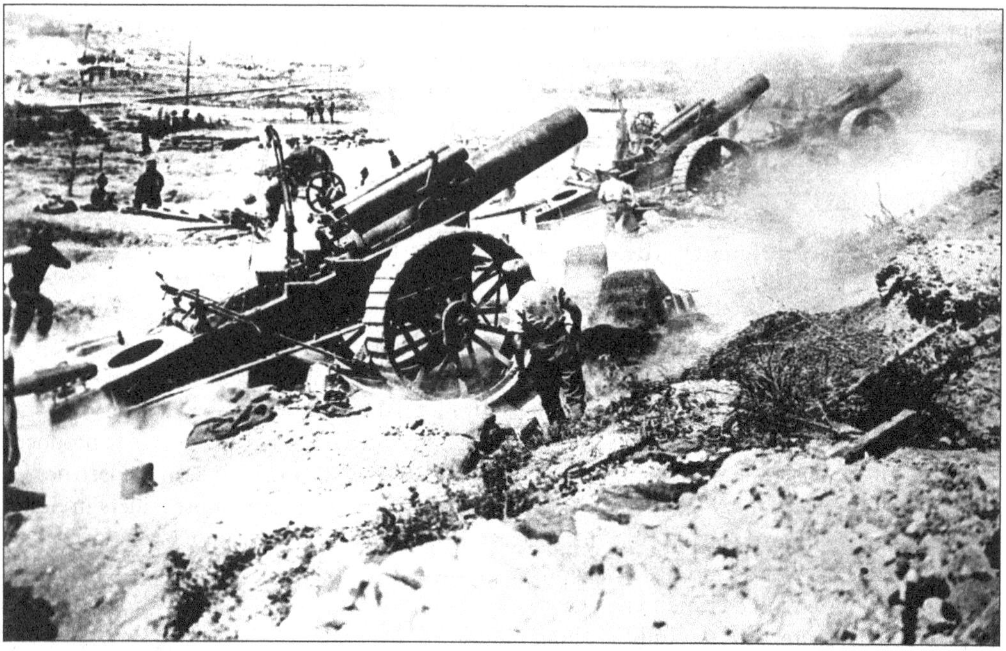

Figure 4.3 Mark V, 8-inch howitzers in action on the Somme, August 1916. Most wounds during the Great War were inflicted by shellfire. Fragments of shell casing of different sizes and shapes caused appalling wounds. (Wikimedia Commons)

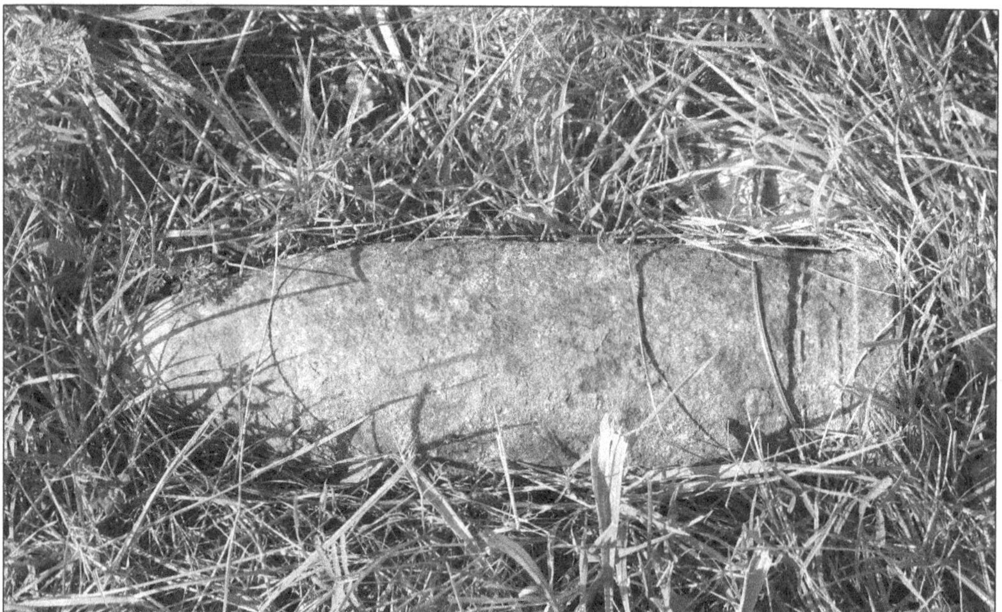

Figure 4.4 High explosive shells were unreliable in the early years of the war. It has been estimated that around one third of shells failed to explode. This shell was fired on the Somme in 1916. (Author's photograph)

his honour. Following the outbreak of war in 1914, Horsley made a request to be posted for active duty on the Western Front and he worked initially at a hospital in Wimereux. In May 1915, he was appointed Director of Surgery of the British Army Medical Service in Egypt and was based at the 21st General Hospital in Alexandria in support of the Dardanelles Campaign. In 1916 he volunteered for field surgery duty in Mesopotamia, where he died unexpectedly of heatstroke at Amara on 16 July 1916.

Most Boer War wounds were caused by bullets and few by high explosive shellfire. The opposite was the case in the Great War, when most wounds were inflicted by fragments of high explosive shell casing and shrapnel balls.

The severity of wounds was accentuated by the stupendous expenditure of energy of the high-explosive shell and hand grenade. The great variation in the shape and size of the fragments from these agents, and their comparatively low velocity, resulted in a very wide range of wounds. Fragments often lodged within the body and lacerated severely. A distinct and very important element in their action was that they almost invariably carried portions of clothing and other matter into the depths of the wound.

Table 4.1 gives a breakdown of wounding agents. This is a 'snap shot' of admissions on a single day (21 September 1917) to casualty clearing stations dealing with the wounded from the Third Battle of Ypres, which began on 31 July and ended on 10 November 1917 with the capture of the ruins of the village of Passchendaele. The date 21 September is significant, because it was the day following a major engagement which subsequently became known as the 'Battle of the Menin Road Ridge' (20-25 September) during which a great many casualties were sustained and 21 September was the busiest day for many of the clearing stations dealing with wounded from Third Ypres.

Table 4.1 Causes of wound in Great War-24 hour 'snapshot 21 September 1917

Wounding Agent	Number of Wounds	Percentage
High Explosive	3,867	35.8
Shrapnel	2,142	19.9
Bullet	2,933	27.2
Hand Grenade	77	0.70
Bayonet	17	0.16
Gas	209	1.94
Uncertain	1,544	14.3
Total	10,789	100

Macpherson, W.G., *History of The Great War based on official documents Medical Services General History Vol. III*, (London: His Majesty's Stationery Office, 1924), pp. 170-171.

The Boer War was fought over the dry grasslands of the Transvaal and Orange Free State, while the Great War on the Western Front was fought in the richly fertilised fields of France and Flanders where dangerous anaerobic organisms lived naturally. Sir Almroth Wright working at General Hospital 13 at Boulogne did a great deal of research into the causes and management of wound infections. Wright believed that the body's own lymph should be used as a purifying agent for wounds. For an explanation of lymph, the reader is referred to Chapter 6:

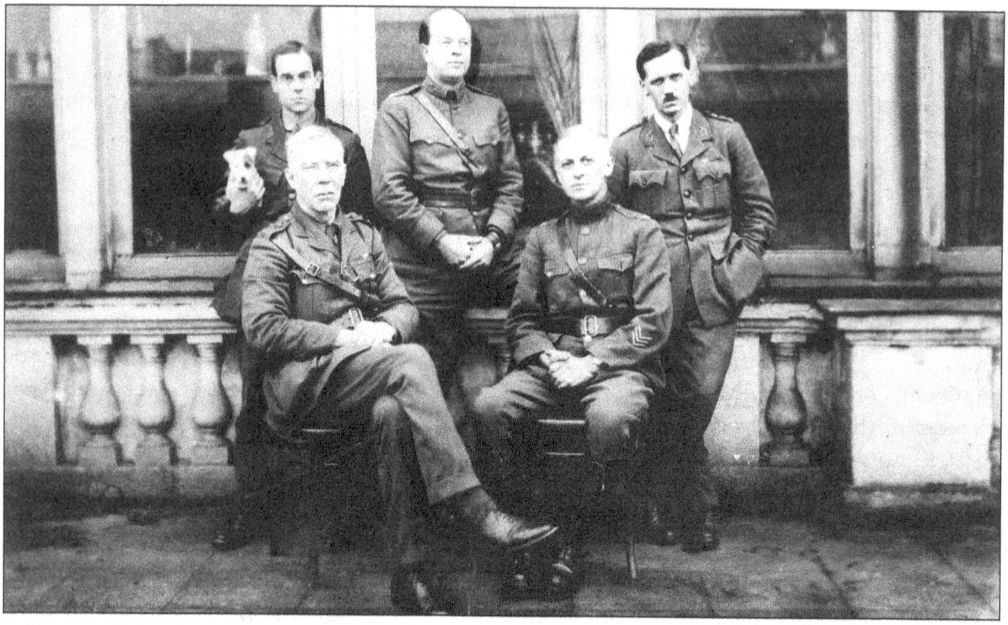

Figure 4.5 Sir Almroth Wright is seated left and American Neuro-surgeon Harvey Cushing is seated right at Base Hospital 13, Boulogne, where Wright carried out vital research work during the war. Standing behind and to the right of Cushing is Alexander Fleming (1881-1955), who would discover the antibiotic properties of penicillin in 1928. (Courtesy Wellcome Library, London)

> Everyone is surprised at the amount of sepsis, not only streptococci and staphylococci but Clostridium Perfringens, Clostridium Tetani, and other anaerobes. The whole fighting area is one of intense cultivation; this may even be called a war of faecal infection-streptococcus and anaerobes. The missile goes through clothes soiled with faeces. Bathing and clean clothes may help to prevent contamination, in conjunction with use of carbolic in the Field Ambulances. Drainage is only the first and crude stage [of treatment], for lymph is the only real purifying agent.[9]

Wright employed hypertonic saline to stimulate lymphatic flow and as the war progressed, he persevered with his laboratory-based research at General Hospital 13 in Boulogne. Figure 4.5 is a photograph of Wright and his team, which includes a young Alexander Fleming, who would discover the antimicrobial properties of penicillin on 28 September 1928. Fleming's research in Boulogne showed that the bacteria responsible for gas gangrene and tetanus were able to grow in the anaerobic depths of the wounds which antiseptics did not reach and which sometimes exacerbated the condition by harming cells that defend the body against invading organisms. Celebrated American neuro-surgeon Harvey Cushing, who was with the "Ambulance Américaine" in Paris in 1915 and who arrived in France in May 1917 with American Base Hospital 5 (Harvard Unit), is also in the photograph. Much more will be said about Cushing later.

9 Butler, *Official History*, p.315.

Surgeons working in the clinical setting of clearing stations and base hospitals, meanwhile, were appalled by what they were seeing and tried to improve matters by making changes to the existing disastrous regime by using all methods which were at their disposal. In October 1914, every wounded man was given a prophylactic dose of Anti Tetanus Serum (ATS) as soon as possible after the infliction of his wound. The incidence of tetanus dropped from 9 cases per 1,000 wounded to 1.4 per 1,000 by December 1914. As will soon become apparent, excision of dead tissue also came to play a significant role in reducing the incidence of tetanus, but since this could not be done early in every single case, ATS was a vital addition and saved lives. If a patient arrived in a clearing hospital and there was doubt about whether a dose of ATS had been given since the infliction of his wound, one was given to make certain. In men wounded for the second or subsequent occasions, the dose was administered slowly in case it precipitated an adverse (anaphylactic) reaction which might cause circulatory collapse or even death. In all serious wounds, administration of ATS was repeated every seven days until the wound was clean and fit for closing.[10]

Surgeons also took steps to change the way in which wounds were dealt with. The disastrous consequence of wound closure in dressing stations of field ambulances became obvious very quickly and immediate suturing of wounds was abandoned. What happened next, however, was that every anti-septic known to mankind was applied to wounds in a fruitless search to find one that worked and improved results, but all those tried were associated with poor outcomes, some worse than others:

> Most (antiseptics) were futile, some grossly harmful. Of the cresol paste and salicylic and boric dusting powder-'Borsal'- devised in February, 1915 by Sir Watson Cheyne, Lister's most ardent disciple, the *British Official History* notes that in cases arriving at the Base 'the wound aperture was often blocked … or a dark evil-smelling discharge was exuding. The limbs were swollen, and acute progressive infection of the tissues was present. When opened up a surface resembling … necrotic liver substance was exposed'.[11]

It would seem from what has been said that Joseph Lister's antiseptic methods were ultimately responsible for the dreadful surgical outcomes in the early months of the Great War. It would be very unfair to blame Lister, however, because he employed antiseptic agents to prevent infection in elective surgically incised wounds and to treat injuries which were genuinely relatively clean, as in the case of the boy run over by a cart (Chapter 2). He never employed antiseptics to cure established deep-seated sepsis caused by particularly virulent bacteria.

Tissue irrigation

The next step after the unsuccessful use of antiseptics was to drain wounds and to wash them, to irrigate them, to flush out bacteria and debris and to allow them to heal up (granulate) from their depths, and perhaps become amenable to suturing after several days. Large drainage tubes

10 Gray, H.M.W., *The Early Treatment of War Wounds* (London: Henry Frowde, Hodder and Stoughton, 1919), pp. 138-139.

11 Butler, *Official History*, p.313

were inserted into grossly contaminated wounds in dressing stations of field ambulances to encourage mechanical drainage. It was suggested that a blunt spoon would be a useful addition to a surgeon's armamentarium to scoop out loose bits of dead muscle to assist in this cleansing process. Alexis Carrel was a distinguished French surgeon who did pioneering work before the war on stitching damaged blood vessels back together and was awarded a Nobel Prize for Medicine in 1912. Henry Dakin was an English chemist who collaborated with Carrel during the Great War. By employing a system of irrigation tubes inserted deep into the recesses of wounds, Carrel delivered high concentrations of Dakin's Solution (an antiseptic agent with sodium hypochlorite as active agent) to the depths of the wounds.

Meanwhile Sir Almroth Wright in Base Hospital 13 continued his research into the physiological irrigation of tissues using hypertonic saline solution to encourage lymphatic flow:

> The ideal of physiological treatment is to give intelligent aid to the organism in combating the bacterial infection. Saline dressings supply a means for evoking, in the infected wound, certain requisite physiological reactions. By their aid we can, while at the same time inhibiting bacterial growth, drain the tissues, resolve infiltration, and promote the separation of the sloughs-besides giving other assistance.[12]

There was much debate about methods of wound cleansing. Some of the more innovative surgeons felt that while irrigation systems were all very well and were a step in the right direction, scooping out bits of debris with a spoon scarcely represented a satisfactory way of dealing with large amounts of dead muscle, the presence of which facilitated the growth of the dangerous anaerobic organisms Clostridium Perfringens and Clostridium Tetani. Wound irrigation and antiseptics had a part to play in the management of wounds with established infection, but only after comprehensively dealing with the wounds surgically, not in a haphazard way with a large spoon, but by employing radical surgery to remove all non-viable tissue. If operative intervention could be carried out in the pre-infective state as soon as possible after the infliction of wounds, then there was a good chance that major wound infections might be avoided.

Wound excision

The definitive surgical procedure involved the systematic removal of *all* foreign material, the radical removal of *all* devitalised tissue and the conversion of the wound into a macroscopically clean one before the organisms colonising the wound had time to become established and cause a wound infection. This became known as wound excision and was the single most important surgical development made during the Great War. Henry Gray from Aberdeen and Edward Milligan from Melbourne pioneered the procedure. The operation relied on common sense and clinical judgement, which Gray and Milligan possessed in abundance.

Henry Gray (1870-1937) was born in Aberdeen and graduated in medicine with honours from the University of Aberdeen in 1895. One of his medical classmates, in what was a very bright

12 Butler, *Official History*, p.319.

year, was Arthur Lister[13] the nephew of Lord Lister, who had first introduced antiseptic surgery in 1867. Gray's first appointment was house surgeon to Professor Sir Alexander Ogston, who is credited with bringing antiseptic surgery to Aberdeen, although he is best known for his "discovery" of the staphylococcus, which was and still is, the most important micro-organism responsible for causing surgical wound infections (Chapter 2). Gray spent three and a half years in France during the war, at first in charge of the surgical activities of a group of base hospitals in Rouen before becoming Consulting Surgeon to the British Third Army in 1917 shortly before the Battle of Arras.

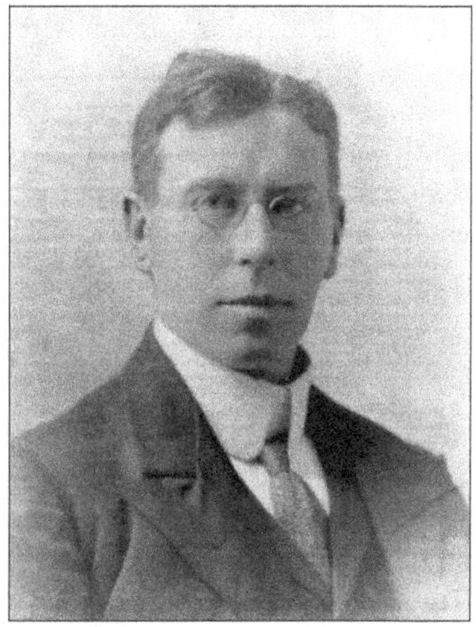

Figure 4.6 Henry Gray (1870-1938) in 1904 after his appointment as Consultant Surgeon to Aberdeen Royal Infirmary. (Courtesy Ann Boyer, Henry Gray's great niece)

Gray was a determined and single minded individual, who did not tolerate opposition and since many of his colleagues were against his radical new methods, it is no surprise that he made enemies amongst his peers. He was, however, extremely supportive of hard working young surgeons who were under his tutorage and he readily acknowledged their contributions to surgery:

> This is a young man's war, in surgery as well as in purely military matters. The progress of events demands that younger men should have every chance in a sphere of action where mental and bodily activity count for so much.[14]

They in turn admired him greatly, because he was always with them in the thick of things, encouraging them and assisting them to do difficult cases.[15] Milligan was a protégé of Gray and was a graduate of Melbourne University. At the outbreak of war he was engaged in special study in England where he joined the RAMC. Gray and Milligan published their accounts of wound excision separately, although the two men undoubtedly collaborated.

Gray as explained was in charge of the surgical activities of a group of base hospitals in Rouen, while Milligan (1886-1972) was working in the dressing station of a field ambulance closer to the front line.[16] Milligan published his work in the British Medical Journal in June 1915,[17] while Gray's paper appeared in the Journal of the Royal Army Medical Corps the same month. Gray went further and proposed excision and primary closure of selected wounds.[18]

13 Obituary, Sir Henry Gray, KBE, CB, CMG, LLD, FRCSEd, *British Medical Journal*, 2:4086 (15 October 1938), p. 814.
14 Gray, *The Early Treatment of War Wounds*, p. x.
15 Scotland, T., Boyer, A., *Henry Gray: Surgeon of the Great War Saving Lives in a Theatre of Destruction* (Edinburgh: Capercaillie Books Ltd., 2015).
16 Butler, *Official History*, p. 326.
17 Milligan, E.T.C., The early treatment of projectile wounds by excision of the damaged tissue, *British Medical Journal*, 1: 2843, (26 June 1915), p. 1081.
18 Gray, H.M.W., The treatment of gunshot wounds by excision and primary suture, *Journal Royal Army Medical Corps*, No. 24 (June 1915), pp. 551-54.

Gray was a senior surgeon with considerable 'clout', whose collaboration with Milligan gave his young colleague much needed support to fend off the inevitable hostility and criticism emanating from surgeons who disagreed with the new concept of wound excision and who continued to pin their hopes on antiseptic agents as the way to resolve appalling wound infections. Milligan needed Gray's help, because he soon found himself in deep water when he began employing this revolutionary technique. Milligan observed:

> Opposition came from three quarters: 1. From the administrative officers of the R.A.M.C.; for it meant increase in staff, alteration of equipment and allotment of work, and more accommodation in order to submit the greater numbers of wounded to anaesthesia and operation. 2. From some consulting surgeons, who felt that it was unjustifiable to submit a man already badly wounded to further trauma even with a scalpel. Undoubtedly confidence in antiseptic treatment, and fear of spread of infection after operative interference, made some surgeons bitterly hostile to the procedure. 3. From junior medical officers who disliked the comparatively uninteresting work of administering the large numbers of anaesthetics required for carrying out excision of wounds.[19]

He continued:

> Opposition was so great locally that I first carried out excision of wounds under local anaesthesia, and general anaesthetics induced by myself and continued by an orderly; and this often at late hours and unknown to those in authority. At the request of a Consulting Surgeon of the Army, who opposed this treatment, my Commanding Officer ordered me to discontinue surgery, and only allowed me to return with the request that I should cease excision of wounds ... Sir Anthony Bowlby, the chief consultant of the B.E.F., expressed himself in agreement with my publication at the time. Sir Henry M. W. Gray, to whom war surgery owes so much, was carrying out the treatment independently at the Base in France, and soon afterwards advocated it energetically at the front. Under pressure of these opinions, and from their own convictions, many surgical specialists now took up the treatment, and the necessary administrative alterations were made by the R.A M.C. for carrying it out.[20]

The necessary administrative arrangements were as follows:

- All early operative work was delegated to the casualty clearing stations which were altered accordingly.
- Surgical specialists and anaesthetists were appointed to organise the surgery of casualty clearing stations.
- Accommodation was made to enable four to six surgeons with their teams to operate at the same time so that large numbers of wounded were dealt with, teams working in shifts night and day during active fighting.

19 Butler, *Official History*, p.328.
20 Butler, *Official History*, p.328.

- The success of all antiseptic treatment depended on the preliminary excision of the wounds; as did also the good results of the Carrel-Dakin treatment … and [it] paved the way for primary and secondary suture of wounds.[21]

By performing surgery early before inflammation (infection) became established, Gray and Milligan were following an important surgical principle laid down by Guthrie and Larrey more than a century before. As already stated, wound excision is a systematic procedure, removing dead skin, dead fat, dead and contused (bruised and/or crushed) underlying muscle and where there are fractures, removing debris and loose pieces of bone which have lost normal soft tissue attachments before thoroughly cleansing and irrigating the tissues. Even apparently minor looking missile wounds might be grossly contaminated on the inside from shell fragments carried into the depths of the wound. Unless all dead and contaminated tissue was completely excised and unless there was nothing left but healthy, bleeding tissue, the operation would fail, with potentially catastrophic consequences for the patient. Under such circumstances, gas gangrene could become established and result in the loss of a soldier's limb or his life. Gray went on to publish his work again in the British Medical Journal in August 1915 to make the method more widely known to the surgical community.[22]

Gray combined wound excision with primary wound closure in carefully selected cases, a technique he first began employing in November 1914. To be successful, surgery *had* to be undertaken early, before the wound began to display the signs of infection with swelling, induration (a woody hardening of tissues) and erythema (redness) of the surrounding skin. After excising every last piece of contaminated and dead tissue, the wound was sutured, allowing healing by first intention, which saved a great deal of time and effort. Wounds treated this way required much less nursing care, pain was diminished, the number of dressings was reduced, and complications of a septic wound were avoided. However, it was absolutely essential that *all* devitalised tissue was removed otherwise wound closure over residual dead or contaminated tissue would inevitably result in major sepsis with the added risk of gas gangrene. The operation had to be performed by a sufficiently experienced surgeon exercising sound clinical judgement.

Sometimes Gray might not have been sure of the completeness of a wound excision to feel confident to proceed with primary closure. Under such circumstances, he would leave the wound open with a salt pack in situ, after the technique of Sir Almroth Wright, and have a second look after 48 hours when it would usually be possible to close the wound if it looked healthy. This is called delayed primary closure.

If too much time had elapsed since wounding and the patient already had established infection when first seen and operated upon, then primary or delayed primary closure was out of the question. Dead and contaminated tissue was surgically removed from the wound, which was left open for 12-14 days before being closed by secondary suture. Anti-septic agents had a role to play in this situation, to assist with the killing of bacteria which had become firmly established within the wound. Sometimes the damage to tissues was so great that in the case of an arm or leg, primary amputation was the only safe course of action.

21 Butler, *Official History*, p.328.

22 Gray, H.M.W., Treatment of Gunshot wounds by excision and primary suture, *British Medical Journal* 2: 2852 (28 August 1915), p. 317.

During 1915, casualty clearing stations began to provide the essential facilities and resources for early wound excision, before patients were sent by hospital train to the base hospitals. It is interesting to reflect that when James McGrigor arrived in Portugal in 1812, one of the first things he did was to arrange for casualties to be admitted to regimental hospitals closer to the front, thereby receiving treatment earlier, rather than subject the wounded to energy sapping journeys to distant base hospitals (Chapter 2).

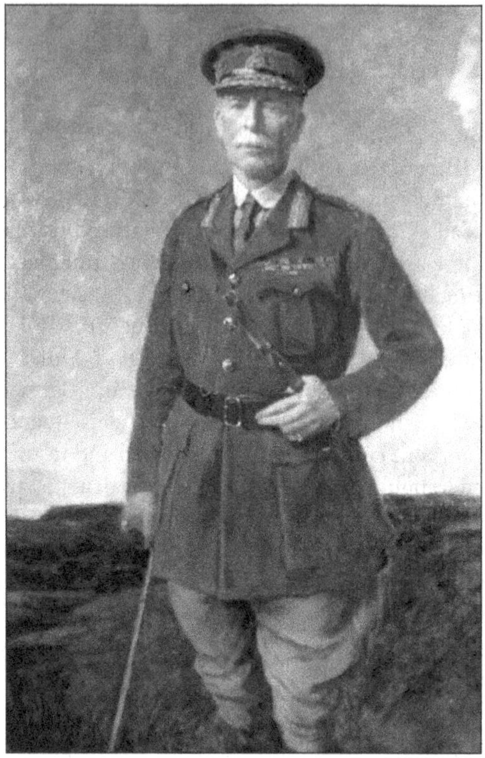

Figure 4.7 Sir Anthony Bowlby (1855-1929) became general adviser at the Front to the Director-General, Army Medical Service, and towards the end of the Great War, he became Adviser on Surgery for the whole of the British area, Front and Base. (Courtesy Royal College of Surgeons of England)

It was in large part due to the pioneering work of Gray and Milligan and to Sir Anthony Bowlby's recognition that wound excision was a most valuable procedure that definitive surgery was performed at casualty clearing stations closer to the front. Sir Anthony Bowlby (1855-1929) was Senior Consulting Surgeon to the British Forces in France and Flanders with the rank of Major-General Army Medical Services. Towards the end of the war he became Advisor on Surgery for the entire British area of operations, both at the front and base. In 1920, he became President of the Royal College of Surgeons of England, a position he held for three years.

The surgeons of all belligerent nations encountered exactly the same problems with wound infections. French and Belgian surgeons began to employ a technique called débridement which had been used one hundred years previously by Dominique Larrey, Surgeon-in-Chief to Napoleon's Army. The term 'débridement' comes from the French verb *débrider* which means to unbridle. Larrey believed that inflammation or injury could produce constriction of tissues within muscle compartments confined or constrained by deep fascia, the strong membrane which surrounds skeletal muscle. Such constriction, if allowed to persist, may result in the death of the underlying muscle as a result of a dangerous build-up of pressure within the muscle compartment. An incision made through the deep fascia unbridles or relieves the pressure on the underlying muscle. Larrey used débridement to remove foreign bodies and to uncover and ligate bleeding vessels within the muscle groups. The procedure fell into disuse until a Belgian surgeon called Antoine Depage (1862-1925) began employing débridement on war wounds in 1914.[23] Not

23 Helling, T.S., Daon, E., The Great War, Antoine Depage and the Resurgence of Debridement, *Annals of Surgery*, Vol. 228, No. 2, (1998), pp. 173-81.

only did he 'unbridle' the wound, by making an incision in the deep fascia, he also excised dead and contaminated tissue beneath, making the procedure equivalent to wound excision. Over the ensuing years, débridement has evolved to include all sorts of different ways of removing devitalised tissues including chemical methods to clean up wounds and the employment of maggots to eat their way through all the dead tissue within a wound. Maggots only eat dead tissue, leaving viable tissue undisturbed. All these developments distort Depage's original concept of débridement and obscure its original meaning and purpose. Wound excision is a much more precise surgical term.

In 1917, during an inter-allied conference on wound management, it was universally agreed that minimal surgery should be carried out in the forward areas of regimental aid posts and field ambulances and the wounded should be transported to casualty clearing stations as quickly as possible for urgent definitive surgery. A clinical research centre for wounds was established at Casualty Clearing Station Number 10 at Remy Siding in 1917, with the aim of evaluating the safety of primary excision and suturing of recently inflicted wounds. When judged not to be safe, packing for 48-72 hours with flavine was performed followed by suture at the end of this period. It was concluded that excision was the essential feature of the operation and the antiseptic used, whatever it happened to be, was of secondary importance.

Hnry Gray's opinion of the place of antiseptics in the management of wounds

Gray noted that much attention was given to the use of a wide variety of antiseptics, in an attempt to kill bacteria within wounds while hopefully avoiding too much direct damage caused by the antiseptic to the surrounding healthy tissues. These methods included the use of salt packs, Bismuth, Iodine, Dakin's Solution (active ingredient sodium hypochlorite), EUSOL (active ingredient chlorinated lime and boric acid), hydrogen peroxide and acriflavine, to give but a few examples.

It has been suggested recently that Alexis Carrel's technique employing irrigation tubes to reach the depths of a wound and using Dakin's Solution as a germicide, was the main reason for reduction in mortality of compound fractures of the femur.[24] Much more will be said about the management of femoral fractures later, but suffice it to say here that this is a complete misperception and it is very important to realise that while antiseptic agents were used extensively, their use was no substitute for adequate surgery. Gray was absolutely clear about this when he wrote:

> It cannot be emphasised too urgently that the use of antiseptics will not make up for inadequate operative treatment. It can safely also be said that the stronger the antiseptic, the worse the result. The fact should be remembered when a particularly soiled wound tempts the use of strong remedies, or when one vaunted antiseptic is tested against another. On the other hand, provided the operation is adequate, one kind of rational after-treatment does not seem to influence the patient's chance of life or limb more than another.[25]

24 Cooter, R., *Surgery and Society in Peace and War* (Basingstoke: MacMillan Press Ltd., 1993), p.111.
25 Gray, *The Early Treatment of War Wounds*, p. 107.

Gray's firmly held beliefs created animosity amongst those of his peers who were not converts to wound excision, given that tact and diplomacy were not Gray's strong points.[26]It wasn't just Gray who took this stance on the use of antiseptics, however, and the Official History of the Australian Army Medical Services clearly summed up matters:

> In practically all severe wounds admitted to C.C.S.s, it is found necessary to give anaesthetics to enable the damaged muscle, fascia, etc, bordering on the wound to be excised and foreign bodies removed, and to enable the surgeon to provide sufficient drainage. This is a preliminary to any form of treatment whether by 'Carrel,' salt pack or any other method of dressing. It is this measure alone which diminishes the danger of severe anaerobic infection.[27]

26 Scotland and Boyer, *Henry Gray: Surgeon of the Great War.*
27 Butler, *Official History,* p. 329.

5

Early anaesthetic disasters and their solutions

Case history

The young medical officer who had been told to give the anaesthetic stood at the top end of the operating table, holding a Schimmelbusch Mask in his left hand. The apparatus had been invented by Kurt Schimmelbusch in 1890 as a convenient way to administer anaesthetic agents including ether and chloroform. The mask was a wire frame covered with several layers of gauze swabs and shaped to fit over the patient's mouth and nose. He held a bottle of chloroform in his right hand and was summoning up the courage to pour some onto the gauze and administer his very first anaesthetic. He wracked his brain for any pearls of wisdom he had gleaned from his undergraduate medical teaching in anaesthesia two years previously, but his efforts were in vain. His patient was a 22-year-old private who had sustained a very bad wound of his left leg involving the lower end of the femur (thigh bone), knee joint and upper tibia. He had lost a great deal of blood. The Second Battle of Ypres had started a couple of weeks previously on 22 April 1915, when the Germans had used chlorine gas for the first time against French Colonial troops around the village of Langemarck, some six miles from Ypres. Heavy casualties had been sustained by both sides in the intervening fortnight. The wounded man was confused and mumbled incoherently. He shivered uncontrollably. The shattered end of his left femur was sticking up at a right angle to the rest of his thigh and his proximal tibia was so smashed that there was nothing in the way of recognisable normal anatomy. The kneecap was in many bits. The inexperienced medical officer persuaded himself that the general condition of the patient was acceptable despite the seriousness of the wound. The soldier's skin was very cold to the touch, which was not surprising, considering that the boy had spent several hours in the bottom of a waterlogged shell hole before the regimental stretcher bearers had managed to extract him after nightfall. Perhaps they should have spent more time warming the wounded man up before bringing him through to the operating theatre. Some hot water bottles had been used by the regimental medical officer and there had been a strategically positioned coke burning stove at the advanced dressing station and another at the casualty clearing station, but they had not had the benefit of a hot air bath to warm the patient more effectively and to raise his core temperature (Figure 5.3). The soldier's pulse was very rapid at around 150/minute and was difficult to feel. His blood pressure was low at 90 systolic, but the young medical officer reassured himself that everything would be alright. Besides, the surgeon was beginning to pace around impatiently and was clearly anxious to be underway. Spinal anaesthesia, involving the injection of a local anaesthetic into the spinal canal to paralyse the lower limbs and abolish sensation, had gained in popularity as a way of dealing with major lower limb trauma. Since neither the surgeon nor the young anaesthetist had any experience of performing it, they decided to keep things as simple as possible and use chloroform, which was well known for its ease of administration, speed of onset of anaesthesia and the small amount required. The anaesthetist made a start and the wounded soldier quickly became unconscious. After a couple of minutes, the surgeon applied a tourniquet to the upper thigh of the shattered limb and began the operation by fashioning flaps for the amputation. After a few minutes, the wounded man's blood pressure began to fall and continued to drop. Quickly, the anaesthetist asked for rectal fluids to be given and an orderly passed a rubber tube through the patient's anus into his rectum and began to run in a litre of saline. The boy's blood pressure rose a little, which provided some relief to both surgeon and anaesthetist, but this improvement was short-lived and the blood pressure fell away again. The anaesthetist inserted a hollow needle into the skin beneath the boy's right axilla (arm pit) and connected it via a length of sterile tubing to a litre bottle of saline and began running it into the subcutaneous tissues. It had no effect whatsoever and the blood pressure continued to fall. It dropped from 70 mm to 50 mm mercury. The patient was now a deathly white colour and his breathing became very irregular. The surgeon completed the amputation as quickly as possible and removed the tourniquet while the anaesthetist discontinued the chloroform, hoping and praying that the wounded boy would show some sign of improvement. Instead, his blood pressure fell to 30mm mercury over the following hour and then became unrecordable. His heart stopped beating, his pupils became fixed and dilated and the young soldier was pronounced dead.

In 1900, the teaching of anaesthesia was not on the curriculum of most medical schools. It wasn't thought to be necessary and there was a widely held belief that anaesthesia had progressed as far as it ever would. During the Second Boer War (1899-1902), doctors on horseback were given a saddlebag containing a bottle of chloroform and base hospitals were each supplied with ten pounds of chloroform and five pounds of ether and anaesthetics were administered by very junior surgeons. It was all very simple. In 1909, a bill proposing that all general anaesthetics should be administered by a medical practitioner failed to get through parliament, although in 1912 the General Medical Council finally accepted that anaesthesia should be the last of 16 subjects on the undergraduate curriculum of all medical schools. It is little wonder that two years later there was a major shortage of trained anaesthetists to deal with the wounded and the job was often given to the most junior medical officer available. After all, there was so much surgery to be done that an experienced clinician could scarcely be spared to administer anaesthetics. Ether and chloroform were available just as they had been during the Second Boer War, and what was good enough for the Boer War was good enough for this conflict.

The reader is reminded that between 1864 and 1901, no fewer than seven committees investigated the potential hazards of chloroform (Chapter 2), but it was not until 1911 that Dr Alfred Goodman Levy demonstrated conclusively that strong stimulation of a patient under light chloroform anaesthesia could cause ventricular fibrillation, a fatal cardiac arrhythmia, proving that chloroform was potentially dangerous in inexperienced hands. As you have just witnessed, the use of chloroform also proved to be very problematic in wounded men who had lost a great deal of blood. Chloroform reduces the pumping action of the heart which was very dangerous in this group of patients. It lowered the blood pressure and aggravated and, in some cases, precipitated surgical shock, a state of circulatory collapse due to underlying excessive major bleeding. The blood pressure often dropped irreversibly, and this resulted in the death of the patient during or immediately after surgery.

There was another form of anaesthesia which had not been available during the Second Boer War and which seemed particularly appealing in 1914 because it could be administered by the surgeon himself without the need for an anaesthetist. This was spinal anaesthesia employing an injection of a local anaesthetic into the spinal canal. Writing in "War Surgery 1914-18, Robertson explained that the first substance noted to have local anaesthetic properties was cocaine, and in 1884 Karl Koller, a German eye surgeon, used a direct application of cocaine to carry out eye surgery. In 1891 the German physician Heinrich Quinke described the technique of lumbar puncture, when a hollow needle was inserted into the fluid which surrounds the spinal cord (cerebrospinal fluid). Seven years later in 1898, one of his former students, August Bier, documented that the injection of small amounts of cocaine into the cerebrospinal fluid of six patients produced sufficient abolition of sensation to allow surgery to be performed. This was the origin of spinal anaesthesia.[1] Cocaine is highly addictive, and searches immediately began for better agents. Stovaine, the brand name for the local anaesthetic amylocaine, was synthesised by French chemist Ernest Fourneau (1872-1949) shortly after he became research director for the pharmaceutical company Établissements Poulenc Frères. On 5 July 1904, at a meeting of l'Académie Nationale de Médecine, French surgeon Paul Reclus (1847-1914) reported the results of a series of successful cases of pain-relieving epidural injections using Stovaine. Within a month or two, this news was documented in British, Canadian and American medical journals. Local anaesthesia was certainly very appealing to clinicians in 1914. An intra-spinal injection of Stovaine administered by the surgeon would cause paralysis and sensory loss of the lower extremities, which on the face of it appeared potentially very useful for the management of major lower limb trauma, leaving chloroform and ether to deal with other clinical situations.

Unfortunately, in practice things did not always work out as anticipated, and just as there were appalling and frequently fatal surgical disasters in the opening months of the Great War, so too there were many unnecessary anaesthetic related deaths. Once again, experience in the Boer War had been inadequate preparation for the types of wound seen in 1914. Most wounds in the Boer War were caused by rifle bullet fired from long range and few were caused by shellfire. The opposite was the case in the Great War when high explosive shellfire caused filthy contaminated wounds associated with much tissue destruction. Wounds were frequently multiple, and patients often reached medical facilities in a state of circulatory collapse due to blood loss. On examination, they were cold, pale and sweaty. Their breathing was shallow, their pulse barely palpable and blood pressure difficult to record. This was the picture of surgical shock. Death frequently occurred during or shortly after surgery. The number of casualties presenting in this shocked state was sometimes overwhelming. One only has to compare casualty figures from the Second Boer War with those of the opening months of the Great War to appreciate this. Table 5.1 shows the battle casualties for the entire South African conflict, which lasted almost three years and those for the first five months of the Great War between August and December 1914.

1 Robertson, A., in Scotland, T. Heys, S., *War Surgery 1914-18*, (Solihull: Helion and Co., 2012), p. 88.

Table 5.1 Battle casualties for the Second Boer War and those for the opening five months of the Great War

Battle Casualties	Second Boer War October 1899-May 1902	Great War August-December 1914
Killed	5,774	13,009
Died of wounds	2,018	3,657
Missing presumed dead	105	6,569
Prisoners of war	102	19,915
Total died	7,999	43,150
Wounded and survived	19,457	55,689

Mitchell, T.J., Smith, G.M., *History of the Great War Medical Services Casualties and Medical Statistics*, (London: His Majesty's Stationery Office 1931).

Mortality figures for Boer War include those who died as prisoners of war. There is no equivalent mortality figure for soldiers who died in captivity in the Great War, so these are excluded from the calculation.

Geoffrey Marshall (1887-1982)

Before the Great War, Geoffrey Marshall was a demonstrator in physiology at Guy's Hospital in London. He was an aspiring physician with an interest in respiratory medicine and the physiology of anaesthesia. Following the outbreak of war in 1914, he joined the Royal Army Medical Corps and was posted to Number 13 General Hospital in Boulogne, where in view of his clinical background he worked as an anaesthetist. Much of his time was spent with surgeon Percy Sargent who had established a neurosurgical unit at General Hospital 13 with his neurologist colleague, Gordon Holmes. Both men came from the National Hospital for Nervous Diseases, Queen's Square, London. More will be said about Holmes and Sargent in Chapter 7, which is devoted to clinical advances in the surgical specialties. Marshall gained much experience in the use of intravenous ether anaesthesia, which enabled him to keep well out of the way while Sargent set about operating on the patient's skull and brain. After a few months, Marshall longed to see a bit more of the action closer to the front and was appointed to take command of a hospital barge of Number 2 Hospital Barge

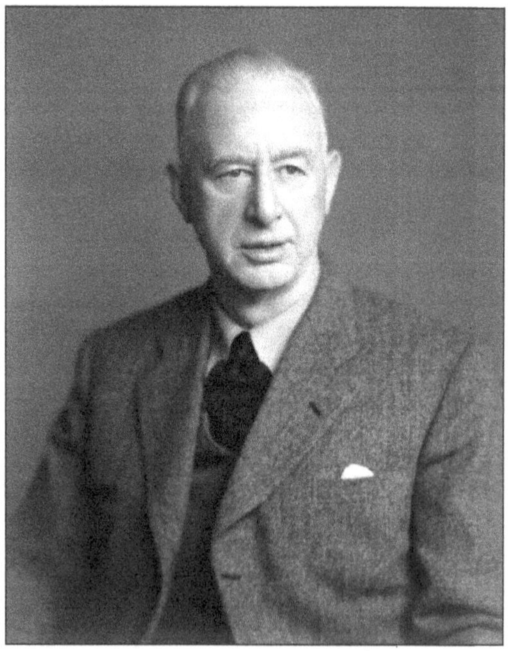

Figure 5.1 Geoffrey Marshall (1887-1982). (Courtesy of National Portrait Gallery, London)

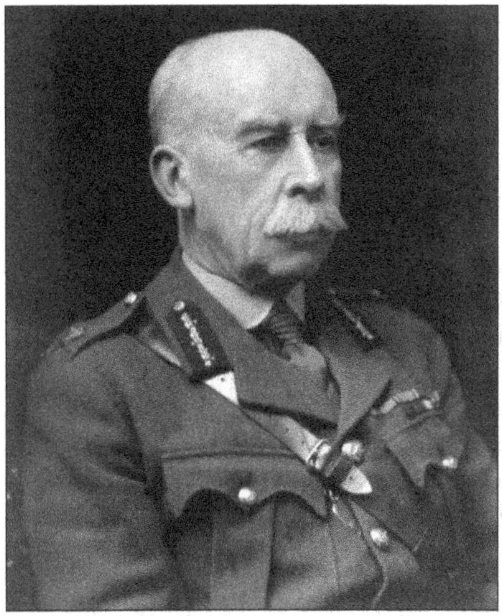

Figure 5.2 Sir Anthony Bowlby (1855-1929). (Courtesy National Portrait Gallery, London)

Flotilla near Bethune in northern France. There were four barges in the flotilla and Marshall's had 20 beds, staffed by two nursing sisters of Queen Alexandra's Imperial Military Nursing Service and four medical orderlies. The barge crew was made up of Norfolk Broadsmen. The four barges were pulled by tugboat along the canal till they got as close to the front line as possible, where they remained moored until they filled up with casualties, mostly head and chest cases, before being tugged back to the base at Le Havre. In quiet times, Marshall borrowed a horse or a motorbike to explore the surrounding countryside. It was, he declared, a perfectly nice job. Unfortunately, after six months this idyllic posting came to an abrupt end. Marshall later recollected:

> Then a dreadful old man, who was the senior consultant Sir Anthony Bowlby, drove up to my barge one day-lovely day-and said, 'Marshall, we are having an awful lot of deaths in the forward hospitals from shock and I want you to come along and see if you can do anything about these chaps'. And so, he hooked me off my perfectly nice barge and sent me to a clearing station (CCS 17 Remy Siding) in the Ypres Salient, which wasn't nearly so peaceful.[2]

Marshall spent the next three years at Casualty Clearing Station 17. When he first arrived, he was confronted by wounded men whose lower limbs had been very badly smashed, most frequently by high explosive shellfire and who urgently needed an amputation but whose general clinical condition was very poor. They were cold and clammy, had a low blood pressure and a rapid, barely perceptible pulse. It may have taken many hours or sometimes even longer to extract them from no man's land and transport them to Remy Siding. Marshall recorded a death rate of approximately 90 percent for patients requiring amputations above the lower third of the femur.[3]

The reader is reminded that between 21 June and 24 December 1813, Peninsular War surgeon George James Guthrie documented an overall operative mortality of 14.8 percent in 128 cases of lower limb amputations performed within a very short time of the infliction of wounds. Surgery was performed without anaesthesia, which had not yet been discovered. At the same time, Guthrie reported a mortality of 58 percent in 255 cases presenting late for lower limb amputation. With the benefit of hindsight, perhaps a contributory factor to the lower percentage operative mortality in Guthrie's cases presenting late in 1813 compared with Marshall's in 1915 was because there were no anaesthetic agents available in 1813 with which to kill patients. Guthrie's

2 Evans, Barbara, A doctor in the Great War-an interview with Sir Geoffrey Marshall, *British Medical Journal*, 285: 6357 (18 December 1982), pp. 1780-1783.

3 Evans, *British Medical Journal*, 18 December 1982.

cases would not all have been through the thigh and most, unlike those of the Great War, would not have been such high energy wounds, but the figures still provide much food for thought.

There were two major problems which Marshall had to contend with. He had to try and improve the patient's general condition by dealing with the shocked state in which the wounded soldier arrived at the clearing station and he had to employ the safest anaesthetic available with which to anaesthetise the severely wounded man. He quickly appreciated that any intervention was quite impossible without first attempting to correct the soldier's surgical shock, which was due to massive blood loss. In 1914-15, there was a very limited amount he could do because there was no clear understanding of what surgical shock was. The next chapter explains how knowledge of the condition gradually improved, but it would be the second half of 1917 before blood transfusion became available in casualty clearing stations. Only subcutaneous or intra-rectal saline infusions were available to Marshall in the first two years of the war to replace fluid and to attempt to restore the circulating blood volume, thereby improving the patient's condition. Administration of subcutaneous saline was completely useless as Marshall demonstrated by post mortem studies shortly after his arrival at CCS 17 in 1915. Saline injected beneath the skin around the upper lateral chest wall was not absorbed into the circulation and was still sloshing around there after the patient died a few hours or a day or two later. Intravenous or intra-rectal saline produced only a fleeting improvement before the patient's condition deteriorated once more. An explanation of this transient improvement is provided in the next chapter. In Marshall's opinion, the single most important measure to combat shock was to warm the patient with hot water bottles and to employ a hot air bath. We now know that the stroke volume (the amount of blood pumped with every contraction of the heart muscle) falls directly with a decrease in body temperature and correspondingly increases as the body temperature rises, better preparing the patient for surgery and improving his chances of survival. However, the longer one waited for an improvement, the greater was the chance of overwhelming infection gaining a firm hold and it was very much a question of balancing the risks and getting the timing of surgery right.

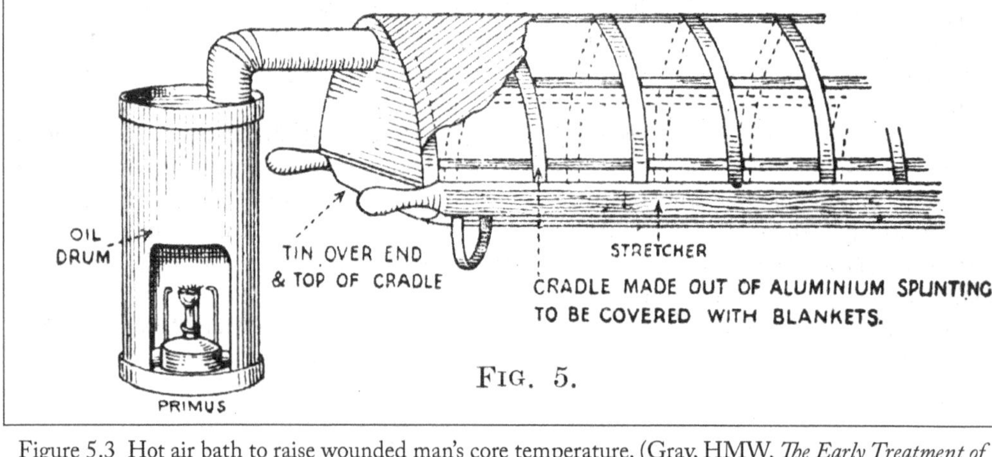

FIG. 5.

Figure 5.3 Hot air bath to raise wounded man's core temperature. (Gray, HMW, *The Early Treatment of War Wounds*, (London: Henry Frowde, Hodder and Stoughton, 1919), p. 21.)

Choice of anaesthetic agent

It was presumed that spinal anaesthesia would fulfil all the anaesthetic requirements for wounds of the lower extremities, but Marshall challenged this belief and looked at what happened to 50 consecutive cases of major lower limb trauma treated in CCS 17, in which spinal anaesthesia with Stovaine was employed. All patients had their haemoglobin levels checked pre-operatively. Patients fell into three distinct groups. Group A were soldiers whose wounds were less than 40 hours old when they underwent surgery and who had a low haemoglobin level indicative of severe haemorrhage. Group B were patients whose wounds were less than 40 hours old when they underwent surgery but who had a normal haemoglobin level, indicating that their blood loss was less severe. Group C were patients whose wounds were older than 40 hours when they underwent surgery. They nearly all had low haemoglobin levels but had had time to adjust haemodynamically. There were 22 patients in Group A, 16 patients in Group B and 12 Patients in Group C.[4]

Figure 5.4 is the anaesthetic chart of a Group A patient. He was a soldier with severe wounds of his buttock and leg. His haemoglobin was 85 percent, the normal being 100-120 percent. Following injection of the spinal anaesthetic, his blood pressure crashed, dropping to 40mm mercury. At the same time, his pulse rate became exceedingly rapid at 170 beats per minute. The patient left theatre after 90 minutes. He died of gas gangrene within 24 hours. Wounds of the buttock were particularly susceptible to gas gangrene, and Marshall also noted that a prolonged spell of hypotension (low blood pressure) during the operative procedure predisposed to the development of the condition, because hypotension resulted in poor blood flow to the tissues and created the ideal anaerobic conditions (without oxygen) upon which the causative organisms for gas gangrene depended for their survival and proliferation.

Figure 5.5 is the chart of a Group B patient, with severe wounds of his thigh, whose haemoglobin level was 102 percent. Following induction of anaesthesia, there was no appreciable change in the patient's pulse and blood pressure. He left theatre after 40 minutes having undergone wound excision. He recovered without mishap.

Figure 5.6 is the chart of a Group C patient with a haemoglobin level of 45 percent. He had an infected wound of his thigh involving damage to his femoral artery. His wound had been sustained 23 days previously and he had developed progressive ischaemic changes of his extremity, with blackening of the skin and muscles of his leg and foot caused by the damage to his femoral artery. Following induction of anaesthesia, his pulse and blood pressure remained steady throughout the procedure. He had an amputation through the lower third of the thigh and recovered.

Group A and Group B patients had a similar clinical appearance. Both groups on admission were cold, pale and clammy. The only way to distinguish between them was by measuring their haemoglobin levels. Group A patients had very poor outcomes with a high operative mortality, while Group B patients usually survived their surgical procedures without mishap. Marshall concluded that administration of a spinal anaesthetic to a recently wounded soldier with a low haemoglobin level was dangerous and should never be employed, although he did not understand at the time why Group A patients suffered such catastrophic falls in blood pressure. His clinical conviction to challenge a prescribed anaesthetic regime certainly subsequently saved many soldiers from death.

4 Marshall, G., The administration of anaesthesia at the front, *British Medical Journal,* 1: 2944 (2 June 1917), pp. 722-725.

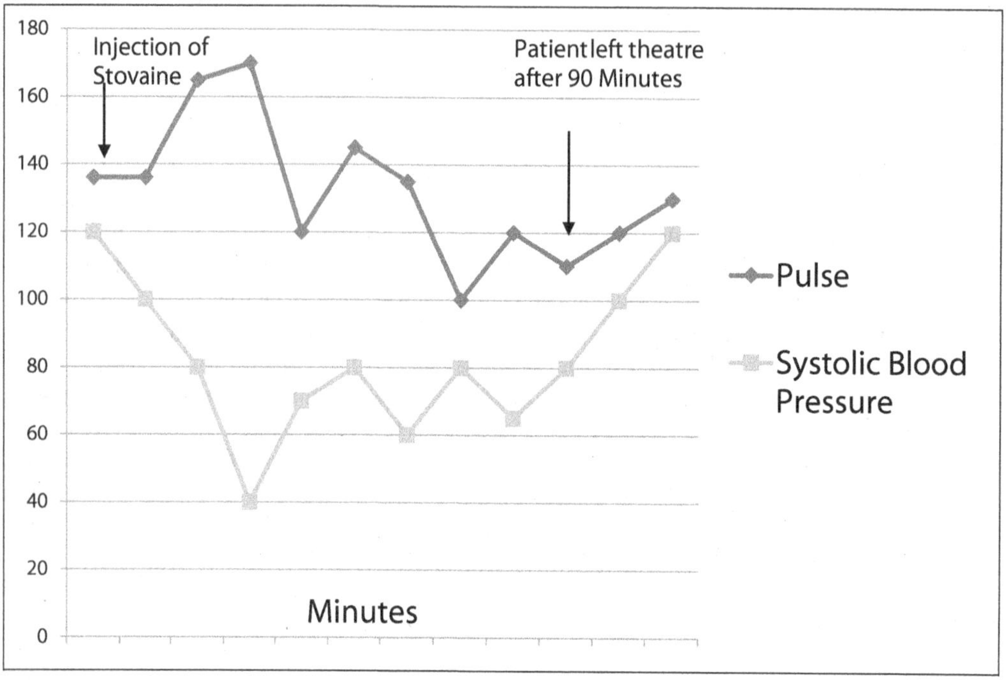

Figure 5.4 Spinal anaesthesia of Group A patient; wound of buttock and leg 21 hours old; haemoglobin 85 percent; attempted limb sparing operation; patient died of gas gangrene 24 hours later. (*British Medical Journal*, 2 June 1917)

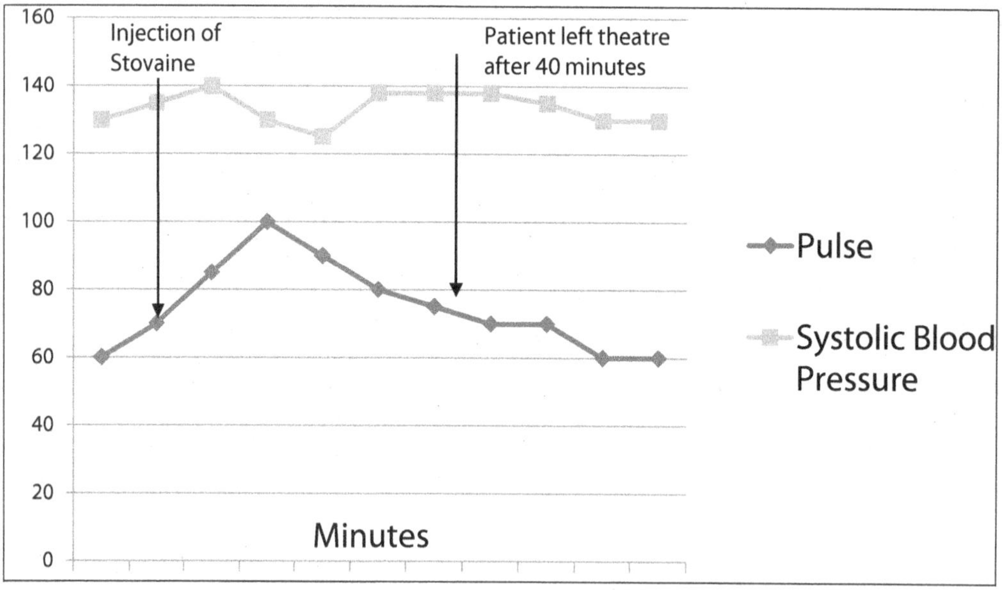

Figure 5.5 Spinal anaesthesia of Group B patient; wound of thigh sixteen hours old; haemoglobin 102 percent; wound excision; patient survived. (*British Medical Journal*, 2 June 1917)

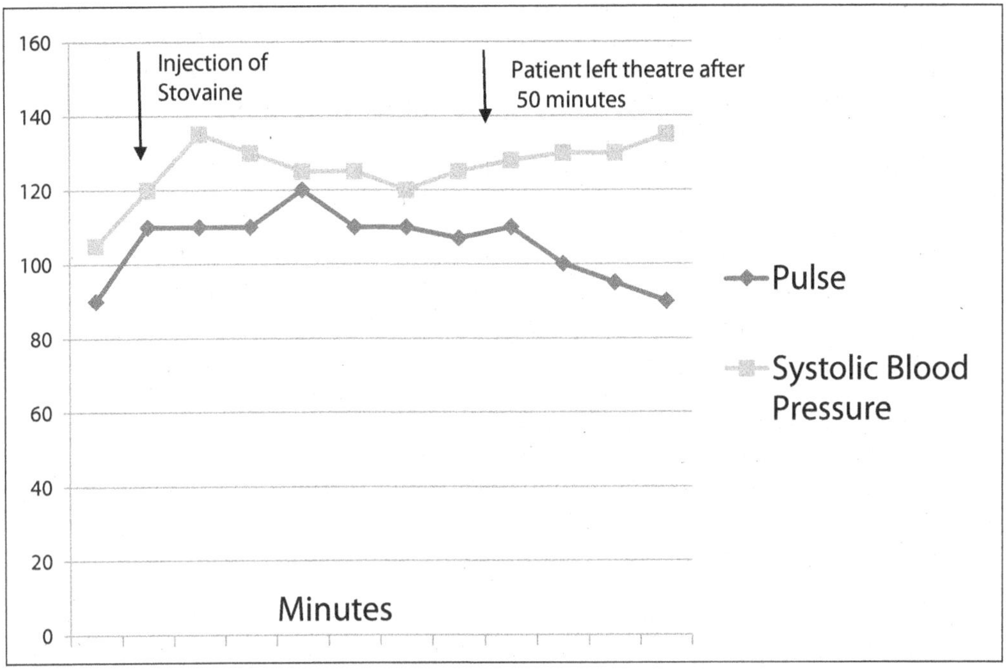

Figure 5.6 Spinal anaesthesia of Group C patient; wound of thigh and femoral artery twenty three days old; haemoglobin 45 percent; marked ischaemic change of leg; amputation through the lower third of thigh; patient survived. (*British Medical Journal*, 2 June, 1917)

Group C patients managed very well with spinal anaesthesia, even when the haemoglobin was 45 percent as in the case described. The critical factor here was the time that had elapsed since the wound had been inflicted. The patient's blood volume had been restored by haemo-dilution and his circulation was in a stable and steady state so that the spinal anaesthetic was safe.

As Robertson pointed out, with the benefit of current knowledge, when a local anaesthetic is injected into the fluid around the spine, it blocks not only the sensory nerves that carry the sensations of touch and pain to the brain and the motor fibres which allow the brain to send impulses to move the limb but also the fibres of the sympathetic nervous system. These sympathetic nerve fibres innervate the small blood vessels in the body to alter their calibre in response to changes in blood volume and to the outside temperature. When a patient is shocked due to blood loss these small vessels constrict to direct blood to the brain and heart in an attempt to preserve the function of these vital organs. If a patient in such a precarious state has a spinal anaesthetic, so that the action of the nerves on the blood vessels is blocked, the compensatory vasoconstriction mechanism that has been maintaining the blood pressure is withdrawn and the peripheral blood vessels dilate uncontrollably. No amount of increase in the pulse rate will counteract the problem, and the blood pressure crashes. It is perhaps a testament to the fitness of youth that some men did survive this experience.[5]

5 Robertson, A., in Scotland, T, Heys, S., *War Surgery 1914-18*, (Solihull: Helion and Company, 2012), pp. 93-94.

Marshall's next problem was to find a safer anaesthetic for Group A patients. The two conventional general anaesthetics, ether and chloroform were unsatisfactory. Chloroform resulted in a progressive fall in blood pressure culminating in the death of the patient, while ether protected the patient during the operation, only for the blood pressure to drop catastrophically post operatively. Present knowledge attributes the protective effect of ether during surgery as sympathometric. Marshall's observations on chloroform led to a decline in the popularity of this anaesthetic agent, except for use in patients with chest wounds, where ether caused troublesome bleeding. [6]

For an extreme case of completely shattered limb or limbs, which left the patient in a collapsed state due to blood loss and pain, Marshall concluded that a gaseous anaesthetic of nitrous oxide and oxygen was the only safe regime to employ after first attending to the general resuscitation of the patient. Nitrous oxide had been used during the 19th century for dental extractions but had never found favour in other clinical situations. Nitrous oxide and oxygen will not render a healthy person unconscious, but if an individual is slipping in and out of consciousness due to severe blood loss, then it will suffice to permit the performance of a quick procedure, such as an amputation. Some of the 90 percent of patients mentioned at the beginning of this chapter would probably have survived if their amputations had been performed using nitrous oxide and oxygen.

So much for quick amputation, but what was to be done if the procedure was a longer and more intricate one? It would be unhelpful to have a patient wriggling around in a semi-conscious state while the surgeon tried to get on with the operation. Marshall noted that a small amount of ether could safely be given with the nitrous oxide and oxygen to enable a longer procedure to be performed. Marshall previously had a chance meeting with American anaesthetist James Gwathney (1863-1944), who in 1912 had developed a nitrous oxide and oxygen machine containing a sight-feed meter to measure the amount of nitrous oxide being delivered.[7] Marshall set about adapting this to make a machine to deliver nitrous oxide, oxygen and ether. He engaged the services of a local French tinsmith to make a machine to his design. Using this method, he reduced the mortality of mangled limbs requiring amputation from 90 to 25 percent.[8] He took his design to the firm of Coxeter in London, which developed a definitive version for him. He later observed:

> So Coxeter developed it for me. I came home on leave and showed them a drawing of what I wanted, which I had had made by the tinsmith out there. So Coxeter made it and then said 'For goodness sake publish this, because some chap has borrowed our blocks'. However, the other gentleman did publish it and that was the origin of Boyle's apparatus. Well, he thought it was alright and I didn't mind, because I wasn't going to be an anaesthetist anyhow.

Captain Henry Boyle (1875-1941) was the 'other gentleman' Marshall referred to. Boyle had met Gwathney in 1912 at the Seventeenth International Congress of Medicine in London.

6 Metcalfe, N.H., The Effect of the First World War (1914-18) on the development of British anaesthesia, *European Journal of Anaesthesia*, 24:8 (24 August 2007), pp.649-57.
7 Metcalfe, *European Journal of Anaesthesia*, 2007.
8 Evans, *British Medical Journal*, 18-25 December 1982.

Boyle persuaded his hospital governors to purchase a Gwathney machine, which he modified by adding some of Marshall's innovations and published his design in 1919.[9]

Geoffrey Marshall's work at CCS 17 at Remy Siding was very important for several reasons. He employed common sense and clinical judgement to solve a major anaesthetic problem which had cost many lives. He established the role of the anaesthetist as the per-operative physician. Dealing with shock and improving the patient's general condition was a vital part of his work before any anaesthetic or operation could be considered. He demonstrated beyond reasonable doubt that a correct choice of anaesthetic was of first importance. The patient's life would be as much imperilled by the faulty judgement of the anaesthetist as by a wrong decision on the part of the surgeon.

As indicated, Marshall spent most of his war at CCS Number 17 at Remy Siding. When the Third Battle of Ypres began on 31 July 1917, there were four casualty clearing stations at Remy Siding which were the biggest on the Western Front. They were British 10 and 17 and Canadian 2 and 3. Because of their size and location they were the sites of much clinical research. Apart from Marshall's work on anaesthesia, there was a wound research centre at Casualty Clearing Station Number 10 which evaluated the safety of primary excision and suture of recently inflicted wounds. Other clinical research work included the evaluation of blood transfusion (Chapters 6 and 7) and performance of pioneering surgery for chest wounds (Chapter 7), both at Canadian CCS Number 2. Table 5.2 shows the numbers admitted to each of the Remy Siding group of clearing stations between 31 July and 10 November 1917. Between 25-30 percent of those admitted had urgent definitive surgery performed at the clearing stations, with a percentage mortality of 3.7 percent.[10]

Table 5.2 Admissions to the four casualty clearing stations at Remy Siding during the Third Battle of Ypres between 31 July and 16 November 1917.

Casualty clearing stations Remy Siding	Number admitted	Number operated on	Percentage operated on
No 2 Canadian	20,497	6,016	29.6
No 3 Canadian	18,721	4,673	25
No 10	17,343	5.002	29
No 17	17,361	5,816	30.02

Macpherson, W.G., *History of the Great War based on official documents Medical Services General History Vol. III*, (London: His Majesty's Stationery Office, 1924), p.169.

Figure 5.7 is an view of Lijssenthoek Military Cemetery, which was the burial ground of the Remy Siding clearing stations. There are 10.821 graves. Had it not been for the work of Geoffrey Marshall and others like him performing vitally important clinical research, there would have been many more.

9 Boyle, H.E.G., Nitrous oxide-oxygen-ether outfit, *Lancet,* No. 1 (1919), p. 226.

10 Macpherson, W.G., *History of the Great War based on official documents Medical Services General History Vol. III*, (London: His Majesty's Stationery Office, 1924), p. 167.

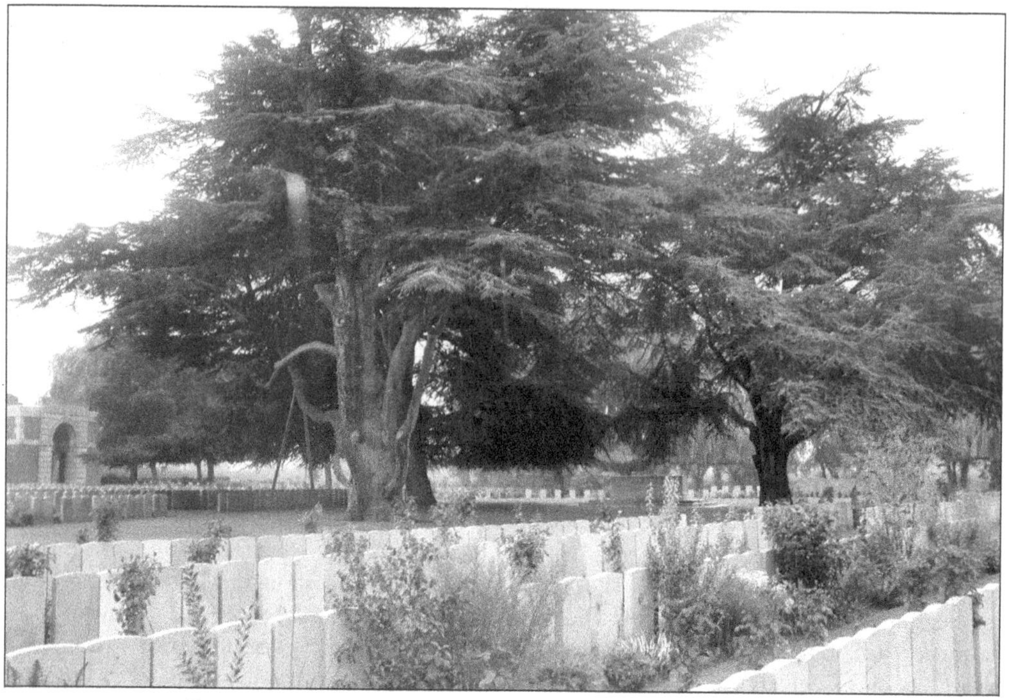

Figure 5.7 Lijssenthoek Military Cemetery. (Author's photograph)

Despite the importance of good anaesthesia, for the most part anaesthetics were not administered by specialist anaesthetists but by officers from various medical units. The importance of the quality and training of personnel at casualty clearing stations became the concern of an American anaesthetist called Arthur Guedel, who believed that young medical officers could not become proficient and safe clinicians while learning on the job. He set up training schools in Chaumont and Contrexville. He realised that these young men needed instruction in basic principles of airway control and depth of anaesthesia. He devised a chart which demonstrated the changes in the reaction of the pupils and certain reflexes under ether anaesthesia so that medical officers could recognize when they had achieved a suitable plane of anaesthesia.[11] To cement this training, he became a well-known figure travelling between casualty clearing stations on a motorbike.

Some specialist anaesthetists were appointed to casualty clearing stations by 1916 but, generally speaking, clinicians gaining experience in anaesthesia had no security of tenure and could be moved to work as regimental medical officers close to the front line. Fortunately this state of affairs came to the notice of Sir Anthony Bowlby, who ordered the presence of a specialist anaesthetist at every casualty clearing station who was able to supervise the training of young medical officers and some of the 200 nurses who were taught to administer anaesthetics in late 1917 and

11 Guedel, A., Third Stage Ether: A sub-classification regarding the significance of the position and movements of the eyeball, *American Journal of Surgery*, 34, (1920), pp. 53-57.

employed to do so early the following year.[12] Unfortunately one of the reasons for training nurse anaesthetists was to enable the release of a corresponding number of medical officers for service closer to the front line. The specialist anaesthetist was also responsible for checking the supply of suitable anaesthetic agents and maintaining equipment. Bowlby realised the importance of the anaesthetist's role in preventing wound shock as well as in administering an anaesthetic skilfully and this helped to cement the anaesthetist's role as the per-operative physician.[13] As knowledge and experience grew during the four years of conflict, the most appropriate anaesthetic agents were employed for each clinical condition to help minimise morbidity and mortality. More will be said about this in Chapter 7 which deals with the development of surgical specialties.

12 Metcalfe, *European Journal of Anaesthesia*, 2007.
13 Whitehead, I.R., *Doctors in the Great War* (Barnsley: Leo Cooper, 1999), pp. 79, 201, 208.

6

Wound shock and its management: a light at the end of a dark tunnel

Wound shock is defined as a condition of circulatory failure due to deficient entry of blood into the heart. We now know it as hypovolaemic or haemorrhagic shock. It was one of the most serious clinical conditions which confronted clinicians during the Great War and was responsible for high morbidity and mortality rates. Its presence delayed and sometimes prevented operative intervention. Patients suffering from wound shock were cold and clammy and had a very rapid pulse rate with a low blood pressure. They usually had impaired conscious levels when they presented at casualty clearing stations and required immediate resuscitation if their lives were to be saved.

This chapter begins by describing the clinical research of two young surgeons who were attached to the British First Army in Northern France during 1915. Captain Ernest Cowell (1886-1971) working at Casualty Clearing Station 23 and Captain John Fraser (1885-1947) based at Casualty Clearing Station 33, collaborated to study wound shock by first measuring the blood pressures of uninjured soldiers in the front line to establish a baseline level. The systolic blood pressure is the pressure within the arteries during contraction of the heart and the diastolic pressure is the pressure within the vessels during the relaxation phase of the heart. These frontline soldiers were frequently exhausted, cold and dehydrated as a result of poor fluid intake, all of which predisposed to the subsequent development of shock in the event of being wounded. Their average systolic blood pressure was found to be slightly raised at around 140 mm Hg compared to the normal value of 110-120 mm Hg (mercury). This was attributable to the stress of being in the front line and to the risk of being killed or wounded. Some soldiers immediately after being wounded had a raised systolic blood pressure of around 180 mm Hg which soon returned to normal, while others had a low blood pressure which continued to fall as they progressed to a state of circulatory collapse with a pressure of 90 mm Hg or less.[1]

The Consulting Surgeon to First Army was Cuthbert Wallace (1867-1944), and he formed a close working relationship with Fraser and Cowell during the conflict. Before the war, Wallace was Consulting Surgeon at St Thomas's Hospital in London, where he had also done his surgical training. He volunteered for service in South Africa during the Second Boer War and served 1899-1900 as surgeon to the Portland Hospital under his friend Sir Anthony Bowlby of St Bartholomew's Hospital. On the outbreak of war in 1914, Wallace once again volunteered

1 Van Der Kloot, W., *William Maddock Bayliss's Therapy for Wound Shock* <http://rsnr.royalsocietypublishing.org/>.

and became Consulting Surgeon to the British First Army after the formation of two British Armies in December 1914. He initially held the rank of Temporary Colonel but was promoted to Major-General in December 1917.

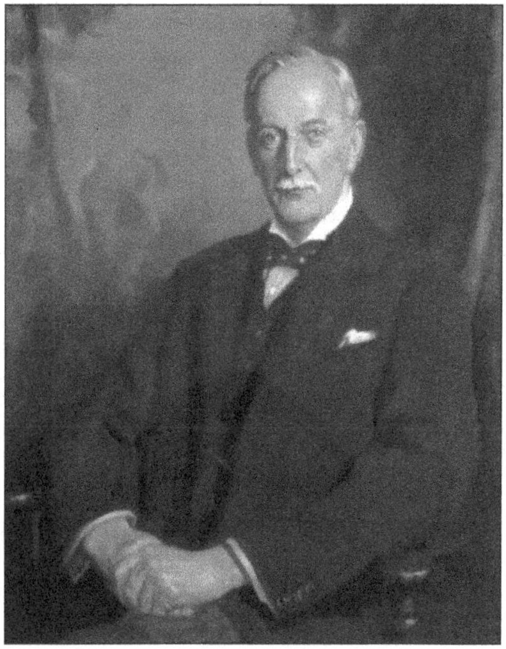

Figure 6.1 Sir Cuthbert Wallace (1867-1944); Consulting Surgeon British First Army. (Courtesy Royal College of Surgeons of England)

Case history

In 1918, Wallace and Fraser published a book entitled *Surgery at a Casualty Clearing Station*, in which they described the characteristic clinical presentation of a soldier suffering from wound shock by considering a hypothetical case. They imagined a fragment of shell casing had penetrated a soldier's thigh without fracturing his femur (thigh bone). The regimental stretcher bearers collecting the patient from no man's land noticed that the wounded man was very pale and sweaty. By the time he was examined by the regimental medical officer (RMO) in the regimental aid post (RAP) close to the front line, his pulse rate was steady and his blood pressure was normal or even slightly elevated despite his appearance. Wallace and Fraser explained that this medical state was primary shock, which was the soldier's immediate response to being wounded.

The wounded man was taken from the RAP to the advanced dressing station (ADS) by wheeled stretcher over open ground. The journey was a very cold and prolonged one and the soldier's condition deteriorated significantly during the transfer. By the time he was examined at the advanced dressing station, he was still conscious and could answer questions but he was very cold and his body temperature was falling. His pulse was rapid and difficult to feel because it was weak. His blood pressure was low and continued to fall during his transfer by ambulance wagon to a designated casualty clearing station (CCS) nearby. By the time he reached the CCS, he was unresponsive, was bathed in perspiration and his pulse was very rapid indeed and barely palpable. His blood pressure was difficult to record, but his systolic pressure was certainly less than 80 mm Hg. Wallace and Fraser explained that this was secondary shock due to severe blood loss and that without treatment it would lead inevitably to the patient's death. [2]

At the time of their clinical research, Wallace, Cowell and Fraser did not understand what pathological changes were occurring within the patient to explain why his condition had seemed to be perfectly reasonable initially, only to deteriorate dramatically to the point of near death by the time he reached the casualty clearing station. With the benefit of present day knowledge, we know

2 Wallace, C.S., Fraser, J., *Surgery at a casualty clearing station*, (London: A&C Black, 1918), pp. 7-22.

what happened. His initial blood loss was significant, probably more than the attending clinicians had appreciated, but because he was young, fit and healthy, he was able to compensate for this blood loss by constricting the blood vessels to his skin, muscles, kidneys and other organs not immediately essential for survival in order to maintain the vital circulation to his heart and brain. This vasoconstriction produced the initial slight rise in blood pressure when the stretcher bearers retrieved him from no man's land. A young man can lose up to 30 percent of his blood volume without any change in blood pressure and only a modest rise in his pulse rate. During his difficult journey to the casualty clearing station, he continued to bleed into his thigh wound and lost much more blood. He also became cold, which made matters significantly worse. His compensatory vasoconstriction was no longer able to cope and his cardiac output fell. The cardiac output is the amount of blood pumped by the heart per minute and is a function of the heart rate and the stroke volume, the latter being the amount of blood pumped out by the heart every beat. By multiplying the heart rate by the stroke volume, a figure is arrived at for the cardiac output. Normally it is between four and eight litres a minute. Two major factors contributed to the fall in cardiac output in the soldier's case, namely continuing blood loss and lowered body temperature. On-going bleeding meant there was less blood returning to his heart and therefore less blood available for the heart to pump out every beat. When the soldier's body temperature dropped, his stroke volume fell as a direct result of the cold and would have done so regardless of whether there had been ongoing bleeding or not. By the time he arrived in the CCS, he was in extremis and unless something was done right away to raise his blood pressure and stabilise his condition, he would die.

If a senior elderly officer had been wounded in a similar way, he would not have reached the casualty clearing station alive. He would have died on the way because his reflex vasoconstriction would have been much less effective than that of the young soldier. His small blood vessels, having lost much of their elasticity, would have been unable compensate for the severe blood loss and he would have passed into a state of circulatory collapse very quickly.

Shock is often reversible if caught in time. In the present day, it is possible to transfuse patients with massive quantities of blood to restore blood volume and pressure and to maintain the perfusion of vital organs. If too much time has passed before resuscitative measures are initiated and the blood pressure has remained low for too long, irreversible tissue damage occurs, the patient fails to respond, and death is the inevitable outcome. This is called irreversible shock. If the blood pressure falls much below 60mms Hg, then the brain is no longer perfused and vital centres within the brain that maintain life cease to function.

In the first two years of the war, resuscitative fluid replacement therapy following wounding was very inadequate. Oral fluids were frequently given, but following a serious wound, they were often poorly tolerated and in penetrating abdominal wounds they were positively harmful. It has already been mentioned that subcutaneous saline and intra-rectal saline were employed to replace fluid in the early months of the war. In 1915, Geoffrey Marshall working at Casualty Clearing Station 17 at Remy Siding (Chapter 5), showed by post mortem studies that subcutaneous saline injected through a hollow needle below the axilla around the upper lateral chest was of no value whatsoever, because it was never absorbed and was still present around the axillary region after the patient had died. One litre of saline inserted via rubber tubing through the anus into the rectum was absorbed into the circulation quite rapidly because the wall of the rectum has a rich supply of small blood vessels. Unfortunately, any slight rise in blood pressure brought about by absorption of the saline into the circulation was transient for the same reason as an intravenous saline infusion (see below) and there was no sustained rise in the blood pressure and no sustained improvement of the patient's general condition. Soldiers with penetrating wounds of the chest were even given intra-rectal coffee sweetened with a tablespoonful of glucose, which of course did nothing to improve matters.[3]

During the Battle of the Somme in 1916, intravenous saline was administered as clinicians attempted to restore blood volume in a more predictable way, or so it was believed. By employing this regime, it was hoped that the blood pressure would respond with a sustained rise. Captains Cowell and Fraser demonstrated that while an intravenous infusion of one litre of saline produced a transient increase in blood pressure, this was not maintained, and the blood pressure quickly fell again.[4] Figure 6.2 is a chart of a young soldier who sustained a severe shell wound. His systolic blood pressure on admission to the casualty clearing station was very low at 30mm Hg. An infusion of one litre of 0.9 percent saline raised his systolic blood pressure to 80mm Hg, but it quickly fell again, where it remained at 25-30 mm until he died less than two hours later.

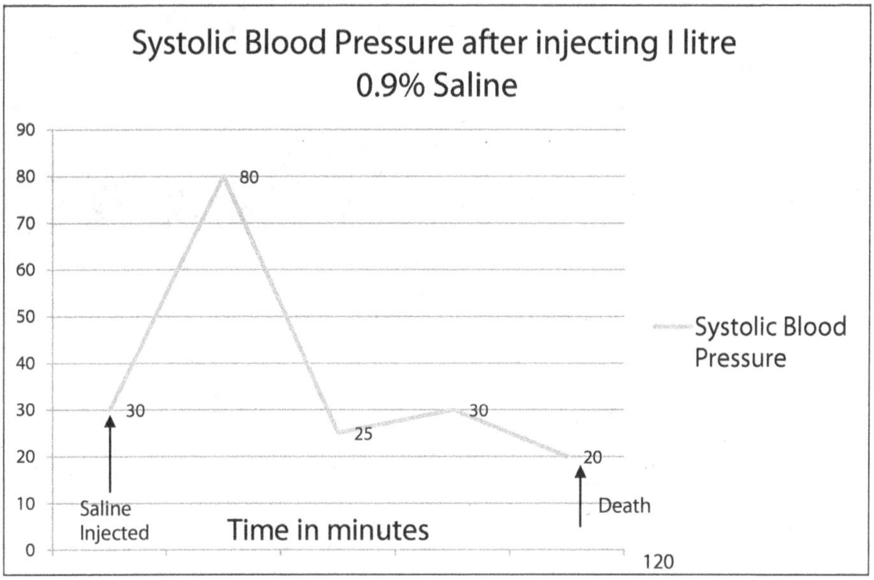

Figure 6.2 Patient of Captains Howell and Fraser admitted with a severe wound caused by a fragment of shell casing; he died 2 hours after administration of one litre of 0.9 percent saline. (Data Van Der Kloot, *William Maddock Bayliss's Therapy for Wound Shock*, p. 8)

The explanation for the transient rise in blood pressure is quite simply because the infused saline does not stay in the circulation. It quickly escapes through microscopic, thin-walled blood vessels called capillaries. The capillaries connect tiny arteries (arterioles) to equally tiny veins (venules). Within these tiny blood vessels are red blood cells which carry oxygen to the tissues and blood plasma which is a straw-coloured fluid containing salts (called electrolytes) and proteins, the most prevalent being albumin. Following an injection of one litre of 0.9

3 Roberts, J.E.H., Craig, J.G., The surgical treatment of severe wounds of the chest, *British Medical Journal,* 2: 2966 (3 November 1917) pp. 576-579.
4 Van Der Kloot, *William Maddock Bayliss's Therapy for Wound Shock.*

percent saline, water and salt are pushed out of the blood plasma inside the capillaries because the hydrostatic pressure of plasma is higher than that of the interstitial fluid which bathes the surrounding cells. The capillary wall functions as a filter, because it does not allow proteins in the blood plasma to pass. Under normal circumstances, the proteins retained inside the capillaries generate a colloidal osmotic pressure, which draws fluid out of the interstitial space and back into the plasma within the capillaries. The opposing forces of hydrostatic and osmotic pressures are almost equal, and a balance is maintained. Any excess fluid in the interstitial space is called lymph and this makes its way back to the circulation by a separate route via thin-walled lymph channels. This mechanism of fluid exchange was worked out by a famous physiologist called Ernest Starling (1866-1927) and is called Starling's Principle. If a litre of saline is introduced into the circulation following a severe wound from which many blood cells have been lost, the plasma is diluted, and the colloidal osmotic pressure which draws fluid by osmosis out of the interstitial space and back into the plasma is decreased, with the result that the hydrostatic pressure effect produced by the added saline is overriding and the saline is soon driven into the interstitial space where it stays and the blood pressure falls as quickly as it rose.

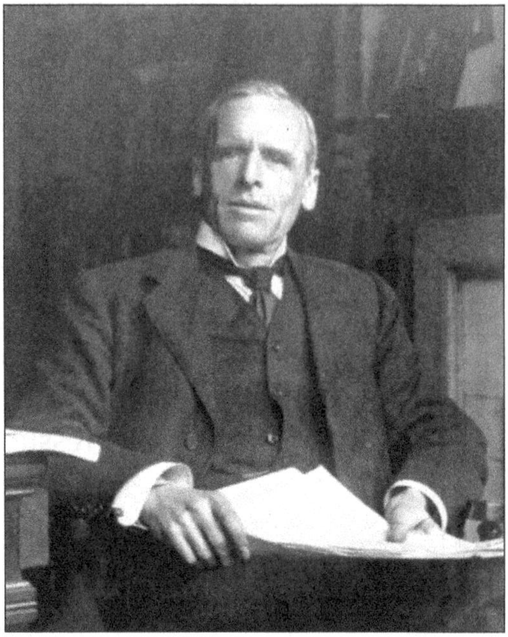

Figure 6.3 Ernest Starling (1866-1927) was a most distinguished British physiologist who made great contributions to scientific progress during the Great War. He chaired the MRC Special Investigative Committee on Wound Shock and Allied Conditions. (Wikimedia Commons)

Ernest Starling was a brilliant physiologist and one of the most outstanding scientists of his era. His discoveries had a major impact on scientific thinking and certainly influenced the outcome of the war as will be explained shortly. Before the war, Starling collaborated with his brother-in-law William Bayliss (see below), who was also a physiologist, to discover the hormone secretin which regulates secretions of the stomach, pancreas and liver. He is also known for Starling's Law of the Heart, which states that the stroke volume of the heart (the amount of blood pumped out of the heart in a given beat) increases in response to an increase volume of blood filling the heart, if other factors remain constant. Conversely, if the volume of blood returning to the heart is reduced, as in wound shock, the stroke volume of the heart decreases. The heart, in effect, is a self-regulating pump. It is important to note the last part of Starling's Law, 'if other factors remain constant', because a decrease in body core temperature will reduce the stroke volume in its own right and will worsen shock brought about by blood loss.

During the war, Starling was initially a commissioned officer, and did a considerable amount of work on the effects of poison gas and on the design of gas masks. He became very frustrated by poor and cumbersome administrative support and was very outspoken to his superiors in the War Office. This is reflected by the award of knighthoods to many of Starling's contemporaries, while he only got a CMG (Companion of the order of St Michael and St George). He resigned from the army in June 1917 and ironically was far better able to help the war effort as a civilian than as a serving officer in the RAMC. Starling became Chairman of the Medical Research Committee's Special Investigative Committee on Surgical Shock and Allied Conditions in August 1917 (see below) and in November 1917 he sat on the Royal Society Food Committee, which was set up to give advice to the recently formed Ministry of Food. Three weeks later, Starling became Chairman of the Food Committee, which did much valuable work in advising the Government on how best to set about feeding the British Nation, so that no man, woman or child went hungry, despite significant food shortages brought about by German U-boat activity which restricted the import of vital grain and other foodstuffs from North and South America. Starling and the Food Committee were instrumental in introducing food rationing in 1918 and their work made a major contribution to winning the war on the home front. Germany had similar food shortages due to the Royal Naval blockade of merchant shipping bound for German ports, but the Germans managed their food shortage problem disastrously, with the result that many German civilians died of starvation.

Special Investigative Committee on Surgical (Wound) Shock

A Special Investigative Committee on Surgical Shock and Allied Conditions was set up to try and solve many of the problems associated with secondary wound shock. The committee first met on 17 August 1917 with Ernest Starling in the chair. Amongst its members were distinguished scientists doing research in the United Kingdom and clinicians who were engaged in more practical aspects of clinical research in the casualty clearing stations on the Western Front.

Definition of wound shock

The Investigative Committee began by defining wound shock as a condition of circulatory failure due to deficient entry of blood into the heart (q.v.). The definition clearly shows Starling's influence and one cannot read the definition without Starling's Law of the heart coming to mind.

The following personnel all served on the Investigative Committee during the war although not necessarily at the same time. Commissioned officers have their rank before their names; Professor W. M. Bayliss, F.R.S.; Captain H.C. Bazett, RAMC, Professor F. A. Bainbridge; Lieut.-Colonel W. B. Cannon, M O.R C., U.S.A; Dr. H. H. Dale, F.R.S.; Colonel T. R. Elliott, F.R.S., R.A.M.C.; Captain John Fraser, R A.M.C.; Colonel H.M.W. Gray, R A.M.C.; Dr. P. P. Laidlaw, F.R.S.; A. N. Richards; Professor C. S Sherrington, F.R.S.: Professor E. H. Starling, F R.S.; Captain K.M. Walker, RAMC; Major-General Cuthbert S. Wallace, A.M.S. (T).[5]

Other clinicians made important contributions at the request of the Advisory Committee without being formally invited to join. The Advisory Committee was a fairly even balance of scientists and clinicians. Table 6.1 shows the activity of the Advisory Committee during its working lifetime.

5 Butler, A.G., *Official History of the Australian Army Medical Services, 1914–1918 Vol. II – The Western Front* (Canberra: Australian War Memorial, 1940), p. 953

Table 6.1 List of Reports of Special Investigative Committee on Surgical Shock and Allied Conditions with date reports submitted

Report	Name of Report	Investigators and dates
No. 1	Intra-venous injections to replace blood	WM Bayliss, 25 November 17
No. 2	Nature and treatment of wound shock and allied conditions	25 December 17
No. 2.1	Clinical study of blood pressure in wound conditions	Captain J Fraser RAMC Captain E Cowell RAMC
No. 2.2	Alteration in the distribution and character of blood	WB Cannon (US Army) Captain J Fraser RAMC Captain E Cowell RAMC
No. 2.3	Acidosis in cases of shock, haemorrhage and gas infections	WB Cannon (US Army)
No. 2.4	The initiation of wound shock	Captain E Cowell RAMC
No. 2.5	A consideration of the nature of wound shock	WB Cannon (US Army)
No. 2.6	The preventive treatment of wound shock	WB Cannon (US Army) Captain J Fraser RAMC Captain E Cowell RAMC
No. 3	Use of intra-venous injection gum acacia in surgical shock	Captain H Drummond RAMC; Captain E Taylor RAMC, 7 January 18
No. 4	Memorandum on blood transfusion	OH Robertson (US Army) 4 April 1918
No. 5		25 April 1918
No. 5.1	Value of haemoglobin and blood pressure observation on surgical cases	Captain HC Bazett RAMC
No. 5.2	Observation on blood pressure in gas gangrene	Captain H Drummond RAMC
No. 6	Memorandum on blood volume after haemorrhage	Oswald Hope Robertson and Arlie Brock 8 August 1918
No. 7	Acidosis and shock	Subcommittee October 1918
No. 8	Traumatic toxaemia in shock	14 March 1919
No. 8.1	Introductory	Major General Cuthbert Wallace RAMC
No. 8.2	Action of histamine Its bearing on traumatic toxaemia as factor in shock	HH Dale, PP Laidlaw, AN Richards
No. 8.3	Supplementary note on histamine shock	HH Dale
No. 8.4	Muscle injury in relation to shock	WB Cannon, WM Bayliss
No. 8.5	Further note on muscle injury	WM Bayliss
No. 8.6	Characteristics shock induced by tissue injury	WB Cannon (US Army)
No. 8.7	Observations on wound shock with regard to muscle damage	Major JW McNee RAMC Captains AF Sladden RAMC Captain JE McCartney RAMC
No. 8.8	Blood volume in wound shock	Captain NM Keith RAMC
No. 8.9	Changes in Central Nervous System in shock	Lt. Col. Mott, FRS, RAMC
No. 9	Blood volume changes in wound shock	NM Keith 14 March 1919

Butler, A.G., *Official History of the Australian Army Medical Services, 1914–1918 Volume II – The Western Front* (Canberra: Australian War Memorial, 1940), p. 953.

A.G. Butler, the Official Historian of the Australian Medical Services, was in no doubt that most of the progress was made by clinicians faced with the harsh reality of treating critically wounded patients suffering from secondary wound shock:

> It was from the domain of clinical, rather than of analytical science that the most important and practical developments in the treatment of the physiological effects of wounding and /or of haemorrhage chiefly derived. Certainly, it is beyond cavil that much the most important contribution to the problem belongs wholly to the clinician. It was made at the end of 1914, by a British provincial orthopaedic surgeon; and was the use of the Thomas knee-splint in gunshot fracture-wounds of the femur; the very type and exemplar of shock-preventers.[6]

The British provincial orthopaedic surgeon referred to by Butler who took Thomas Splints to France was Alexander MacCormick (1856-1947), who was born in Argyllshire, Scotland. He was a graduate of the University of Edinburgh and in 1883 he emigrated from Scotland to Sydney, Australia. According to Butler, MacCormick took some Thomas Splints to France in 1914 but failed to persuade his surgical colleagues of their value in immobilising fractures of the femur. More will be said about MacCormick later in the chapter, but it was surgeon Robert Jones from Liverpool who is credited with introducing Thomas Splints to the casualty clearing stations on the Western Front and Henry Gray from Aberdeen who ensured their use in clinical practice during the Battle of Arras during April-May 1917 (Chapter 7). The Thomas Splint was described by George Washington Crile of the 4th American Base Hospital as the most important device used for the prevention of wound shock because it immobilised fractured femurs so effectively that it reduced blood loss significantly and saved many lives.[7]

One of the most important scientific contributions was made by Professor William Maddock Bayliss, whose work will be considered at length. Some of the scientific research by others was well wide of the mark and contributed little to the advance in knowledge of surgical shock.

Professor William Maddock Bayliss (1860-1924)

Professor Bayliss was Ernest Starling's brother-in-law and was a key figure on the Advisory Committee. He was elected a Fellow of the Royal Society in 1903 and became Professor of Physiology at University College, London in 1912. He was knighted for his contributions to medicine in 1922. While at University College, he made a discovery that would prove to be of great practical value in the latter stages of the war. He experimented with an infusion of Gum Arabica, which unlike saline, stayed in the blood plasma of experimental shocked animals and maintained the blood pressure. He thought this might be of value in a clinical setting. In 1916, Bayliss injected experimental animals with salt solutions containing 5 percent Gum Arabica, or Gum Acacia, as it is also known. Gum Arabica comes from two species of the Acacia tree which grow in Egypt, the Sudan and sub-Sahara Africa. Gum Arabica is a complex polymer of polysaccharides and glycoproteins with large and inert molecules which do not cross the filter in

6 Butler, *Official History of the Australian Army Medical Services*, Vol. II, pp. 946-47.
7 Jones, R., Crippling due to fractures: its prevention and remedy, *British Medical Journal*, 1: 3359 (16 May 1925), pp. 909-13.

the capillary wall referred to above and have a definite osmotic pressure. In his experiments, Bayliss injected Gum Arabica solution into haemorrhaged animals, restored their blood pressure and successfully maintained it. This was a potential breakthrough, because with Gum Arabica, clinicians working in France might now have a biophysical treatment for wound shock which could be tested on moribund patients who had no other hope.[8]

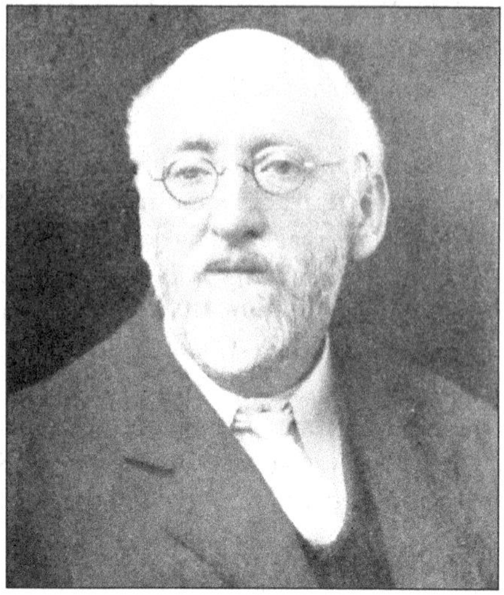

Figure 6.4 Professor William Maddock Bayliss (1860-1924) was a very influential Figure on the Special Investigative Committee on Surgical Shock and Allied Conditions. He discovered that infusion of a 6 percent solution of Gum Arabica in 0.9 percent saline in shocked experimental animals resulted in a rise in blood pressure which was maintained. (Courtesy Wellcome Library, London)

In 1917, Bayliss visited France to see what clinicians were doing to treat wound shock. He went to Casualty Clearing Station 23 in Northern France where he met Captain Ernest Cowell, who informed him about the clinical management of shock. Cowell stressed the very important relationship between cold and secondary shock. Soldiers who had lain in no man's land awaiting rescue and who were hypothermic were much more susceptible to the effects of shock. Warming patients was of great importance and Cowell had designed a special blanket covered with a waterproof sheet to help keep patients warm and to prevent the blanket from becoming saturated with muddy water. Stretcher bearers were instructed on how to wrap patients in three of these blankets, since by keeping them warm, shocked patients had a better chance of survival. This was a very sensible method to combat shock introduced by a practical clinician of great experience. During the war, various measures were introduced to warm wounded soldiers during their journeys to casualty clearing stations. Some of these have already been discussed. In the later stages of the war, ambulance wagons could be kept warm by using a heat exchange mechanism from the vehicle's exhaust system.

Bayliss next visited Casualty Clearing Station 33, where he met three men who would be invited to join the MRC Shock Subcommittee. They were Colonel Cuthbert Wallace, Consulting Surgeon to the British First Army, and his very capable young colleague, Captain John Fraser from Edinburgh, both of whom had an interest in surgical shock. Both men had extensive experience in treating patients with penetrating wounds of the abdomen, many of whom were suffering from wound shock as a result of major bleeding from vessels within the abdominal cavity (Chapter 7). Also present at CCS 33 was American Walter Cannon (Figure 6.5) from Harvard University. Cannon came to France with the American Base Hospital Number 5, the Harvard Unit, and had a particular interest in wound shock, having read all about it before he came to France. He was an extremely enthusiastic and very confident American with definite ideas about the cause of wound shock and gave the impression that he would soon sort everything out.

8 Van Der Kloot, *William Maddock Bayliss's Therapy for Wound Shock.*

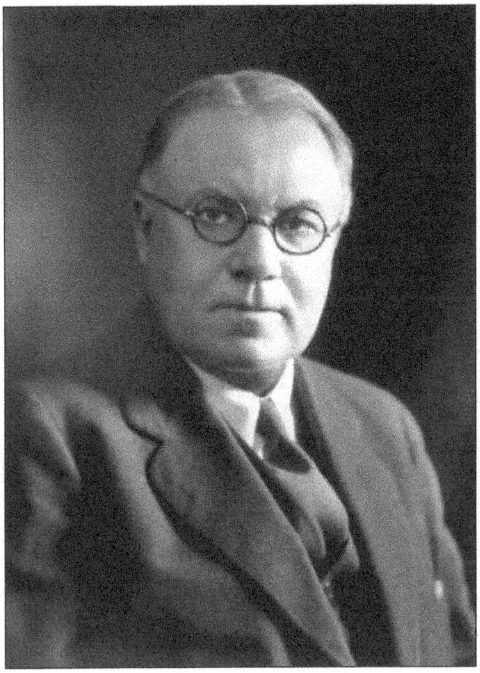

Figure 6.5 Walter Cannon (1871-1945), Professor of Physiology, Harvard. (Courtesy Wellcome Library, London)

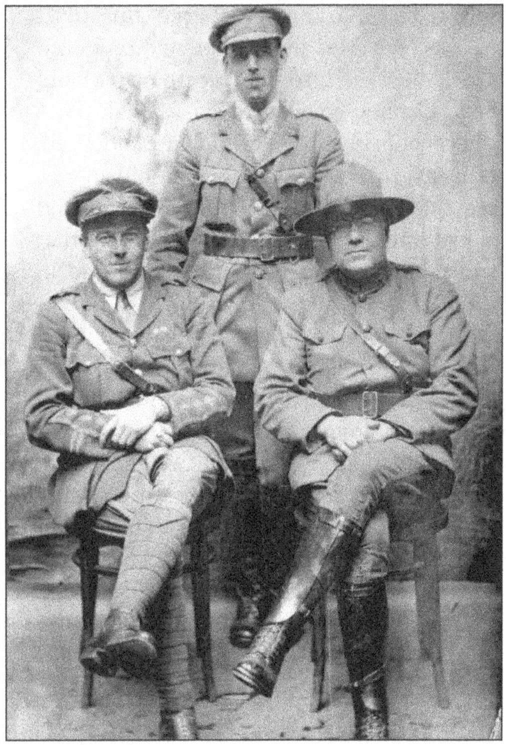

Figure 6.6 Seated left to right, Captain John Fraser, RAMC; Lieutenant-Colonel Walter Cannon, MORC (Medical Officers Reserve Corps) USA; standing Captain AM Hooper, RAMC; Cannon joined Fraser and Hooper at CCS 33 where they were doing clinical research into shock. Unlike Cannon, Fraser and Hooper were very practical individuals. (Courtesy Harvard Medical Library in the Francis A Countway Library of Medicine)

Unfortunately, Cannon was not a particularly practical individual and although a qualified doctor had never practised clinical medicine. He was Chairman and Professor of Physiology at Harvard Medical School. He declared that soldiers suffering from secondary shock must have pooled their blood somewhere within the body to explain the catastrophic and sustained fall in blood pressure which had occurred. Cannon thought the answer was obvious. If the blood had left the systemic circulation, it must be hiding away in the splanchnic circulation. In other words, it must have pooled in engorged blood vessels around the patient's bowel and liver. He obtained permission from Cowell to inject pituitary extract into the abdominal cavities of shocked patients which caused the gut vessels (vessels of the splanchnic circulation) to contract and if he was correct, blood would be diverted into the main circulation, the blood pressure would rise, and the patient would be cured. Unfortunately, it didn't work and post mortem studies showed that the splanchnic circulation was most certainly not engorged; quite the opposite in fact, but this came as no surprise to the experienced clinicians who had to deal with these patients on a daily basis.

Undeterred by this setback, Cannon fired off in another direction. He had acquired apparatus to measure the blood gases of patients and noted that the bicarbonate level in shocked patients was reduced. Cannon believed this must have been caused by acid. If acid produced shock, then surely sodium bicarbonate would help. Cannon concluded that the administration of baking soda would cure shock. As things turned out, baking soda did in fact prove to be helpful.[9] Further experimental work some time later, however, revealed that while bicarbonate did help wound shock, Cannon had things the wrong way round. Acid did not cause shock. It was produced as a result of shock. We now know that in patients suffering from wound shock, blood is diverted from skeletal muscle to maintain vital supplies to the heart and brain. Metabolism in muscle switches from using oxygen (aerobic metabolism) to not using oxygen. The latter is called anaerobic metabolism and it produces lactic acid. It is what happens when athletes run in a 400-metre race and their muscles are worked so hard that they don't get enough oxygen and have to switch to anaerobic metabolism. Lactic acid builds up causing pain in the muscles.

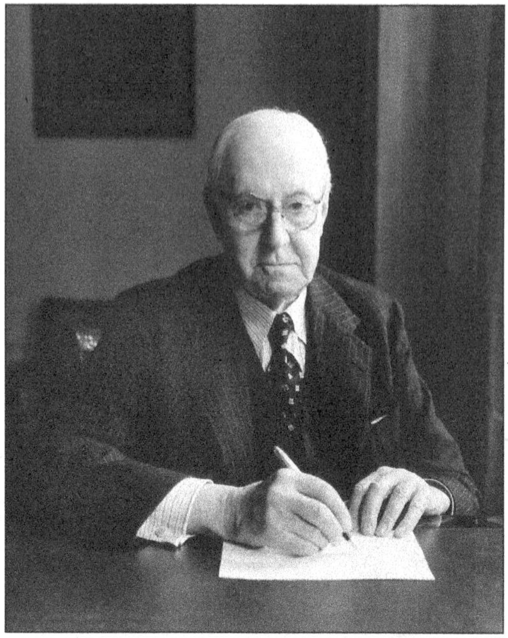

Figure 6.7 Henry Hallet Dale (1875-1968) was Director of the Department of Biochemistry and Pharmacology at the National Institute for Medical Research in London. (Courtesy Wellcome Library, London)

Colonel Sir Almroth Wright at Base Hospital 13 in Boulogne picked up on Cannon's error and published a paper in the Lancet in 1918.[10] Work had already been done showing that muscles working without oxygen produced lactic acid and Wright concluded quite rightly that this was the same process as occurred in shock when diminution of the circulation to muscle cut of the supply of oxygen to the tissues and metabolism switched to the anaerobic variety which resulted in the production of lactic acid. Concerning treatment of shock, Wright paid particular attention to the warming of patients. Ideally, he said, prevention of heat loss was better than cure and the giving of hot drinks and application of warmth as early as possible was advisable. However once shock was established then too rapid resuscitation by warmth would convey large amounts of lactic acid from the muscles into the blood stream once the circulation was re-established. He suggested treating patients with sodium bicarbonate before beginning thermal resuscitation, thus avoiding large amounts of lactic acid being liberated into the bloodstream and subjecting patients to surgery before the alkalinity of the blood was corrected.[11]

9 Cannon, W.B., Acidosis in cases of shock, haemorrhage and gas infection, *Journal of American Medical Association,* 70 (23 February 1918), pp. 531-35.

10 Robertson, A., in Scotland, T., Heys, S., *War Surgery 1914-18,* (Solihull: Helion and Company, 2012), pp. 105-06.

11 Wright, A.E., Colebrook, L., On the Acidosis of Shock and Suspended Circulation, *Lancet* 1:191 (1 June 1918), pp. 763-65.

Henry Hallet Dale (1875-1968)

In 1914, Henry Dale (Figure 6.7) was Director of the Department of Biochemistry and Pharmacology at the National Institute for Medical Research in London, where he identified the substance acetylcholine as a possible neurotransmitter. For this work, he was awarded the Nobel Prize for Medicine jointly with Otto Loewi in 1936. He also discovered the substance histamine a few years before the start of the Great War.[12] When injected into the circulation, histamine causes a dramatic fall in blood pressure. It is the same thing that happens in anaphylactic shock, when a sensitized individual is stung by a wasp or a bee. Anaphylactic shock is associated with histamine release within the body from specialised cells which cause a profound dilation of blood vessels and subsequent complete circulatory collapse because the pooling of blood in greatly dilated peripheral vessels prevents it from getting back to the heart and thence to the brain with vital oxygenated blood. Histamine makes capillary walls more permeable, so that proteins can escape from the blood plasma into the interstitial space. Because collapse due to wound shock bore a superficial resemblance to circulatory collapse secondary to histamine injection, Dale was convinced that there must be a substance like histamine acting as an agent to produce wound shock. This belief resulted in Dale directing his efforts to finding such a substance.

Dale collaborated with Professor Patrick Playfair Laidlaw (1881-1940), Professor Alfred Newton Richards (1876-1966) and Francis Arthur Bainbridge (1871-1924), all of whom had done research work using histamine. Laidlaw was Professor of Pathology at Guys and Richards was Professor of Pharmacology at the University of Pennsylvania. Bainbridge was Professor of Physiology at St Bartholomew's Hospital in London. Apart from his collaborative work with Dale, Bainbridge showed that an increase in pressure on the venous side of the heart resulted in an increase in the heart rate. This is called the Bainbridge Reflex.

Dale's research would lead his team of workers up a blind alley, however, because circulatory collapse from wound shock is quite different from that due to histamine injection. In wound shock there is complete peripheral vasoconstriction to maintain blood flow to the vital centres of the heart and brain. In contrast, histamine injection causes a profound and potentially fatal peripheral vasodilatation which prevents sufficient blood getting back to the heart. Injection of adrenaline into a patient with histamine-related shock causes vasoconstriction and cures the problem. Injection of adrenaline into a patient suffering from wound shock changes nothing, because the blood vessels are already fully constricted.

The Advisory Committee also asked the Dale group to establish if the injection of acid caused a fall in blood pressure, inducing shock. In the fullness of time they found that it did not, calling Cannon's hypothesis into serious question. The Committee investigated the relationship between cold and wound shock and found experimentally that whilst cold itself did not cause shock, it required the removal of significantly less blood from experimental animals to precipitate the condition. In other words, cold made the animals more susceptible to the effects of shock. Ernest Cowell would have been able to tell the members of the Advisory Committee this from his own clinical experience treating wounded soldiers suffering from wound shock in

12 Van Der Kloot, W., *Great Scientists Wage the Great War* (United Kingdom and United States: Fonthill Media, 2014).

the casualty clearing stations on the Western Front. In fact, he had already done so when he spoke to Bayliss when the latter visited CCS 23 in France.

From the experimental work done, there was no doubt that the most hopeful line of research from a practical point of view was Bayliss's work on Gum Arabica in Ringer's Solution, the latter being a solution of various salts. Much time had passed since his initial observations on experimental animals in 1916 and it was not until a meeting in November 1917 that the Advisory Committee learned that 5 percent Gum Arabica in Ringer's Solution had been used in France and had helped to save lives on the Western Front. Cannon was at the meeting and in view of his research in France where he showed that sodium bicarbonate had a beneficial effect in the treatment of wound shock, Cannon argued that a bicarbonate solution would be better than Ringer's. Cannon, of course, mistakenly believed that acid caused shock and bicarbonate cured it, although his error had not been picked up on at that point in time. Unfortunately, the Advisory Committee agreed to Cannon's proposal, and decided to have 5 percent Gum Arabica in 3 percent sodium bicarbonate manufactured and sent to France to treat patients. This proved to be impossible, unfortunately, because Burroughs's Wellcome Enterprise, the company charged with manufacturing the infusion, was unable to keep the gum dissolved in bicarbonate solution. It was not until 25 March 1918 that the Advisory Committee finally issued a memorandum that 6 percent Gum Arabica in 0.9 percent saline should be issued and sent to France forthwith. It was 104 days since they had learned of the value of treating shocked patients with Gum Arabica in saline, and almost two years since Bayliss's original experimental work. [13] Many lives had been lost which otherwise might have been saved. By that time, Cannon had been ordered back to France, which was probably just as well for him.

Colonel TR Elliott (1877-1961) RAMC was a clinician working with the Third Army. After Gum Arabica in 0.9 percent saline had finally been made available and was in clinical use, he and Captain Kenneth Walker reported back to the Advisory Committee in London, noting that it was quite effective if given to shocked men very soon after their admission to a casualty clearing station, but if its administration was delayed for eight to twelve hours, then blood transfusion was much better. Elliott eventually became Professor of Medicine at University College London, and Walker a distinguished urologist and the author of many books. Walker was working at Casualty Clearing Station No 3 at Gézaincourt, where Consulting Surgeon to the British Third Army, Henry Gray (Figure 6.8), had established a shock centre.

Shock Centre at CCS 3, Gézaincourt

Gray was a pioneering clinician who had great experience in dealing with patients suffering from wound shock. In 1915 while in charge of surgical activities of a group of base hospitals in Rouen, he and Australian surgeon Edward Milligan had pioneered wound excision (q.v.). As Consulting Surgeon to the British Third Army at Arras in 1917, he ensured that all compound fractures of the femur were immobilised effectively using Thomas Splints. Patients arrived in casualty clearing stations in good clinical condition and fit to undergo the necessary wound excision to save their limbs and their lives. The reader is referred to Chapter 7, which deals

13 Van Der Kloot, *William Maddock Bayliss's Therapy for Wound Shock.*

with developments in surgical specialties, to learn more about the history and use of the Thomas Splint in clinical practice.

While Gray had the necessary 'clout' to insist on the use of Thomas Splints, he was not the first person to try to use the device. As already stated, Alexander MacCormick (1856-1947) was born in Argyllshire, Scotland. He was a graduate of the University of Edinburgh and in 1883 he emigrated from Scotland to Sydney, Australia. On the outbreak of war in 1914 MacCormick returned to Britain and joined the Royal Army Medical Corps in November. As a colonel and consulting surgeon he served in France at a base hospital in Boulogne. He took with him a supply of Thomas knee splints and in vain urged their use by field ambulances.[14] Butler, the Official Historian of Australian Army Medical Services observed:

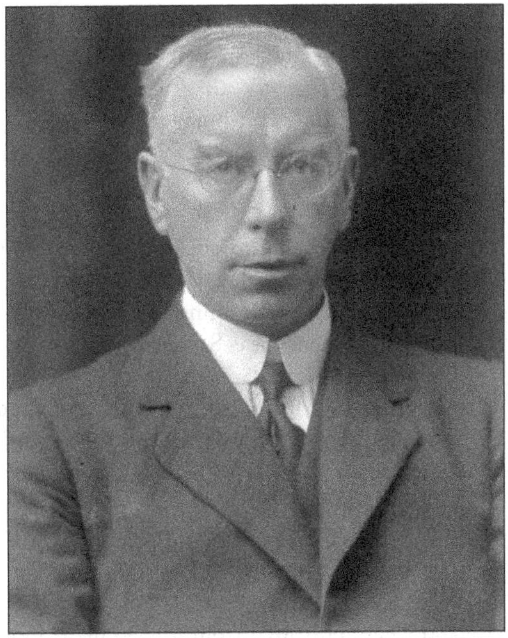

Figure 6.8 Henry Gray, Consulting Surgeon British Third Army; Gray was one of the first to describe wound excision in 1915; he was recognised as an outstanding orthopaedic military surgeon in France and opened a shock centre at CCS 3 at Gézaincourt in 1917. This photograph was taken in 1919. (Courtesy National Portrait Gallery, London)

> It is interesting to note that Sir Alexander MacCormick was one of the first, if not the first, to advocate strongly in the Great War the use of the Thomas knee splint for the transport of patients with fractures of the femur due to gunshot wounds. It is claimed that he actually bought and took across to France, early in 1915 the first Thomas knee splints used for transport purposes in this war.[15]

Nevertheless, MacCormick failed to persuade his colleagues to use the Thomas Splint and he left France for Lemnos in 1915 after being commissioned into the Royal Australian Army Medical Corps. Things got no better for him there since he wasn't given any operating to do and so he went home to Australia totally frustrated and demoralised, feeling that his skills as a surgeon had not been put to good use.

Gray's extensive experience with femoral fractures made him an obvious choice to be on the Advisory Committee and with the help of his enthusiastic young colleague Captain Kenneth Walker, he established a shock centre at CCS 3 at Gézaincourt. Gray paid full tribute to Walker's contributions in his book *The Early Treatment of War Wounds.*[16] Given that Gray had many other commitments as Consulting Surgeon to the Third Army, the day to day running

14 Miller, D., *MacCormick, A., (1856-1947),* Australian Dictionary of Biography, Vol. 10, 1986.

15 Butler, *Official History of the Australian Army Medical Services,* Vol. II, p. 349.

16 Gray, H.M.W., *The Early Treatment of War Wounds*, (London: Henry Frowde, Hodder and Stoughton, 1919), pp. 80-104.

of the shock centre was left very much in the hands of Captain Walker, who wrote most of the chapter on wound shock in Gray's book.

Kenneth Walker was an Anglo-Scot who originally planned to study medicine at the University of Edinburgh but was advised to go to Cambridge instead. Dr. George Ogilvie, a Scottish consultant working in London, suggested to him that he really ought to go to Cambridge:

> They are beginning to object in London to what they called the 'Celtic invasion', and a degree from Cambridge will carry more weight than one from Edinburgh. Mind you, I'm not saying that the training in Cambridge is any better than in Edinburgh, but it's more canny to humour these Sassenachs.[17]

Walker's undergraduate clinical years were spent at St Bartholomew's Hospital in London, where he met Sir Anthony Bowlby, who would become Consulting Surgeon to the BEF in 1914. He became Bowlby's junior house surgeon and then senior house surgeon. Walker greatly admired his chief:

> Anthony Bowlby was not only a good surgeon, but he was also a wise man, and would have made a name in any profession or business he had cared to take up. He became my model and I have borrowed from him so many movements, mannerisms, inflexions of the voice and methods of speech that I fear I should stand mute in my consulting room if by some magic all that I learned from Bowlby were suddenly to be removed.[18]

Following the outbreak of war, Walker went to France under the auspices of the Red Cross before becoming Temporary Captain Walker, RAMC. Thanks to the intervention of his patron, Sir Anthony Bowlby, Walker was spared a dull occupation at the base and spent a year working at an advanced operating centre in a château in the village of Habarcq near Arras, where he dealt with soldiers who were so badly wounded that they would not have survived a longer journey to casualty clearing stations. In 1916 he pulled strings and got a 'joy ride' in an aeroplane over the Somme battlefield. He managed to create a job for himself as an unofficial consultant to the front, which gave him a free hand to go where he liked and to where he felt he would be most useful. During the Battle of Arras in April/May 1917 he dealt with many of the wounded, demonstrating to regimental medical officers that a Thomas Splint could very easily and effectively be applied over battle clothing.

Around that time, the British 3rd Division to which he was attached, was withdrawn from the Arras sector and transferred to the Ypres Salient, whereupon a safe job at the base once again threatened to interfere with Walker's future. Walker needed a reason to stay at the front in his unofficial capacity as roving consultant. He desperately wanted to stay put and hit on the idea of studying wound shock as a way of doing so:

17 Walker, K., *I talk of dreams: An experiment in autobiography* (London: Jonathan Cape, 1946), p. 34.
18 Walker, *I talk of dreams*, p. 98.

> If I were to retain my unscheduled post of consultant to the front area, I must justify it by means of some new line of research. There were two new ideas worth considering, namely the study of the onset of wound shock and an examination of the possibility of protecting certain vital areas of the body by means of some form of light armour.[19]

Walker was summoned to a meeting in Grévillers, where Consulting Surgeon to the British Third Army, Henry Gray had called a meeting to discuss the subject of wound shock, with a view to establishing a shock centre. Gray had heard about Walker's activities at the front and was very impressed. Gray appointed him to be in charge of investigations into shock in the Third Army forward area. Walker would be given a laboratory at CCS 3 at Gézaincourt which he could use as his base. Otherwise he was free to go where he liked to conduct his clinical research. More will be said of this enterprising officer's activities at CCS 3 in Chapter 8.

The establishment of a shock centre in the autumn of 1917 allowed for the education and instruction of medical officers with little or no experience in the management of shock and for the dissemination of knowledge through conferences. Its functions can be summarised as follows:

- To co-ordinate work in the CCS with units in forward area and to foster co-operation;
- To collect reports from Medical Units of the Army;
- To test practicability and utility of remedial measures before general release;
- To provide materials (grouping sera etc) to units which would otherwise have difficulty obtaining them;
- To liaise closely with MRC Advisory Committee;
- To act as training centre for divisional officers from other units, making them familiar with methods of examination and treatment;
- To carry out scientific investigations as required with special laboratory equipment;
- To issue reports from time to time of the shock work done in the army.

The shock centre acted as a focal point for those interested in the subject and was an ideal place where well motivated clinicians could go to exchange ideas and learn from each other. One such person was Captain Oswald Hope Robertson (1886-1966) of the US Army, who had acquired much experience in blood transfusion. Another was Major Holmes à Court of the 4th Australian Field Ambulance, whose ground-breaking work following his visit to CCS 3 is discussed in Chapter 8.

Blood transfusion

The first transfusions for acute haemorrhage were carried out in 1818 by James Blundell, a London obstetrician who had seen women dying of post-partum bleeding. Four of the ten transfusions that he carried out were successful which is remarkable given that he didn't understand the presence of different blood groups or how to stop blood clotting on its route from one person to another.

19 Walker, *I talk of dreams*, p.190.

While blood transfusions were very occasionally performed in the 19th century, bleeding or blood-letting, where blood was removed from a wounded soldier with the intention of removing 'bad blood', was standard practice for any wound in the first half of the century, only gradually becoming less popular as the years progressed.

In the early 20th century, Landsteiner described the four blood groups which went on to become groups A, B, AB and O. It is very important to test donors and recipients for blood group compatibility, otherwise transfusion reactions may occur. The most frequent reactions are fever, chills, severe itch, or urticaria (also known as hives or weals), which typically resolve without specific treatment or complications. Other adverse clinical features associated with a blood transfusion, such as severe shortness of breath, red urine, high fever, or loss of consciousness may be the first indication of a more severe and potentially fatal reaction. Red urine appears because the recipient's plasma may contain an agglutinin causing the red blood cells of the donor to cling together in clumps which then fall to pieces, releasing haemoglobin which turns the urine red and causes serious kidney damage when it is excreted. During the war, blood tests for checking the compatibility of donor and recipient were sometimes not performed for reasons which will be explained. Table 6.2 is a simplified summary of the blood groups and their transfusion compatibility.

Table 6.2 Transfusion compatibility of the four blood groups

		Recipient serum or plasma			
		O	A	B	AB
Donor red blood corpuscles	O	–	–	–	–
	A	+	–	+	–
	B	+	+	–	–
	AB	+	+	+	–

+ = Agglutination
- = No Agglutination

Walker, K., *The Story of Blood*, (London: Herbert Jenkins Ltd., 1958), p. 153.

From the table it can be determined that blood corpuscles from any group on the vertical column can be injected into veins of a member of the AB group without causing reaction in the recipient's serum. Individuals who are of the group AB are therefore called universal recipients. Moreover, from Figure 6.2, corpuscles of the Group O can be injected into the serum of any recipient without causing agglutination. Individuals belonging to Group O are therefore called universal donors. This means that Group O blood can be transfused into patients of any blood group without causing serious transfusion reactions.[20] This was of great practical value during the war, because by using Group O donor blood, there was no need for cross-matching and much time was saved.

20 Walker, K., *The Story of Blood*, (London: Herbert Jenkins, 1958), pp. 152-53.

George Washington Crile (1864-1943) is credited with carrying out direct blood transfusions some years before the Great War by connecting an artery in a donor's wrist to a vein on the inside of a recipient's elbow. Procedures were carried out without cross matching or anti-coagulation to stop the blood clotting. By using a very short tube to connect the two he managed to overlap the two vessels and thus prevent clotting.[21]

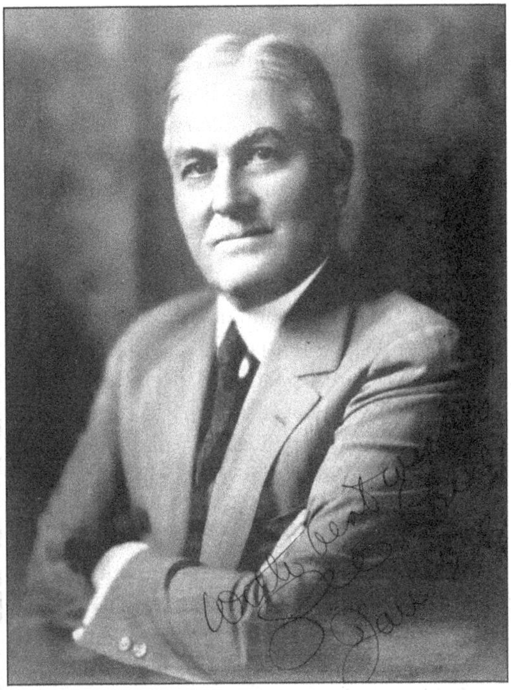

Figure 6.9 George Washington Crile (1864-1943) was the first to carry out direct blood transfusion before the war by connecting an artery in the donor's wrist to a vein on the inside of the recipient's elbow. (Courtesy Wellcome Library, London)

Crile was Professor of Surgery at Cleveland, Ohio. He went to France with the 4th American Base Hospital, the Cleveland Unit, in 1917. Crile had a long-standing interest in shock, having proposed the kinetic theory of shock some years before the war. He believed that the brain became bombarded with stimuli from a wound or from an operation or as a result of fear. He proposed that the continuation of such stimulation led to exhaustion of the part of the brain that controls the peripheral blood vessels (vasomotor centre) with subsequent dilatation of vessels and a fall in blood pressure. He advocated that painful stimuli should be abolished by an injection of local anaesthetic and that nitrous oxide be given to eliminate fear. He called this technique anoci-association.

Lawrence Bruce Robertson (1885-1923)

Blood transfusion during the Great War was first reported by a Canadian Medical Officer called Lawrence Bruce Robertson, who graduated in medicine from the University of Toronto in 1909. He trained for a year and a half in paediatric and orthopaedic surgery at Bellevue Hospital in New York City before spending six months as a house surgeon at the Children's Hospital in Boston. In 1913 he returned to Toronto as an assistant in both clinical surgery and pathology at the Sick Children's Hospital and as a demonstrator in clinical surgery at the University of Toronto.[22]

During his time in New York, Robertson learned about indirect blood transfusion, employing a sterile syringe and cannula to extract blood from a donor and inject it into a recipient. The

21 Robertson, A., in *War Surgery 1914-18*, p. 108.

22 Lawrence Bruce Robertson, Dictionary of Canadian Biography <http://www.biographi.ca/en/bio/robertson_lawrence_bruce_15E.html>.

syringe was coated with liquid paraffin to prevent clotting. Following the outbreak of war, he became a medical officer with the Canadian Expeditionary Force and pioneered this procedure in warfare at Number 14 Canadian General Hospital in the autumn of 1915. Donors were selected from soldiers who had sustained minor wounds. Robertson treated four patients suffering from secondary haemorrhage, a dangerous, potentially life-threatening condition where infection had eroded into large blood vessels causing major bleeding. Robertson did not check his patients and donors for blood group compatibility. His reason for not doing so was because he maintained these cases were so urgent that there was no time, since death was imminent. The seriousness of the bleeding outweighed any risks associated with blood group incompatibility. Two patients survived who would probably not have done so without blood transfusion. One died of septicaemia and one died of acute haemolysis due to a major transfusion reaction.[23]

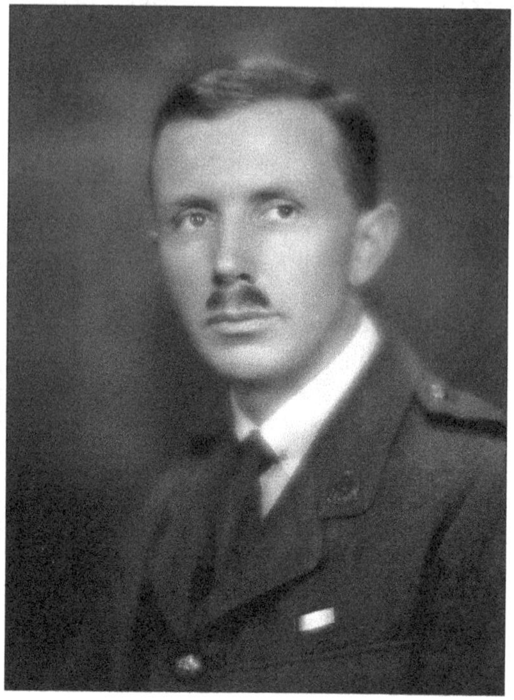

Figure 6.10 Lawrence Bruce Robertson (1885-1923) was a Canadian Medical Officer who pioneered blood transfusion in France, both in a base hospital (1916) and a casualty clearing station (1917). He employed a syringe-cannula method using uncross-matched blood. (Courtesy Archives of Ontario)

In 1917, Roberson was posted to Canadian Casualty Clearing Station 2 at Remy Siding near Poperinghe, where he was stationed during the Third Battle of Ypres and where he performed blood transfusions on recently wounded soldiers in severe shock using the syringe-cannula technique.[24] The amount of blood transfused was 700-1,000cc, a small volume by present day transfusion standards. Nevertheless, many patients in a state of circulatory collapse improved dramatically following transfusion. Robertson reported on the results of transfusion in 36 severely wounded patients in surgical shock, who in his opinion would not have survived without being given blood. His results are shown in Table 6.3. Once again, Robertson used uncrossmatched blood and two patients died as a result of severe transfusion reactions.

23 Robertson, L. Bruce, The transfusion of whole blood, *British Medical Journal*, 2: 2897 (8 July 1916), pp. 38-40.

24 Robertson L.B., Gordon Watson, C., Further observations on the results of blood transfusion in war surgery, *British Medical Journal*, 2:2969 (24 November 1917), pp. 679-83.

Table 6.3 Results of Lawrence Bruce Robertson's 36 transfusions in cases of primary haemorrhage

Effects of transfusion	No. of casualties
Life saving (evacuated to base hospital in good condition)	22
Immediately beneficial but died from infection or operation:	9
No benefit	3
Harmful (haemolysis)	2

Robertson, L.B., Gordon Watson, C., Further observations on the results of blood transfusion in war surgery, *British Medical Journal* 2: 2969 (November 24, 1917), pp. 679-83.

Consulting surgeon Colonel Gordon H Watson added a note to Robertson's publication. He was in no doubt that blood transfusion had saved the lives of those soldiers in the series who had survived. Watson justified the use of uncrossmatched blood by writing:

> Precautions should be taken when the circumstances of the case permit. At the front, particularly during the periods of heavy fighting, time does not permit of tests to eliminate syphilitic taint, nor, indeed, to ascertain if the blood of the donor is incompatible with that of the patient. Such risk as there is must be run if the urgent need of the patient is to be met promptly.[25]

While lives were undoubtedly saved by these transfusions, it should not be forgotten that two soldiers died from severe reactions as a result of blood group incompatibility. Robertson balanced this against the probable death of all patients had transfusion not been immediately performed. Henry Gray, on the other hand, maintained that blood transfusion should not be undertaken without first establishing the blood groups to which the donor and recipient belonged.[26]

In summary, Lawrence Bruce Robertson's notable contribution to medical science demonstrated the value of blood transfusion as a therapeutic measure for combating shock secondary to blood loss and established its importance in resuscitation. His pioneering work resulted in the more widespread use of blood transfusion in the management of severely wounded men:

> During the first two years of the war, transfusion was only performed by a few especially experienced surgeons, and was regarded more as an interesting curiosity than as a practical measure in the treatment of shock. It is only in the last two years that it has been adopted as a recognised part of the treatment of a severely wounded man.[27]

Oswald Hope Robertson (1886-1966)

The limitations of indirect blood transfusion employed by Lawrence Bruce Robertson in a war zone became more problematic the further forward transfusion was likely to be administered.

25 Robertson, L.B., *British Medical Journal* 1917, pp. 679-83.
26 Gray, *The Early Treatment of War Wounds*, p. 94.
27 Gray, *The Early Treatment of War Wounds*, p. 93.

If blood could be made available in bottles like saline, transfusions could be given more easily in field ambulances or even closer to the front line. Preserved blood provided this opportunity. United States Army clinician Oswald Hope Robertson developed and tested this at British Third Army Clearing Stations in 1917.

Robertson was born in London and emigrated from England to America with his parents when he was a year and a half old. He went to France with the 5th American Base Hospital (Harvard Unit) in May 1917. His work on blood transfusion during the war was of enormous importance, since it enabled blood to be stored, ready to be transfused with minimal delay into badly wounded soldiers. It was Oswald Hope Robertson who established the first blood bank in France. Blood transfusion was employed increasingly during the latter part of 1917 and 1918 and was evaluated by the Advisory Committee on Surgical Shock when the latter came into being.

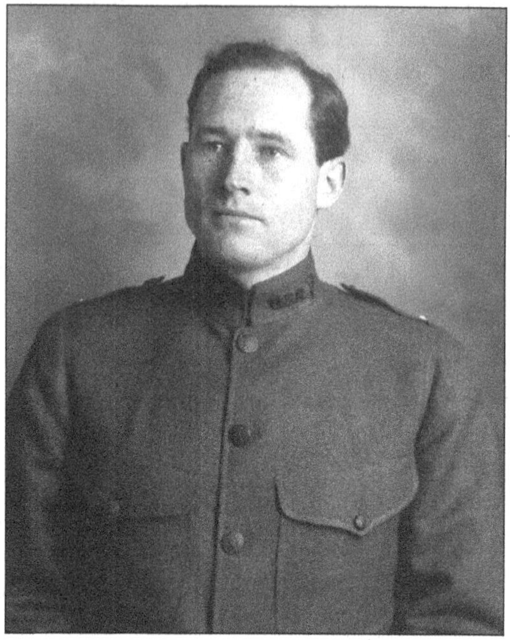

Figure 6.11 Oswald Hope Robertson (1886-1966) M.O.R.C., USA. (Courtesy Rockefeller Archives Centre)

Robertson employed blood from group O donors, which could be transfused into badly wounded soldiers of any blood group without risk of transfusion reactions. The technique used by Robertson to collect blood was first to prepare a preserving solution of 350cc of isotonic sodium citrate solution, which is an anticoagulant to stop the blood clotting and 850cc of isotonic dextrose to provide nutrition for the red blood cells. Both were autoclaved separately before mixing them in a sterile Winchester bottle which was used as the collecting bottle for blood. Blood was removed from the donor using a hollow needle inserted into a vein in the antecubital space and connected by sterile rubber tubing to the sterile collecting bottle. A tourniquet was applied to the donor's arm above the elbow and inflated to 60 mm Hg to allow 500 cc of blood to flow freely into the collecting bottle. An ice box was essential for storing the blood. The red blood cells gradually settled to the bottom over the course of a few days, leaving a supernatant fluid. When blood was prepared for transfusion, the supernatant fluid was drawn off by means of a siphon apparatus. Once all the supernatant had been removed, a 2.5 percent solution of gelatine in normal saline was added to bring the volume up to 1,000cc. The blood cell suspension was then gently agitated and poured through two layers of sterile gauze into a transfusion bottle sterilised by autoclaving.

It can be appreciated from the above description that the preparation of preserved blood involved many steps which depended on absolute sterility to prevent harmful bacteria gaining access and causing devastating infections in recipients. Blood could be stored for up to 26 days, although most was transfused within ten days to a fortnight. Robertson targeted soldiers who would probably have died without a transfusion and yet had a chance of recovery if given blood.

If venous access proved difficult in a shocked patient with collapsed veins, then a cut down procedure was performed to identify a suitable vein and insert the needle under direct vision. Much of Robertson's work was undertaken at the shock centre at CCS 3, Gézaincourt.

In November 1917, during the Battle of Cambrai, Robertson made an ice chest from two ammunition cases and used blood stored in them to resuscitate Canadian soldiers who were too shocked for immediate surgery.[28] He reported the results of 22 transfusions given to twenty patients. Eleven were discharged to the base recovering and nine died, representing a mortality of 45 percent. One patient with profound anaemia died just after being transfused and four died of gas gangrene within 48 hours. The remaining four died of gas gangrene after intervals ranging between two and six days. Without transfusion, all patients would have died. The length of time the blood had been stored appeared to have had no impact on its beneficial effect. [29]

The major advantage of preserved blood was to have large quantities immediately available for transfusion during a busy spell. Soon after one particular engagement began, twenty pints of preserved blood were used for fourteen transfusions. It would have been difficult to obtain fresh blood, because there was a scarcity of suitable donors. Disproportionately large numbers of early admissions to the casualty clearing station had sustained major wounds and were not suitable donors. Preserved Group O blood was administered and since no compatibility blood tests were required, some time was saved. Robertson maintained that during battles when great numbers of wounded were being dealt with, early transfusion using fresh blood would have been impossible, except during lulls.[30]

He reported that it was perfectly feasible to transport blood for six to eight miles over rough roads in an ambulance wagon without damaging the red cells, provided it was kept cold in an ice box. The main disadvantage of this method was the accidental introduction of bacteria leading to infection in the recipient as a result of the multiple steps involved in the preparation of the preserved blood and the practical difficulties of keeping it cold, particularly close to the front line.[31]

Citrated blood

There was a further method of blood preparation developed by Robertson in 1917 which involved its withdrawal from a donor and direct transference into a vessel containing an isotonic solution of sodium citrate to prevent clotting. It was particularly useful because blood could be collected beforehand and kept for up to two hours before use. It did not involve the many steps required

28 Blair, J.S.G., Captain Oswald Hope Robertson, *Journal Royal Army Medical Corps*, 150:4 (1 December 2004), pp. 291-92.
29 Robertson, O.H., Transfusion with preserved red blood cells, *British Medical Journal* 1: 2999 (22 June 1918), pp. 691-95.
30 Robertson, O.H., *British Medical Journal 1918*, pp. 691-95.
31 Westhorpe, R., The introduction of a mobile resuscitation service-1918, in Fink, B.R., LE Morris L.E., & Stephen, C.R. (eds.), *The History of Anaesthesia: Third International Symposium*, (Illinois: Wood Library, Museum of Anaesthesiology, 1992), pp. 438-39.

in the preparation of preserved blood and was a method favoured by personnel of the Australian Field Ambulance Resuscitation Teams in 1918 (Chapter 8).[32]

Henry Gray certainly appreciated the value of blood transfusion, but he issued a cautionary warning about its use too close to the front line:

> Although early transfusion is a valuable asset when it is feasible, it must always merely supplement, and never replace, sound general treatment. To transfuse a man in a forward dressing station, and then send him down with a shattered limb on which a tourniquet is applied, is unsound treatment, since it leaves unremedied the chief cause of his shock. The limb must be amputated, and the tourniquet removed.[33]

Captain Norman Guiou of the Canadian Army Medical Corps had experience of grouping and transfusing patients in advanced dressing stations. He described the transfusion of a particular patient admitted to an advanced dressing station with a compound gunshot fracture of the femur with a tourniquet applied to control severe bleeding. Guiou attempted to resuscitate the patient with 5 percent Gum Arabica and sodium bicarbonate. The wounded man was blood group O and a lightly wounded soldier offered to donate blood. On testing the volunteer, however, his blood group was incompatible. Another donor was sought and this time a lightly wounded corporal volunteered who had the same blood group as the seriously wounded man. A pint of blood was withdrawn from the donor and transfused using the syringe cannula technique. The patient's condition improved briefly, and he was put in an ambulance wagon and sent to the casualty clearing station. He deteriorated and died before he got there. In retrospect, Guiou wondered if the man might have survived if he had been given more blood and warmed up for longer before being sent back.[34]

Gray would almost certainly have disapproved of the way this patient had been managed. Much valuable time had been lost finding a suitable donor and definitive surgical management was delayed while the patient remained cold and in a shocked state. The wounded man should have been put in a heated ambulance wagon straight away and transported to the casualty clearing station as quickly as possible, where further resuscitative measures could have been initiated, including blood transfusion. If he had responded sufficiently, then rapid and definitive surgery using safe anaesthesia (see below) might just have saved his life.

When was it safe to operate on a shocked patient?

The question of when exactly to operate on a patient suffering from the effects of shock was a very difficult one and a balance had to be struck. On the one hand, if an anaesthetic was administered to a severely shocked patient with a very low blood pressure, the chances of the wounded man surviving the anaesthetic never mind the operative procedure were negligible. On the other

32 Holmes à Court, A., Intravenous injections in the treatment of haemorrhage and shock, *The Medical Journal of Australia,* Vol. II, No. 2, (July 10, 1920), pp. 25-30.

33 Gray, *The Early Treatment of War Wounds*, p. 100.

34 Guiou, N.M., Blood transfusion in a field ambulance, *British Medical Journal* 1: 2999 (22 June 1918), pp. 695-696.

hand, if too much time was spent resuscitating the patient to make his clinical condition as good as possible, then the inevitable delay enabled infecting organisms to become established and to 'gain the upper hand.' Operative intervention should not be postponed for any longer than absolutely necessary. Gray subsequently observed:

> A blood pressure of 85 or over will generally allow a previously shocked patient to face an anaesthetic and an operation, provided the anaesthetic is suitable and the operation a rapid one. In performing the operation, two aims should be kept in view: the first, rapidity, and the second, completeness in dealing with sepsis. When the ultimate saving of a limb is of doubtful achievement it should be sacrificed without hesitation. The patient must be left with the minimum possibility of septic absorption, for the danger that lies in front of him is death from the toxaemia of sepsis.[35]

Geoffrey Marshall's work at Remy Siding in 1915 demonstrated that the only safe anaesthetic in a severely shocked patient was nitrous oxide and oxygen. A successful outcome was achieved by a rapid and definitive operative procedure which minimised the risk of sepsis overwhelming the wounded man and resulting in his death. It is noteworthy that in Oswald Hope Robertson's series of patients, eight of the nine deaths were due to gas gangrene, clear examples of infection gaining the upper hand.

35 Gray, *The Early Treatment of War Wounds*, p. 101.

7

Life saving advances in surgery 1914-18

The single most important advance in the surgical management of wounds during the Great War was wound excision, which involves the early removal of all devitalised tissue and foreign material from filthy, contaminated wounds and their conversion into macroscopically clean ones. First described by Henry Gray and Edward Milligan in 1915 (Chapter 4), wound excision was applied to different types of wound, with the aim of reducing the incidence of major infection and its associated high percentage mortality. It was applicable to wounds of the musculoskeletal system and also underpinned the management of wounds of the skull and brain, the chest wall and the thoracic cavity, although direct damage to vital structures often dictated whether the patient lived or died. The Great War was the first conflict in which perforating wounds of the abdomen were submitted to surgery with some success. Expectant treatment had been the order of the day in the opening months of the conflict, as it had been in the Second Boer War, but the mortality was so high that in 1915 a determined effort was made to perform early surgery on these wounds.

By referring to the medical literature, this chapter sets out to show that soldiers sustaining specific wounds in 1918 had a much better chance of surviving them than those with similar wounds in 1914. Improved results were attributable to a number of factors including better surgery, better anaesthesia and a better understanding of shock and how to combat it. The importance of blood transfusion discussed in the previous chapter cannot be overestimated. There were so many casualties that the Great War was a catalyst for many surgical developments. Throughout the 19th century, wounds of the musculoskeletal system were responsible for most of the surgeon's workload. In the absence of anaesthesia in the first half of that century, wounds of the arms and legs were readily accessible and could be dealt with very quickly, often by amputation. Wounds of the chest and abdomen were not considered part of the surgeon's remit. It would have been impossible, for example, to perform an operation to open up the abdominal cavity (laparotomy) and deal with a perforated segment of bowel without employing anaesthesia. Even when general anaesthetic agents became available by the time of the Crimean War, nothing really changed. Wounds of the chest and abdomen were still not dealt with surgically and wounds of the musculoskeletal system remained the principal concern of the surgeon. By the end of the century, abdominal operations were occasionally performed during the Second Boer War by a few enterprising individuals but these procedures were generally discouraged because of the mistaken belief that patients with abdominal wounds were more likely to survive if left well alone. In contrast, head wounds were managed very aggressively during the Second

Boer War. It was noted that while most soldiers shot through the head from a short distance were killed or died within a few hours, those hit from longer range had a greater chance of survival. Many in the latter group had skull fractures with depressed bone fragments and were frequently neurologically intact without any obvious underlying brain damage. These wounded men underwent very invasive surgery to elevate the bone fragments to relieve pressure on the underlying brain.[1] Good results for operative intervention were claimed, although given the relatively uncontaminated nature of the wounds in South Africa it is very likely that many or perhaps most of these cases would have done just as well without such extensive procedures.

Penetrating wounds of the skull and brain during the Great War

Gordon Holmes and Percy Sargent

In 1914, two clinicians from the National Hospital for Nervous Diseases in London called Gordon Holmes and Percy Sargent opened a neurological unit in General Hospital 13, which was housed in a converted casino in Boulogne. Gordon Holmes (1876-1965) was an Irish neurologist who graduated in medicine from Trinity College, Dublin in 1899. Following the outbreak of war he volunteered for overseas service but he was turned down initially because of poor eyesight. Frustrated and disappointed by his rejection, he joined the staff of a Red Cross hospital just behind the front line in France where his impressive work persuaded the War Office to renegotiate his disqualification.[2] Holmes is credited with the standard neurological examination and in the absence of sophisticated methods of investigating patients with neurological disturbances which are available to clinicians today, an accurate clinical examination was very important to establish the extent and severity of a brain injury pre-operatively and to detect the onset of complications post-operatively. Holmes also did a great deal of very useful clinical research involving the study of wounds affecting the visual cortex of the brain and the cerebellum. From late 1915, British soldiers wore the Brodie pattern steel helmet, which did not provide any protection for those parts of the brain because it was deficient at the back. The German M16 stalhelm, in contrast,

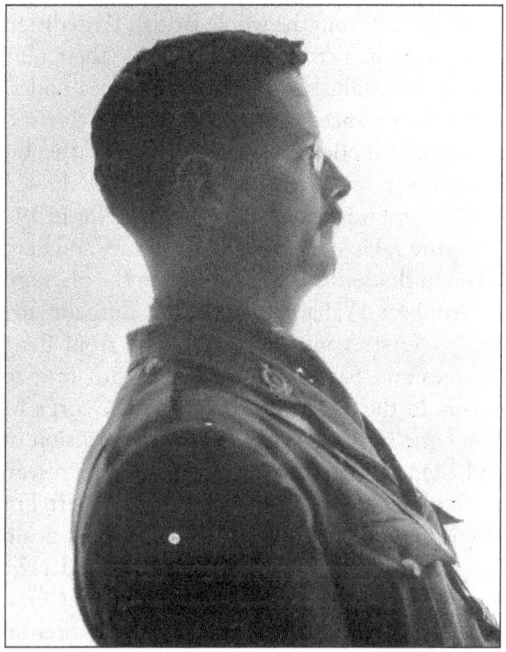

Figure 7.1 Gordon Holmes (1876-1965). (Courtesy Wellcome Library, London)

1 Stevenson, W.F., Surgical Experiences from the Boer War, *Journal Royal Army Medical Corps*, Vol. 1, No.2, (1 August 1903), pp. 89-95.

2 Pearce, J.M.S., *Historical Note Sir Gordon Holmes* <j.com/content/75/10/1502>.

protected the entire brain by its design. Holmes was awarded the CMG in 1917, the CBE in 1919 and was knighted in 1951.

Percy Sargent (1873-1933) was surgeon to the National Hospital for Nervous Diseases in London. Following the outbreak of war, he was gazetted Captain in the Royal Army Medical Corps and went to France. His qualities as a specialist were quickly seized upon, and with the rank of Temporary Honorary Lieutenant-Colonel from 13 December 1914, he was directed to form a small neurological unit in Boulogne with Gordon Holmes, to which all difficult neurological cases could be sent from the whole British Expeditionary Force area in France and Flanders. Their clinical work was invaluable to their colleagues and their research advanced knowledge about the localization of function in certain areas of the brain. Sargent was awarded the DSO in 1917, the CMG in 1919 and was made a Knight Bachelor in 1928.[3]

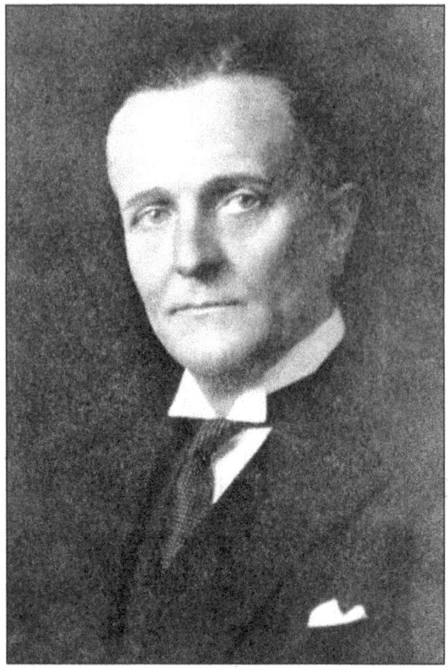

Figure 7.2 Percy Sargent (1873-1933). (Courtesy Wellcome Library, London)

Figure 7.3 is a photograph of Holmes and Sargent taken in Boulogne in 1915. Also, in the photograph is Cuthbert Wallace, Consulting Surgeon to the British First Army, who had come from his base near Bethune in northern France to visit Holmes and Sargent in their specialist unit to assess the work they were doing. The fourth person in the photograph is surgeon George Makins, who spent a short time with Sargent in Boulogne before taking over the supervision of newly established hospital centres at Camiers and Étaples. At Étaples, he established a research centre, where trials were carried out on new methods of wound treatment. Makins left France in July 1917 and became President of the Royal College of Surgeons of England, a position he held until 1920. Makins was awarded a knighthood in 1918[4] and Wallace received a similar award in 1919.

Holmes and Sargent developed a regime for the surgical management of penetrating wounds of the skull and brain and published a preliminary report in the British Medical Journal in 1915.[5] They documented that when a bullet or fragment of shell casing penetrates the skull, it fractures the skull with variable bone loss and displacement before lacerating the thick protective membrane beneath called the dura mater which covers the brain. The missile carries contaminated debris and battlefield filth into the wound and damages the brain beneath, causing the brain to swell up. This brain swelling is called cerebral oedema. Because the brain is confined

3 Sargent, Sir Percy William George, *Plarr's Lives of the Fellows Online*, Royal College of Surgeons, <https://livesonline.rcseng.ac.uk/biogs/E004573b.htm>.

4 Makins, Sir George Henry, *Plarr's Lives of the Fellows Online, Royal College of Surgeons*, <https://livesonline.rcseng.ac.uk/biogs/E000223b.htm>.

5 Sargent, P., Holmes, G., Preliminary notes on the treatment of the cranial injuries of warfare, *British Medical Journal*, 1:2830 (27 March 1915), pp. 537-41.

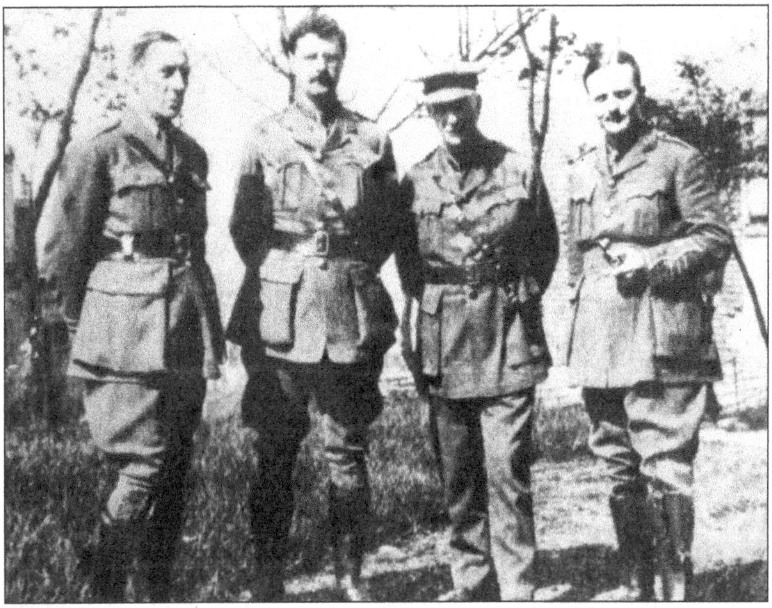

Figure 7.3 Photograph taken in Boulogne in 1915; left to right George Makins, Gordon Holmes, Cuthbert Wallace and Percy Sargent. (Courtesy Wolters Kluwer/ Lippincott, Williams & Wilkins)

within a rigid box of bone, its volume cannot increase and consequently the pressure within the swollen brain increases with the result that brain tissue immediately beneath and adjacent to the defect in the skull is squeezed out through the hole like toothpaste. Because the hole is usually small, the extruded brain is compressed against the sides of the hole and is strangulated. This is called a fungus cerebri and many patients admitted to the neurological unit in Boulogne had a fungus cerebri at presentation (Figure 7.4).

Sometimes when the wounded man arrived in Boulogne, he had already undergone surgery at a main dressing station or a casualty clearing station. The operation had been performed by a clinician not accustomed to dealing with head injuries but who felt he ought to try to do something. Often an inexperienced surgeon made too small an opening through the skull (craniotomy), which only made matters worse as it served as a further defect through which a fungus cerebri could squeeze. As more and more brain tissue was extruded through the limited defect in the skull, parts of the brain not damaged by the initial wound suffered secondary destruction, resulting in the death of the patient (Figure 7.5).

The regime developed by Sargent and Holmes saved lives but required a very extensive operation by a bold and experienced clinician to remove a sufficiently large amount of the skull to successfully decompress the brain beneath and prevent secondary brain damage from a fungus cerebri. Once Sargent had made big enough holes in the skull and in the dura mater beneath, the patient's brain, or what was left of it, was safe from further secondary damage. While the brain might still protrude, it now did so uniformly through a large defect in the dura and skull, with no risk of strangulation. This is called a hernia cerebri and Sargent and Holmes were careful to distinguish it from a fungus cerebri. Here is a summary of Sargent's operative procedure:

- The surgical aim is to comprehensively decompress the brain, limiting the brain damage and removing devitalised contaminated tissue (wound excision).

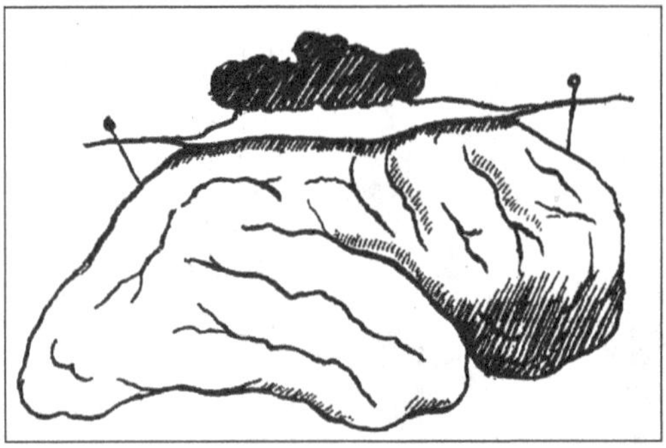

Figure 7.4 This diagram shows a fungus cerebri. (From Sargent, P., Holmes, G., Preliminary notes on the treatment of the cranial injuries of warfare, *British Medical Journal*, 1:2830 (27 March 1915), pp. 537-41)

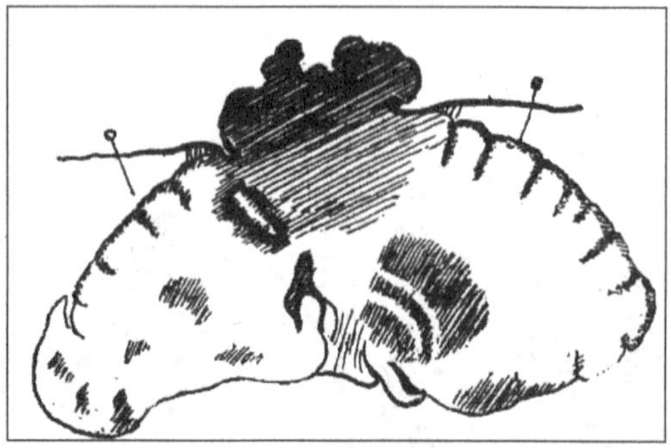

Figure 7.5 This diagram shows secondary destructive effects resulting from a fungus cerebri. (From Sargent, P., Holmes, G., Preliminary notes on the treatment of the cranial injuries of warfare, *British Medical Journal*, 1:2830 (27 March 1915), pp. 537-41)

- A big enough scalp flap must be used to permit the widest craniectomy required to decompress the brain.
- As much bone as needed is resected to permit as wide excision of dura mater as required, both of which are necessary to adequately decompress the brain.
- Necrotic contaminated brain is removed as part of wound excision.
- Foreign bodies are removed when safe to do so.
- Closure of the skin wound is sometimes difficult; it is essential to cover brain tissue. Sometimes Sargent used a dural flap and sometimes a pericranial flap (flap made from lining membrane or periosteum of the skull bone) to cover brain tissue, leaving part of scalp flap open. This does not matter provided the part of the scalp flap left open does not overlie exposed brain tissue.
- That part of the scalp flap left open heals up spontaneously by secondary intention after two to three weeks.

In September 1916, Sargent and Holmes reported on the late outcome of 610 patients who returned to Britain and who had sufficiently detailed case records to make worthwhile outcome[6] observations:

- Many patients returned to Britain with scalp wounds still open, but these quickly healed up.
- 6 percent of patients suffered from fits; they had all sustained severe compound fractures with much damage to the dura.
- 120 patients had a cerebral hernia and 24 percent of them died.
- Sargent and Holmes concluded that the operative procedures they had developed in France to deal with penetrating wounds of the skull and brain had been adequate.

6 Sargent, P., Holmes, G., Report on the later results of gunshot wounds of the head, *Journal of the Royal Army Medical Corps*, Volume 27, No. 3 (September 1916), pp. 300-11.

- Efforts should be made to avoid cerebral hernia if possible. (This would have been easier said than done).
- Sargent and Holmes noted that late improvements could occur.
- Cases of serious mental disturbances or insanity necessitating confinement were very rare.

Harvey Cushing (1869-1939)

On 30 May 1917, American Base Hospital Number 5 (the Harvard Unit) arrived in France. The United States of America had declared war against Germany on 6 April 1917 after the re-introduction of unrestricted submarine warfare by Germany which began on 1 February and resulted in the sinking of American merchant ships and the loss of American lives. With American Base Hospital 5 came Harvey Cushing.

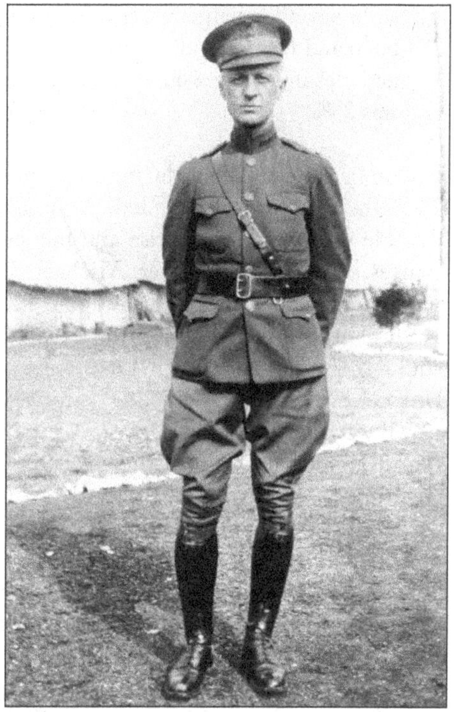

Figure 7.6 Harvey Cushing (1869-1939). (Courtesy of Cushing/Whitney Medical Historical Library)

Harvey Cushing studied medicine at Harvard University and graduated in 1895. He did his internship at the Massachusetts General Hospital before doing a surgical residency at the John Hopkins Hospital in Baltimore, where he became associate Professor of Surgery and specialised in surgery of the central nervous system. He became Professor of Surgery at Harvard in 1912, by which time he was established as his country's leading neurosurgeon. Cushing first went to France in 1915 when he headed the Harvard Unit at the *Ambulance Américaine* in Paris. In May 1917 he worked with the British Expeditionary Force because it would be more than a year before American soldiers reached France in significant numbers. Cushing could be petty and arrogant and was very difficult to work alongside. He was a 'prima donna', and as America's leading neurosurgeon, he expected the British to provide him with 'red carpet treatment'. Instead, the Harvard Unit was allocated British General Hospital Number 11, which was a soggy rat-infested tented hospital at Camiers, just north of Étaples. A staffing level planned for 500 patients ended up looking after as many as 1,800 casualties. Cushing was absolutely disgusted. He complained bitterly about the facilities and the conditions. Most of all he complained about his hosts: "I am driven to distraction by the British dilatoriness, the everlasting stopping for meals. Someone is eating all day long."[7]

On 7 June 1917, the British Second Army attacked and captured the Messines Ridge south of Ypres. This was a necessary preliminary step before the Third Battle of Ypres which began on

7 Bliss, M., *Harvey Cushing: A Life in Surgery* (Oxford: Oxford University Press, 2005), p. 324.

31 July. Cushing assisted in the management of head cases, which were dealt with at the New Zealand Stationary Hospital in Hazebrouck. Three teams of surgeons in two operating theatres worked in shifts:

> The majority of cases had compound fractures of the skull without dural penetration. X-rays were used in all cases. The operative methods adopted consisted in: excision of the scalp wound, enlargement of the opening in the skull, removal of depressed fragments of bone and foreign bodies where accessible; arrest of haemorrhage, the application of BIP and closure of the wound without drainage. The immediate mortality of the head cases was 25%.[8]

It soon became apparent during this time that Cushing was a very slow operator- far too slow, given the numbers of wounded. At home, he was accustomed to doing one major head case a day. He was really too precise and meticulous to be operating on patients under such circumstances. A recent biographer, Michael Bliss, said this of him: "Harvey Cushing doing brain surgery at a casualty clearing station is like a master chef working at McDonalds."[9]

Sir Anthony Bowlby, Senior British Consulting Surgeon wondered what he could do about this and spoke with Dr George Crile from American Base Hospital 4 (Cleveland Unit). Crile was a friend of Cushing's who happened to be in the vicinity. He advised Bowlby to allow Cushing to carry on and act as a model for perfect surgery and let others round about him handle the overflow and basically do most of the work. For his part, Cushing was determined to increase the number of major cases he did to eight a day. On 31 July 1917, the opening day of the Third Battle of Ypres, Cushing played a major role in delivery of of neurosurgical services for the British Fifth Army. All head cases were done at Casualty Clearing Stations 12, 46 and 64 at Mendinghem (Figure 7.7), which were much closer to the front and therefore reached much more quickly than base hospitals in Boulogne or Camiers. Cushing himself worked at CCS 46:

> Operating from 8.30 am one day till 2.00am the next; standing in a pair of rubber boots, and periodically full of tea as a stimulant, is not healthy. It's an awful business, probably the worst possible training in surgery for a young man and ruinous for the carefully acquired technique of an oldster. Finished up an hour ago with an extraction of a large piece of shell from a man's badly infected ventricle with a magnet. A lot of wounded must have drowned in the mud.[10]

Despite the many hardships, Cushing successfully increased the number of cases he did per day and modified his surgical technique as he went.[11]

8 Carberry, A.D., *The New Zealand Medical Services in the Great War based on official documents.* (Auckland: Whitcombe and Tombs Ltd., 1924), p. 304.
9 Bliss, *Harvey Cushing*, p. 314.
10 Bliss, *Harvey Cushing*, p. 323.
11 Cushing, H., Notes on penetrating wounds of the brain, *British Medical Journal*, 1:2982 (23 February 1918), pp. 221-26.

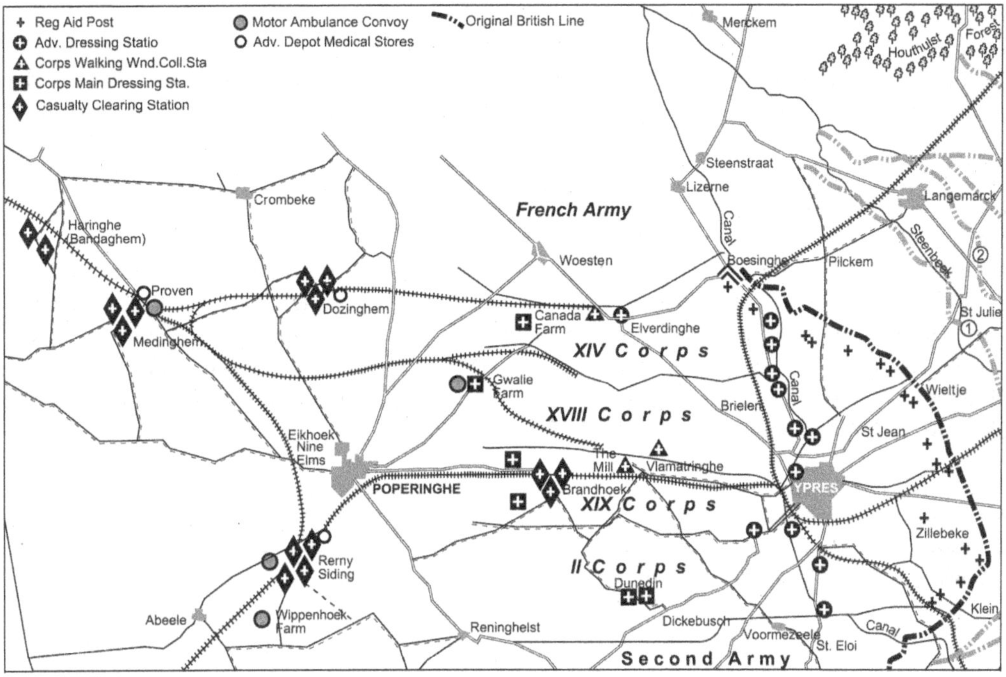

Figure 7.7 The reader's attention is drawn to the three Casualty Clearing Stations at Mendinghem. They were numbers 12, 46 and 64 and dealt with all serious wounds affecting the skull and brain. (Macpherson, W.G., *History of the Great War based on official documents Medical Services General History Vol. III*, London: His Majesty's Stationery Office, 1924, p. 138)

- He employed local rather than general anaesthesia (see below).
- He used a tripod incision which was easier to close over the brain (Figure 7.8).
- He removed the cranial area to be removed en bloc, making excision of devitalised tissue more complete. This involved making a series of interconnected holes in the skull adjacent to the defect caused by the missile and joining them up, then lifting away the entire bone flap.
- Necrotic brain was removed using a suction catheter. Cushing declared: 'We must recognise that the surgical profession contains its little Jack Horners and it is better, on the whole, for us all to keep our fingers out of the brain for so far as is possible'.
- He used a magnet to remove metallic foreign bodies when possible.
- He employed an antiseptic, Dichloramine T, once the surgical procedure was complete.

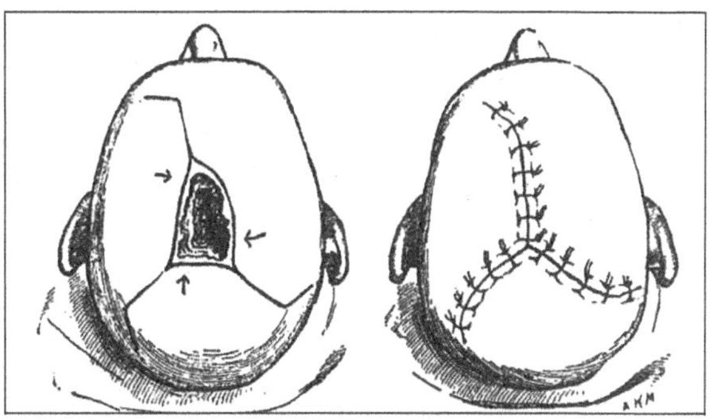

Figure 7.8 This diagram shows Cushing's scalp incision for penetrating wounds of the brain. (Cushing, H., Notes on penetrating wounds of the brain, *British Medical Journal*, 1:2982 (23 February 1918), pp. 221-26)

Anaesthesia for head wounds

Cushing first administered omnopon (a narcotic agent and derivative of morphine) to the patient just before shaving the entire head. Twenty minutes before surgery, the scalp was infiltrated with 1 percent novocaine with adrenaline along the lines of the proposed skin incision. Adrenaline causes vasoconstriction and reduced blood loss from the skin edges once the incision had been made. Cushing indicated that there was a difference of opinion regarding the relative merits of a general versus local anaesthesia for cranial operations. He was in no doubt that local anaesthesia was preferable, since general narcosis increased bleeding from the scalp and encouraged the use of rougher methods which a patient under local anaesthesia would not tolerate. General anaesthesia encouraged speed at the expense of delicacy and threatened to enhance respiratory difficulties for patients in whom inhalational problems were prone to occur. Close observation of every head injury case recovering from a general anaesthetic in a busy casualty clearing station was quite impractical[12]

Table 7.1 Outcome of 133 patients (admitted to CCS 46) with wounds involving penetration of dura between August and October 1917.

Month	Number of cases	Number who died	Percentage mortality
August	44	24	51
September	44	18	41
October	45	13	29

Cushing, H., Notes on penetrating wounds of the brain, *British Medical Journal*, 1:2982, (23 February 1918), pp. 221-26.

Cushing published his surgical results for penetrating wounds of the skull and brain carried out at CCS 46 during the months of August, September and October 1917 (Table 7.1) and these showed a significant and progressive improvement, which Cushing attributed to refinements in his surgical technique and to his clinical expertise. There was 55 percent mortality in August 1917 falling to 29 percent mortality in October.[13] His results were published in the British Medical Journal in February 1918, but Cushing wanted much more. He was determined to stamp his authority on the treatment of penetrating wounds of the skull and brain, and to achieve this, in April 1918, he published a comprehensive account of his wartime surgical experience in the British Journal of Surgery in an article extending to 126 pages.[14] This had many detailed case histories and drawings so that the world would know that Harvey Cushing was unquestionably the greatest neurosurgeon to grace the surgical stage on the Western Front.

Cushing got himself into potentially serious trouble in April 1918 when the British censor intercepted a letter Cushing had written to his wife which also contained extracts of his diary in which he was very critical (again) of the British war effort. He had to write a grovelling letter of

12 Cushing, H., Notes on penetrating wounds of the brain, pp. 221-26.
13 Cushing, H., Notes on penetrating wounds of the brain, pp. 221-26.
14 Cushing, H., A Study of a Series of Wounds involving the Brain and its Enveloping Structures, *British Journal of Surgery*, No. 5 (April 1918), pp. 558-684.

apology. Arrogant he may have been, but Cushing was a great surgeon and his contribution was a very important one. By the end of the war he was exhausted, having developed a toxic neuritis secondary to Spanish Flu which for a time deprived him of the use of his hands and the ability to operate. He had done his very best and subsequently observed:

> The capacity of man himself is only revealed when, under stress and responsibility, he breaks through his educational shell, and he may then be a splendid surprise to himself no less than to his teachers[15]

Penetrating wounds of the chest wall

Throughout the 19th century, surgeons rarely operated on penetrating wounds of the chest, and if they did it was usually to remove a broken sword or lance blade which was protruding from the chest wall and to trim broken ribs before stitching up the wound as quickly as possible. During the Peninsular War, one hundred years before the Great War, George James Guthrie made good use of clinical examination to ascertain if there was any accumulation of fluid (serous, blood or pus) within the chest cavity and employed a trocar and cannula when necessary to drain the collection and alleviate the patient's breathing.[16] He said this of puncture wounds of the chest caused by sword or lance:

> The advantages derived from the closure of punctured wounds of the chest in former times led to the practice of sucking them by the mouths of irregular practitioners, generally the drum major of the regiment, when the patient was a soldier and the consequences, although in some cases miraculous, were in others quite unfortunate. Sucking of a small wound which is unattended by bleeding, does good by attracting the natural fluid to the parts and thus causing them to swell so as to be placed in apposition in the most advantageous manner for their reunion. Punctured wounds of small size may be sucked chirurgically, if anyone be willing to do it, after which a bit of dry lint should be placed on the wound.[17]

Whilst sucking of chest wounds had fortunately gone out of fashion, chest surgery in 1914 was not far removed from Guthrie's practice in the Peninsular War. During the first two years of the Great War, very little was done for these wounds. The patient was put to bed and was given morphine. If infection took hold, as it frequently did, and there was a collection of pus in the chest cavity (empyema), it was drained by resecting a segment of rib and sticking a wide-bored tube into the pleural cavity, allowing the pus to continue draining until it either dried up or the patient died. During the Second Boer War, it was believed that it would be fatal to open the chest cavity without some kind of pressure chamber and that any handling of the lung

15 Harvey Cushing <https://allauthor.com/quotes/124386/>.

16 Guthrie, G.J., *Commentaries on the Surgery of the war in Portugal, Spain and the Netherlands* (Philadelphia: J.B. Lippincott, 1862), pp. 414-442.

17 Guthrie, *Commentaries on the Surgery of the war in Portugal, Spain and the Netherlands*, pp. 414-415.

would cause rapid and fatal bleeding.[18] These misperceptions persisted and adversely influenced management of chest wounds in 1914-15.

George Gask (1874-1951)

George Gask qualified in medicine from St Bartholomew's in 1898 and by 1914 he was an established consultant. He went to France in 1916, was mentioned in despatches four times and won the DSO in 1917. He spent much of his time working in Casualty Clearing Station Number 5 with Major Gordon Gordon-Taylor (see below), where he gained a great deal of experience operating on chest and abdominal wounds. During the Third Battle of Ypres, fought between 31 July and 10 November 1917, he was transferred to Canadian Casualty Clearing Station Number 2 at Remy Siding where he became renowned for his management of penetrating chest wounds. He was appointed Consulting Surgeon to the British Fourth Army in 1918 and was created CMG in 1919 for his services to war surgery. In 1919, Gask became Professor of Surgery at the University of London with his surgical unit at St Bartholomew's Hospital.[19]

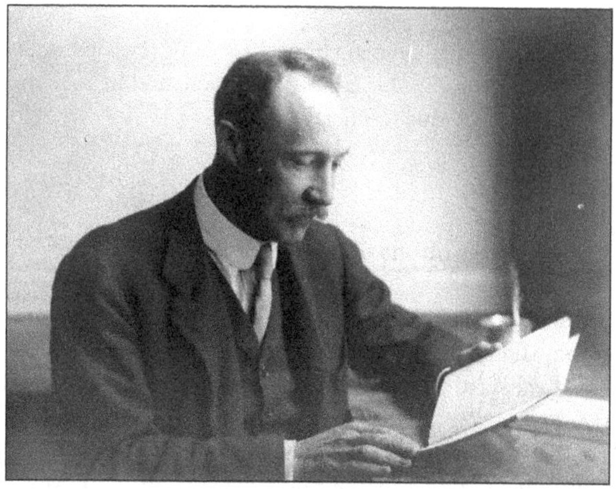

Figure 7.9 George Gask (1875-1951). (Courtesy National Portrait Gallery, London)

The principle of wound excision described by Gray and Milligan in 1915 applied equally to wounds of the chest which were contaminated by metallic foreign bodies, clothing and battlefield debris. Delay in treatment resulted in major sepsis of the chest wall and of the underlying chest (pleural) cavity, where any accumulation of blood or serous fluid acted as a potential breeding ground for bacteria and focus for infection. Just as soldiers with wounds of the extremities arrived at base hospitals in 1914 with overwhelming sepsis, so too did those with penetrating chest wounds. It was essential to operate on these patients much earlier in casualty clearing stations, to excise their wounds and minimise the risk of major sepsis in order to give them the best possible chance of survival.

Gask reported on a series of 500 patients with penetrating wounds of the chest, many of whom he treated at Canadian Casualty Clearing Station Number 2 at Remy Siding in 1917 (Figure 7.7). There were four casualty clearing stations at Remy Siding, British 10 and 17 and Canadian 2 and 3. Gask published his work in the British Medical Journal and extended his thanks to Lieutenant-Colonel J.E. Davey, Commanding Officer of Canadian CCS 2.[20]

18 Gask, G., Gunshot wounds of the chest, *British Medical Journal*, 1:4089 (20 May 1939), pp. 1043-1045.

19 Gask, George Ernest (1875-1951), Plarr's Lives of the Fellows Online, Royal College of Surgeons <ps://livesonline.rcseng.ac.uk/biogs/E004155b.htm>.

20 Gask, G.E., Wilkinson, K.D., Penetrating gunshot wounds of the chest and their treatment, *British Medical Journal*, 2: 2972 (15 December 1917), pp. 781-784.

Many soldiers who sustained penetrating chest wounds died on the battlefield or very soon afterwards, depending on whether vital structures within the chest had been damaged. Deaths amongst those who survived long enough to reach the casualty clearing station were either early or late. Early deaths were due to extensive and severe wounds which could seldom be aided surgically, for example wounds of the heart and great vessels. Deaths occurring a few days after admission to the CCS were always due to sepsis, as were deaths occurring after patients had been transferred to base hospitals. Gask pointed out that treatment must be directed towards the prevention of infection if lives were to be saved.

Missile wounds penetrating the chest wall carried clothing and splinters of rib into the chest (pleural) cavity. Air was often sucked into chest wounds during respiration which invariably led to infection. This was an absolute indication to temporarily suture the chest wound to stop this movement of air and to make the patient more comfortable. Gask expressed the view that all such 'sucking' wounds should be sutured without anaesthetic as quickly as possible in advanced dressing stations. The reader will no doubt remember that one of the main reasons why so many wounded soldiers died in the opening months of the war was because their wounds had been closed at advanced dressing stations before being sent on the long journey to base hospitals on the French coast for definitive surgery (Chapter 4). The immediate suture of a chest wound was in a quite different category. It was a first aid measure which was far more effective than plugging the hole in the chest wall with a dressing to stop air being sucked in. Definitive wound excision was carried out as soon as possible at a designated casualty clearing station located close by. X-ray examination was employed to locate metallic foreign bodies to get an idea of their size and position. The aim of surgery was to reduce the probability of sepsis, thereby reducing the number of avoidable deaths. There was no need for any pressure chamber, as had been feared in 1914. Gask's indications for early surgery were as follows:

- Ragged dirty wound of soft parts chest wall; all necrotic tissue excised, converting a filthy contaminated wound into a clean one;
- Compound fracture of ribs; all loose and dead pieces of bone excised;
- Bleeding from the chest wall; bleeding intercostals vessels tied off to stop bleeding. If lung damaged, the damaged section of lung removed without significant bleeding; lung should always be sutured to prevent organisms passing from lung to pleural cavity;
- Suction of air into the chest cavity; suture after wound excision;
- Removal of large foreign body in accessible position;
- Pain due to in driven splinters of bone; remove splinters;
- Rapidly increasing and potentially fatal pneumothorax called a tension pneumothorax (air forced into the chest cavity causing the lung to collapse and the entire contents of the chest pushed towards the other side) due to valve action of pleural flap; immediate surgery essential to relieve pressure and repair chest wall.

Anaesthesia for chest wounds

Gask believed every patient on whom an intrathoracic operation was performed should have a general anaesthetic by administering chloroform through a Shipway's apparatus.[21] Sir Francis E. Shipway (1875-1968) was a leading specialist in anaesthesia who developed an apparatus in 1916 to deliver a continuous flow of warm anaesthetic vapour. Ether or chloroform was pumped through a vacuum flask containing a coiled tube in hot water. It was very important to use warm vapour otherwise excessive heat was lost from the body which would have aggravated surgical shock.

Wallace and Fraser (see below) noted that local anaesthesia had the advantage that it did not irritate the opposite and possibly undamaged lung, and also that the patient could assist at the end of the operation by partly expanding the injured lung prior to final suture. They used 1 percent Novocaine with adrenaline to infiltrate the wound margins and block the intercostal nerves behind the angles of the ribs. They thought it advisable to use a general anaesthetic during the intrathoracic stage of the operation and recommended nitrous oxide and oxygen. In cases of multiple wounds, a general anaesthetic was essential throughout the entire procedure. Nitrous oxide and oxygen or chloroform and oxygen through a Shipway apparatus were satisfactory, Ether, which aggravated pulmonary haemorrhage, was contraindicated.[22]

If infection became established despite the measures taken, it was essential to carry out an effective operation to remove any accumulation of infected blood (haemothorax) and/or pus (empyema) from within the chest cavity by open operation as opposed to aspiration through a wide bored cannula. After resecting a segment of rib to gain access and thoroughly cleaning out the chest cavity, a wide drainage tube was inserted into the pleural cavity and the chest closed in layers. Streptococci or anaerobic organisms (including causative organism of gas gangrene) were most commonly incriminated. There were, of course, no antibiotics, since they had not yet been discovered. All being well, the drain was removed after a few days once the patient had improved.

Gask dealt with 365 patients at Canadian CCS 2 at Remy Siding. There were 76 deaths, giving a mortality of 20 percent. Forty-five of the deaths were associated with other abnormalities (Table 7.2).

Table 7.2 Casualty clearing station and base hospital deaths of 45 patients with chest wounds associated with other complications

Chest and head	6
Chest and abdomen	14
Chest and spine	4
Chest and heart	4
Chest and great vessels	2
Chest and multiple wounds	14
Chest and gas gangrene	1

21 Gask, G.E., Wilkinson, K.D., Penetrating gunshot wounds of the chest and their treatment, pp. 781-784.

22 Wallace, C.S., Fraser, J., *Surgery at a casualty clearing station*, (London: A&C Black, Ltd., 1918), pp. 199-200.

If the 45 patients with other system involvement are put to one side, then 31 or 9.6 percent of patients died exclusively as a result of their chest wounds (Table 7.3). Wounds caused by shell casing fragments with both entry and exit wounds were associated with the highest percentage mortality (47 percent) and shrapnel ball the lowest (10 percent).

Table 7.3 Causes of death in 31 patients suffering from chest wound only.

Shock and haemorrhage	19
Sepsis	10
Bronchitis	2

Gask, G.E., Wilkinson, K.D., Penetrating gunshot wounds of the chest and their treatment, *British Medical Journal,* 2: 2972 (15 December 1917), pp. 781-84.

Figure 7.10 is a photograph taken in 1917 of Gask performing a chest operation in one of the operating theatres of Canadian CCS 2 at Remy Siding. He and his surgical team are wearing sterile gowns which have been autoclaved to remove bacteria. All are wearing rubber gloves and the surgical instruments have also been autoclaved to reduce the risk of introducing harmful bacteria into the surgical field. If he had been performing an elective procedure by making an incision in the chest wall to operate on the underlying lung, he would have been employing an aseptic surgical technique. Gask's patient, however, has a filthy contaminated chest wound caused by shellfire and Figure 7.10 does not show an aseptic surgical procedure. Gask is removing devitalised muscle from the chest wall, trimming broken ribs and removing any fragments of foreign material, before inspecting the underlying lung and resecting any damaged pulmonary tissue along with accessible foreign bodies. He is attempting to convert a recently inflicted filthy contaminated wound into a macroscopically clean one. If successful, he will probably save the patient's life by preventing infection gaining a foot hold.

The reader will remember from Chapter 6 that Canadian doctor Lawrence Bruce Robertson was engaged in clinical research into blood transfusion at Canadian CCS 2 at the same time. Robertson published the results of transfusion in 36 wounded soldiers who were in extremis when he transfused them. Without blood transfusion, they would almost certainly have all died.[23] Three of them were operated on by George Gask:

> *Case 25 GSW chest, femoral vein and knee joint; evacuated to base in good clinical condition:*
> Dr CJB; admitted in a very grave condition under the care of Major G. Gask, DSO RAMC; Penetrating wound of chest; tear of left femoral vein; penetrating wound of right knee joint. After operation the patient was blanched and collapsed. The pulse was 180 and barely perceptible; blood pressure 60mm Hg. Blood transfusion started, but before 60cc had been injected, death was imminent. The patient's lips were bloodless, pulse imperceptible, breathing slow and jerky; 80cc of very hot saline and 1cc of pituitrin were now given intravenously and transfusion continued. When 400cc of blood had been injected,

23 Robertson, L.B., Gordon Watson, C., Further observations on the results of blood transfusion in war surgery, *British Medical Journal,* 2: 2969 (24 November 1917), pp. 679-83.

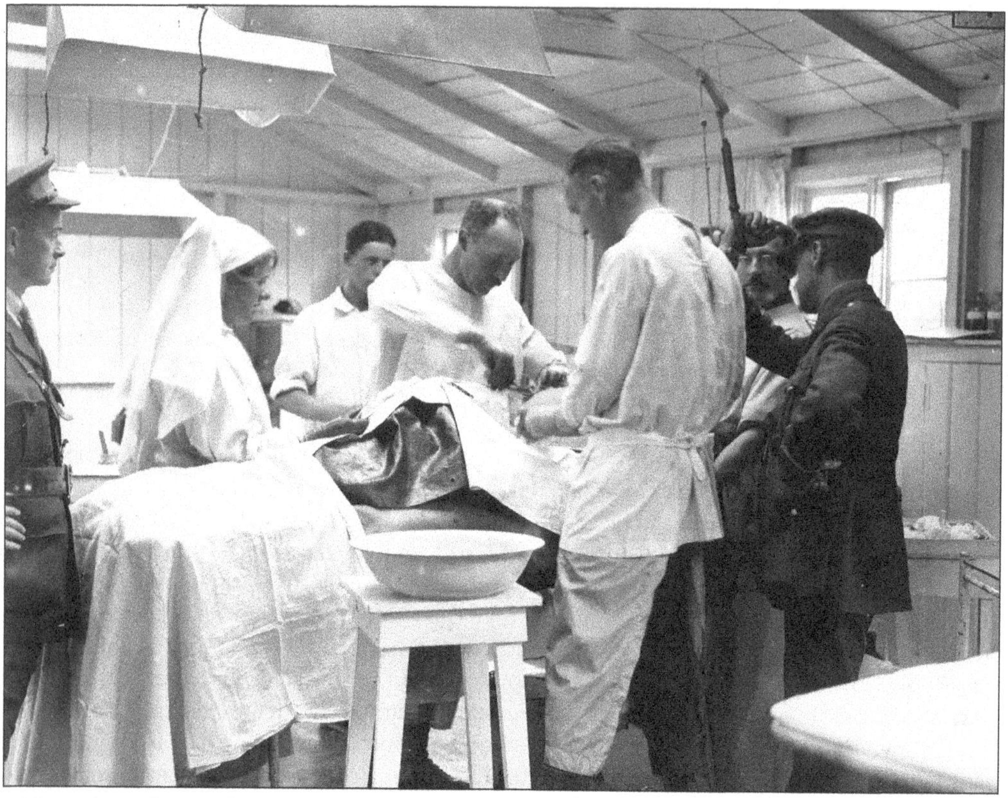

Figure 7.10 George Gask operating on a patient at Canadian Casualty Clearing Station Number 2 in 1917; he is performing a thoracotomy. (Courtesy Archives of Ontario)

the breathing had improved greatly. At the end of the transfusion (1,200cc), the face was flushed, the pulse strong and the patient was attempting to clear his throat. After transfusion, the pulse was 108, blood pressure 144, and further progress uneventful. He was evacuated to base seven days later. Two weeks later he had been evacuated to England in good condition.[24]

Case 26 GSW chest, Haemothorax and laceration of lung; death
Gunner EG, wounded early that morning, was admitted in a very collapsed state under the care of Major Gask, DSO, RAMC, on July 17th, 1917; severe penetrating wound of the chest; extensive damage to lung; blood transfusion (700cc); slight response lasting a very short time. Death occurred some five hours later; necropsy showed gas gangrene infection in haemothorax (blood in chest cavity) and severe laceration of lung.[25]

24 Robertson, L.B., Further observations on the results of blood transfusion in war surgery, pp. 679-83.
25 Robertson, L.B., Further observations on the results of blood transfusion in war surgery, pp. 679-83.

Case 29 GSW Chest, recovery
2nd Lieut. A. J. D. Admitted July 29th, 1917, under the care of Major G. E. Gask DSO, RAMC, in a collapsed condition; severe penetrating wound of chest, from which there had been a large amount 6f bleeding; condition inoperable. Blood transfusion (740 c.cm.) carried out. After 100cc had been injected operation was begun; thoracotomy, removal of shell fragments, irrigation of pleural cavity, closure of chest wall; further progress good; Evacuated to base nine days later in good condition.[26]

Penetrating abdominal wounds

Case history

The patient was anaesthetised using warm ether with a Shipway Apparatus. The surgeon made a long paramedian (longitudinal, a short distance from and parallel to the midline) incision, extending from just below the ribs to just above the pubis and swabbed away a large quantity of blood using a long roll of dry gauze to clear the view. His incision incorporated the hole made by the fragment of shell casing responsible for the wound, which he duly excised. When bleeding was severe, he always packed the peritoneal cavity with gauze to bring the bleeding under control, but this case wasn't too bad. He picked up the caecum (the first part of the large bowel) to identify the terminal small bowel attached to it and then worked his way rapidly but methodically along the whole length of the small intestine, looking for perforations in the bowel as well as for tears in its mesentery which carried blood vessels to and from the bowel. The mesentery was intact, but he found several holes in the small bowel. He marked each by wrapping it in a small moist swab with a length of tape tied to one side of the swab. He then passed the tape through the mesentery and doubled it twice round the segment of bowel covered by the swab. He was careful to examine the whole length of small bowel to make sure he had found all the perforations. He next examined the duodenum and stomach and felt the pancreas while examining the posterior aspect of the stomach. He examined the liver and spleen, before palpating both kidneys to ensure they were intact. He examined the large bowel, confirming it to be intact, before examining the pelvic viscera. He had to clear away residual blood in the pelvis to get a good view. All was well. He found the fragment of shrapnel alongside the mesentery of the small bowel. The problem confronting him was multiple perforations of small bowel which were all quite close together. He had two options. He could either stitch up each perforation individually, or he could resect the entire affected segment of bowel before stitching the ends of the remaining small intestine back together. Experience had taught the surgeon that resection of the damaged segment of bowel was frequently associated with an intense degree of shock, which was infinitely greater than that following the individual suture of multiple perforations and carried a significantly higher percentage mortality. Multiple sutures carried the risk of causing narrowing of the bowel, which was potentially troublesome. Multiple sutures also carried the risk of necrosis of the adjacent bowel which may have been damaged slightly by the shrapnel. This complication was more likely to occur in large bowel than in the small intestine.

26 Robertson, L.B., Further observations on the results of blood transfusion in war surgery, pp. 679-83.

On balance therefore, he decided his better option was to repair all the defects, which he did using linen thread. He closed the abdomen. The patient went on to make a good recovery.

When the Great War started, penetrating abdominal wounds were treated conservatively just as they had been during the Second Boer War. Senior Consulting Surgeon to the BEF, Sir Anthony Bowlby, remarked in 1914:

> The abdomen is to a great extent protected in the trenches, and abdominal wounds are not as relatively common as they were in South Africa. They have, however, been more common in the recent fighting, and I have seen, I suppose, between fifty and sixty. The conclusions of recent wars are confirmed-namely, that they should not as a rule be operated upon. The minority of those I have seen have recovered, although some of them have had such rigidity and vomiting as to make one feel sure of some peritonitis. Wounds through the upper part of the abdomen do better than those below the umbilicus and bullets through the liver do not generally do much harm, although I have seen severe vomiting follow haemorrhage into the peritoneum and have seen fatalities from bleeding. [27]

At the time of writing, Bowlby like many others had not wakened to the fact that the majority of patients with penetrating abdominal wounds died without surgery, especially those who had sustained penetrating injuries involving bowel (see below). Damage to blood vessels within the abdominal cavity often resulted in massive bleeding and the development of surgical shock, which in the most severe cases proved to be fatal. It was estimated that approximately 5 percent of patients with penetrating abdominal wounds died from massive haemorrhage before reaching casualty clearing stations.[28] When bleeding was not sufficiently severe to cause immediate or early death and if small or large bowel was damaged, leaking intestinal contents invariably caused infection within the abdominal cavity (peritonitis) and resulted in death from sepsis after a couple of days. It can be appreciated therefore, that deaths occurring within minutes or hours of injury were caused by bleeding and later ones, after a day or two, by infection.

The key to saving lives was to operate on penetrating abdominal wounds early to stop all bleeding, thus reducing the likelihood of early deaths from haemorrhage and to deal with damaged abdominal viscera, which in cases with perforated bowel involved resecting or repairing the affected bowel to reduce the probability of late deaths from sepsis.

The first successful bowel resection was performed on 18 March 1915 by a surgeon called Owen Richards in Casualty Clearing Station Number 6.[29] The patient was a Canadian Scot who was wounded by a shell fragment in an enemy trench and walked back to his own line holding his intestines which had protruded through a large wound in his anterior abdominal wall. He wanted to die among his friends. Richards removed six feet of damaged small bowel soon afterwards and the soldier survived.[30]

27 Bowlby, A., The work of the clearing hospitals in the last six weeks, *British Medical Journal,* 2:2816 (19 December 1914), pp. 1053-54.

28 Wallace, C.S., Fraser, J., *Surgery at a casualty clearing station,* (London: A&C Black Ltd, 1918), p. 154.

29 Till, A.S., Gordon-Taylor, war surgeon and historian, *Annals of the Royal College of Surgeons of England,* Volume 54 (1974), pp. 33-47.

30 Gordon-Taylor, G., *The abdominal injuries of warfare,* (Bristol: John Wright and Sons, 1939), pp. 23-24.

Cuthbert Wallace (1867-1944)

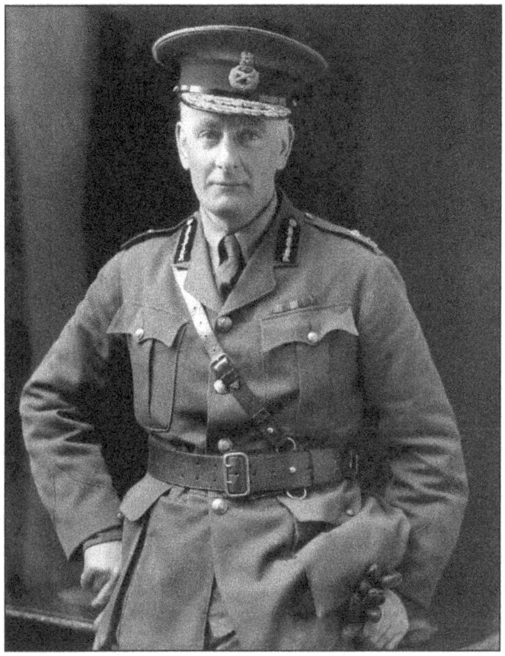

Figure 7.11 Sir Cuthbert Wallace (1867-1944). (Courtesy National Portrait Gallery, London)

Cuthbert Wallace, mentioned previously in connection with surgical (wound) shock, was a key figure in the treatment of penetrating abdominal wounds, and as already indicated a consultant at St Thomas's Hospital in London. During the Second Boer War, he served from 1899-1900 as a surgeon to the Portland Hospital under his friend Anthony Bowlby of St Bartholomew's Hospital. His experience in the surgery of war wounds in South Africa stood him in good stead following the declaration of war in 1914, when Wallace once again served with Bowlby. When two British Armies were formed in December 1914, Bowlby became responsible for the Second Army around Ypres, while Wallace looked after the First Army in Northern France. Wallace's principal interest was the management of penetrating abdominal wounds and in 1918 he published a book *War Surgery of the Abdomen.*[31] He also published *Surgery at a casualty clearing station*[32] with John Fraser after working closely with him for the duration of the conflict. Wallace was created C.M.G in 1916, C.B. in 1918, and promoted K.C.M.G. in 1919. He was mentioned several times in despatches and was awarded the American Distinguished Service Medal.[33]

John Fraser (1885-1947)

Another key figure in the management of penetrating abdominal wounds was John Fraser who came from Tain in the north of Scotland. He graduated in medicine from the University of Edinburgh in 1907 and became house surgeon, then assistant surgeon, to Harold Stiles, Professor of Surgery at the University of Edinburgh. Following the outbreak of war, Fraser joined the Royal Army Medical Corps and worked in the casualty clearing stations of the British First Army near Bethune in northern France, where the Consulting Surgeon was Cuthbert Wallace. Both Wallace and Fraser soon acquired reputations for their work on the management of penetrating abdominal wounds, as well as for their treatment of surgical (wound) shock.

John Fraser was one of the most capable young surgeons working on the Western Front and he and a colleague Hamilton Drummond proved that early operative intervention for penetrating abdominal wounds reduced the overall percentage mortality from more than 80 to 60

31 Wallace, C.S., *War Surgery of the Abdomen* (London: J&A Churchill, 1918).
32 Wallace, C.S., Fraser, J, *Surgery at a casualty clearing station.*
33 Wallace, Sir Cuthbert Sydney (1867-1944), *Plarr's Lives of the Fellows Online, Royal College of Surgeons*, <https://livesonline.rcseng.ac.uk/biogs/E000228b.htm>.

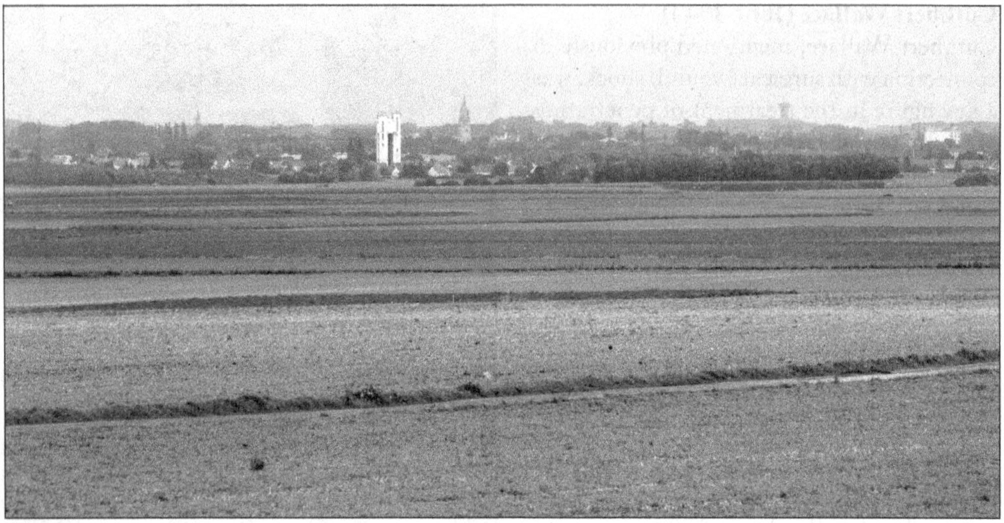

Figure 7.12 The battlefield at Loos looking north towards la Bassée; it was here that John Fraser undertook valuable clinical research on surgical (wound) shock at considerable risk to himself and won a Military Cross. It was also from these fields in 1915 that soldiers with penetrating abdominal wounds were taken to a First Army advanced operating centre where Fraser performed urgent surgery to save their lives.

percent.[34] By present day standards, 60 percent is still a high mortality, but the figure must be viewed in context. There were thousands of wounded soldiers in need of treatment during the Great War with limited resources and facilities. Given that this was the first time British military surgeons had treated abdominal wounds surgically, a 20 percent reduction in mortality represented a significant improvement.

Wallace and Fraser documented that timing of surgery was critical and if a period of six hours or less had elapsed, the chances were in favour of the patient recovering. It is important to appreciate that casualties who had sustained catastrophic haemorrhage, for example from a ruptured inferior vena cava, would have died almost immediately and never reached medical services. Wounded soldiers surviving for six hours were potentially salvageable. After six hours, the position was reversed, and with every hour of delay the chances of recovery grew smaller. Early operative intervention revolutionised war surgery of the abdomen.[35]

Between 1 July 1915 and 30 September 1917, 2,127 patients with penetrating abdominal wounds were documented by Wallace and Fraser. There were 420 moribund patients who were kept comfortable and put aside to die. The total percentage mortality excluding the 420 moribund cases was 50 percent, and total percentage mortality including the 420 moribund cases was 60 percent. A total of 1,707 cases were considered for surgery. Operation was deemed unnecessary in 102 cases. A total of 1,605 operations were performed. The total operative mortality was 53 percent.[36]

34 Fraser, J., Drummond, H., A clinical and experimental study of three hundred perforating wounds of the abdomen, *British Medical Journal*, 1:2932 (10 March 1917), pp. 321-29.

35 Wallace, C.S., Fraser, J, *Surgery at a casualty clearing station*, p. 144.

36 Wallace, C.S., Fraser, J, *Surgery at a casualty clearing station*, p.156.

Wallace and Fraser listed the important factors which influenced the prognosis:

- Time since wounding was critical and was the single most important factor;
- Type of projectile; fragments of bombs and grenades were associated with the lowest mortality and fragments of shell casing with the highest;
- Variety of wound; simple wounds of the small intestine (requiring suture only) had the lowest mortality and complex wounds of small intestine (with involvement of mesentery and requiring bowel resection) had the highest mortality; wounds of solid viscera e.g. liver, kidney did next best after simple small intestinal wounds;
- Wounds of the upper abdomen did better than wounds of the lower abdomen. The latter were associated with a higher incidence of perforated small and large intestine;
- Pulse rate of 100 usually associated with a better prognosis; pulse rate of 120 associated with a poor prognosis; pulse rate >120, few survived (Table 7.4).

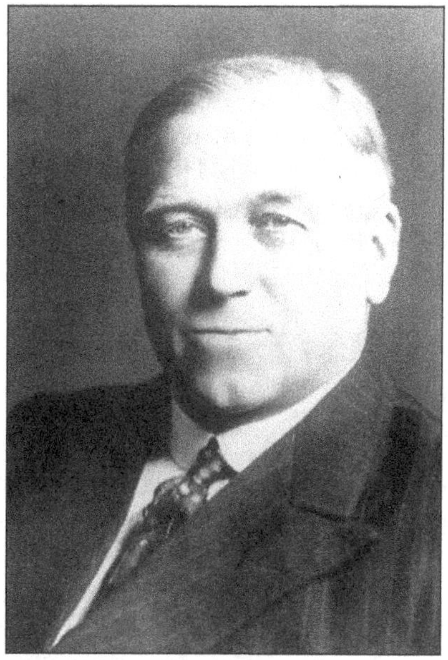

Figure 7.13 This photograph shows Sir John Fraser (1885-1947) in later life. (Courtesy Royal College of Surgeons of Edinburgh)

Table 7.4 Effect of the pulse rate on the prognosis of penetrating abdominal wounds

	Pulse up to and including								
	60	**70**	**80**	**90**	**100**	**110**	**120**	**130**	**140**
Survived to base	1	7	23	30	108	27	37	7	9
Died	1	2	13	18	39	38	88	37	92
Total	2	9	36	48	147	65	125	44	101

Wallace, C.S., Fraser, J., *Surgery at a casualty clearing station*, (London: A&C Black, Ltd., 1918), p. 159.

Anaesthesia for abdominal wounds

Warm ether was used extensively for abdominal wounds. Geoffrey Marshall (Chapter 5) reduced ether induced bronchitis from 54 to 14.7 percent using Shipway's apparatus.[37] Heat loss from coils of bowel was a potential serious problem, and when several feet of bowel were laid outside the abdominal cavity, the blood pressure fell. Marshall recommended surgeons

37 Metcalfe, N.H., The effect of the First World War (1914-1918) on the development of British anaesthesia, *European Journal of Anaesthesia*, 24:8 (2007), pp. 649-57.

should make a large incision and work within the abdomen. Excessive manipulation of the bowel or pulling on the peritoneal lining of the abdomen caused the heart rate to slow and the blood pressure to fall.[38]

Fraser had a 'very successful war', both for his work in clinical surgery, at which he excelled and for his research. His experience in the management of surgical shock has been dealt with in Chapter 6. After the war, he returned to Edinburgh and became Regius Professor of Surgery when (the by then) Sir Harold Stiles retired in 1927. Fraser was knighted in 1937, was created a baronet in 1942 and became Principal of the University of Edinburgh in 1944.

Provisions made to deliver early surgery for abdominal wounds

Following the recognition of the importance of early operative intervention, steps were taken to deliver surgery as quickly as possible after the infliction of abdominal wounds to improve the chances of survival. During the Battle of Loos, advanced operating centres were established to deal with abdominal wounds and patients were taken to these centres as a matter of urgency. Surgeons from casualty clearing stations staffed the advanced centres, and Captain John Fraser went to an advanced centre at Bac St. Maur, while Captain Owen Richards went to a centre at Noeux-les-Mines.[39] In subsequent battles, the formation of specially staffed advanced operating centres for the early treatment of penetrating abdominal wounds became standard practice. During the Battle of the Somme, advanced operating centres were established by field ambulances at Warloy and Authui and specialised teams of surgeons from casualty clearing stations who were experienced in the management of abdominal trauma staffed them. The centre at Authui was located in a small but well- equipped civilian hospital with 75 beds, supplemented by accommodation for 375 other wounded in tents, huts and other buildings. There were three surgeons and nine nursing sisters at Warloy.[40] During the opening weeks of Third Battle of Ypres, which began on 31 July 1917, there were three casualty clearing stations located at Brandhoek (Figure 7.7) which dealt exclusively with penetrating wounds of the chest and abdomen and compound fractures of the femur. These were the wounds most in need of urgent surgery. British CCSs 32, 44 and Australian 3 at Brandhoek were closer to the front line than any other casualty clearing stations. CCS 32 opened first in preparation for the forthcoming battle and Sister Kate Luard, who was in charge of nursing services there, wrote:

> Friday July 27th
> Yesterday everything went so well one knew it couldn't last. The hospital had only been pitched since last Saturday and it was already splendid. This venture so close to the Line is of the nature of an experiment in life-saving, to reduce the mortality rate from abdominal

38 Robertson, A., in Scotland, T., Heys, S., *War Surgery 1914-18* (Solihull: Helion and Company, 2012), p. 96.
39 Macpherson, W.G., *History of the Great War based on official documents Medical Services General History Vol. II* (London: MacMillan, 1923), p. 457.
40 Macpherson, W.G, *History of the Great War based on official documents Medical Services General History Vol. III* (London: His Majesty's Stationery Office, 1924), p. 20.

and chest wounds. Their chances of life depend, except when the injuries are such as to be beyond any hope of recovery, on the length of time between the injury and the operation.[41]

Luard pointed out in her diary that the experiment in saving lives employing the three casualty clearing stations at Brandhoek was Sir Anthony Bowlby's idea, who had clearly kept an open mind about the changing surgical management of penetrating abdominal wounds.

The Third Battle of Ypres commenced on 31 July 1917. Sister Luard wrote:

> Everything has been going at full pitch, with the twelve teams in the theatre only breaking off for hasty meals ... Of course, a good many die but a great many seem to be going to do. We get them one hour after injury, which is our raison d'être for being here.[42]

Figure 7.14 is a photograph of Brandhoek New Military Cemetery near Ypres which has 530 Commonwealth burials and 28 German. The cemetery opened in late July 1917 and closed a month later. All those buried here had penetrating wounds of the chest or abdomen or had compound gunshot fractures of the femur. By this stage in the war, the mortality of compound femoral fractures had been reduced to around 20 percent (see below), so the majority of those buried in this cemetery died from abdominal and/or chest wounds. One interred here is Captain Noel Chavasse, VC and Bar, Regimental Medical Officer to the 10th King's (Liverpool Scots). He won his first VC on the Somme at Guillemont on 9 August 1916 and his second near Wieltje between 31 July and 2 August 1917, the opening days of the Third Battle of Ypres. He was very badly wounded by a fragment of an exploding shell on 2 August which penetrated his anterior abdominal wall and damaged his bowel. He was taken to CCS 32 where he underwent an exploratory laparotomy. The surgeon was a Major Fagge, who repaired several holes in his small bowel. Chavasse failed to rally post-operatively and died on 4 August, almost certainly from peritonitis and septicaemia.[43] The citation for his first VC, for valour on the Somme, stated:

> Captain Noel Godfrey Chavasse, M.C., M.B., Royal Army Medical Corps
> For most conspicuous bravery and devotion to duty;
> During an attack he tended the wounded in the open all day, under heavy fire, frequently in view of the enemy. During the ensuing night he searched for wounded on the ground in front of the enemy's lines for four hours. Next day he took one stretcher-bearer to the advanced trenches, and under heavy shell fire carried an urgent case for 500 yards into safety, being wounded in the side by a shell splinter during the journey. The same night he took up a party of twenty volunteers, rescued three wounded men from a shell hole twenty-five yards from the enemy's trench, buried the bodies of two officers, and collected many identity discs, although fired on by bombs and machine guns. Altogether he saved the lives of some twenty badly wounded men, besides the ordinary cases which passed through his hands. His courage and self-sacrifice were beyond praise.[44]

41 Stevens, J. and C., Editors, *Unknown Warriors, The letters of Kate Luard, RRC and Bar, Nursing Sister in France* (History Press, 2014).
42 Stevens, J & C, *Unknown Warriors.*
43 Clayton, A., *Chavasse, Double VC* (Barnsley: Pen and Sword, 1992), p. 206.
44 *The London Gazette*, Supplement, No 29802, 26 October 1916.

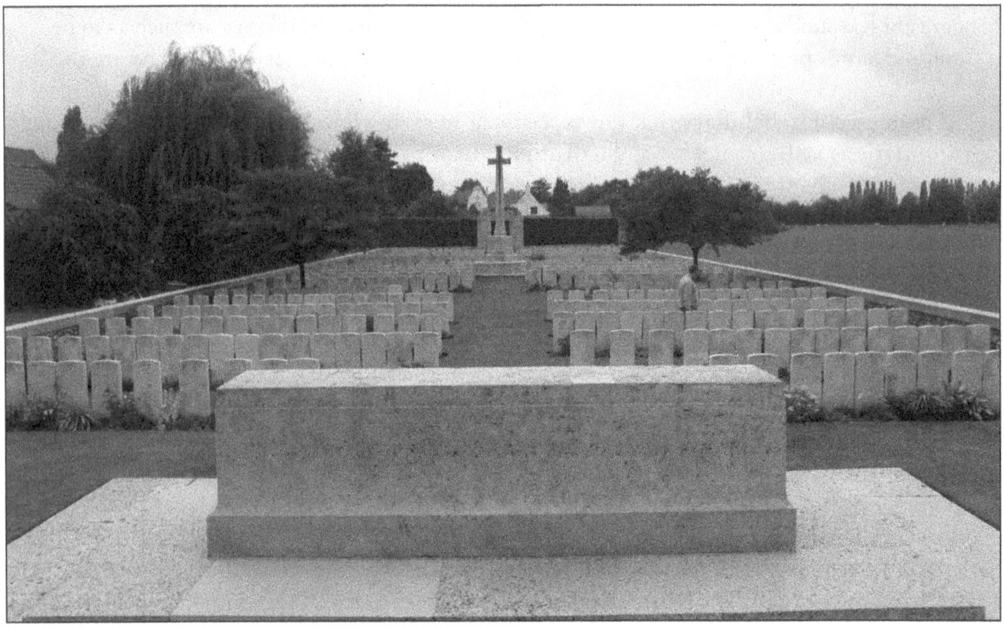

Figure 7.14 Brandhoek New Military Cemetery; it contains the remains of men who died from penetrating wounds of the chest and abdomen and compound fractures of the femur. (Author's photograph)

Chavasse's second award was made during the period 31 July to 2 August 1917, at Wieltje. The full citation was published on 14 September 1917:

> War Office, September 1917.
>
> His Majesty the King has been graciously pleased to approve of the award of a Bar to the Victoria Cross to Capt. Noel Godfrey Chavasse, V.C., M.C., and late R.A.M.C., attached. L'pool R. For most conspicuous bravery and devotion to duty when in action; though severely wounded early in the action whilst carrying a wounded soldier to the Dressing Station, Capt. Chavasse refused to leave his post, and for two days not only continued to perform his duties, but in addition went out repeatedly under heavy fire to search for and attend to the wounded who were lying out. During these searches, although practically without food during this period, worn with fatigue and faint with his wound, he assisted to carry in a number of badly wounded men, over heavy and difficult ground. By his extraordinary energy and inspiring example, he was instrumental in rescuing many wounded who would have otherwise undoubtedly succumbed under the bad weather conditions. This devoted and gallant officer subsequently died of his wounds.[45]

The three Brandhoek casualty clearing stations had always been at risk because they were considerably further forward than other clearing stations. Fears proved to be justified because

45 *The London Gazette*, Supplement, No 30284, 14 September 1917.

on Thursday 16 August, a Medical Officer and corporal were killed by an exploding shell at Australian CCS 3, then on 21 August 1917, Staff Nurse Nellie Spindler working at CCS 44 was killed, also by an exploding German shell. This was the last straw and it was decided immediately to remove the nursing staff and evacuate all the wounded by hospital train. Unfortunately, the adjacent railway platform came under shellfire and the plan had to be abandoned. The patients were taken instead by ambulance wagons to Remy Siding, three miles further west. Two patients suffering from abdominal wounds with multiple perforations of the bowel and three suffering from chest wounds who had all undergone surgery that day were taken to CCS 10 without mishap.[46] CCS 44 was the first Brandhoek clearing station to reopen at Nine Elms near Poperinghe practically straight away. Australian CCS 3 was parked at Remy Siding till the end of August before it too re-opened at Nine Elms. CCS 32 remained at Brandhoek to treat lightly wounded.

Gordon Gordon-Taylor (1878-1960) and combined wounds involving the chest and abdomen

Gordon Gordon-Taylor joined the RAMC in 1914, was gazetted Major in 1915 and was posted to Casualty Clearing Station Number 5, where he remained for most of the war.[47] Like his colleagues Owen Richards, Cuthbert Wallace and John Fraser, he was a vigorous advocate of early surgery for abdominal wounds, which had to be performed quickly and effectively:

> Speed is the handmaiden of success in the operative treatment of gunshot wounds of the belly. There is no place for the surgical sluggard on the floor of the operating theatre of the casualty clearing station. As captain of a surgical team handling abdominal injuries, the surgeon who dawdles is wasteful of the time of others as well as his own. By reason of his very slowness, he will compass the death of many wounded men who might have been saved by an operator of quicker turn of speed.[48]

Personnel at CCS 5 soon acquired well deserved reputations for their excellent management of penetrating abdominal wounds and during the Third Battle of Ypres, Gordon-Taylor was posted to the casualty clearing stations at Brandhoek where he joined friends and colleagues who had similar interest and expertise in the treatment of such wounds.

Between the Battle of Cambrai in November 1917 and August 1918, Gordon-Taylor operated on 75 patients with wounds affecting both chest and abdomen. His recovery rate was 64 percent. In the autumn of 1918, he collected the results of 207 operations for abdomino-thoracic wounds (which included his own) performed by six surgeons attached to the Fourth Army, when the overall recovery rate was 66.6 percent. Individual results depended on the involvement of hollow and solid abdominal organs, the latter having a better prognosis. In 1916, only 18 percent of thoraco-abdominal cases were saved, while in 1917 Sir Anthony Bowlby reported

46 Macpherson, *History of the Great War Vol. III*, p. 155-156.
47 Till, A.S., Gordon-Taylor, *Annals of the Royal College of Surgeons of England*, Vol. 54 (1974), pp. 33-47.
48 Gordon-Taylor, G. *The Abdominal Injuries of Warfare* (Bristol: John Wright and Sons Ltd., 1939), p. 6.

a recovery rate of 49 percent.[49] According to Gordon-Taylor, the improved prognosis was in no small measure attributable to the enterprising surgery of his friend and colleague from CCS 5, Major George Gask, who helped to show others the way. Growing clinical experience and expertise, better anaesthesia, better resuscitation and blood transfusion were also very important factors. Gordon-Taylor declared:

> The results of surgical treatment of abdominal wounds did not improve in spectacular fashion when operation became orthodox until blood transfusion came to aid the victim; but some men are, from the very first, mortally wounded.[50]

Orthopaedic wounds

Case history

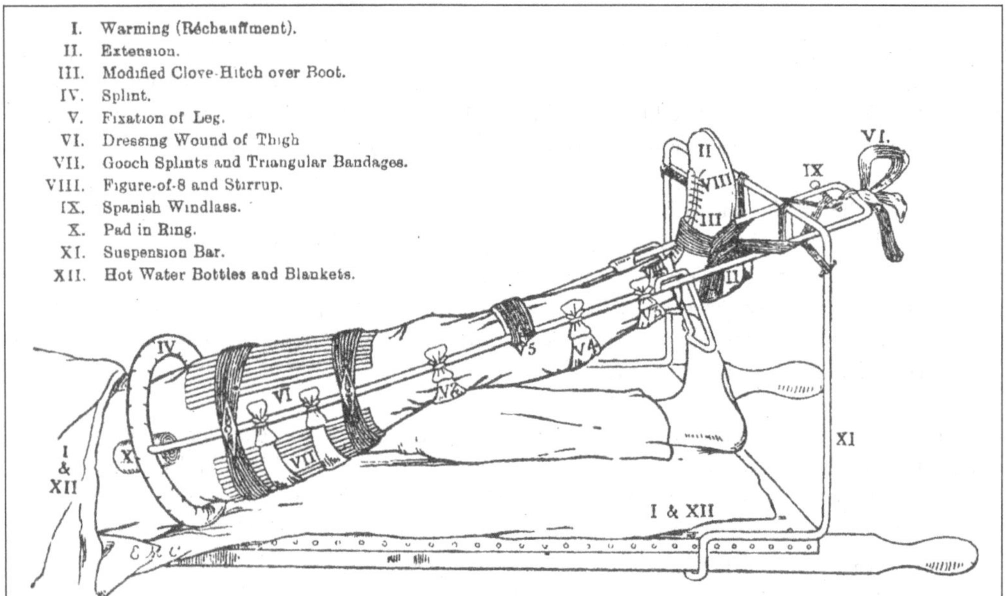

A Front Line Application of the Thomas Splint

Figure 7.15 This diagram is of a Thomas Splint as applied in the field for compound fracture of the femur. (Wallace, C.S., Fraser, J., *Surgery at a casualty clearing station* (London: A&C Black, Ltd., 1918), p. 105.)

The two regimental stretcher bearers who were following up behind the attack soon reached a badly wounded soldier lying in a shallow shell hole with a grossly deformed right thigh. He was bleeding heavily from a wound in the outer aspect of the thigh and it was clear that he had

49 Gordon-Taylor, G., The abdominal injuries of warfare II, *British Medical Journal*, 2:4099 (29 July 1939), pp. 235-38.
50 Gordon-Taylor, G., *The Abdominal Injuries of Warfare*, p. 87.

sustained a compound fracture of his femur. The first stretcher bearer turned him onto his back while the second exerted traction on the wounded man's limb by holding the heel and foot of the casualty's boot and pulling firmly, keeping the fracture under control to relieve pain. Then the first gave him an injection of morphine before slitting open his trousers to expose the wound, to which he firmly applied a field dressing to control bleeding and then four small pieces of Gooch splinting round the fracture site. No disturbance of the casualty's clothing was necessary, other than slitting his trousers to apply the dressing. He reached for the Thomas Splint they had brought with them, which had been prepared beforehand in the regiment aid post by slinging a series of three-inch flannel bandages across from one side of the splint to the other and arranged so that they would support the posterior surface of the thigh and calf with the splint in position. He gently manoeuvred the splint over the wounded soldier's foot and ankle, slipping it up the leg, over the knee and up to the groin. During this time, the second stretcher bearer maintained a strong and sustained pull on the limb, leaning back and straining as hard as he could. The first stretcher bearer then took an eight-foot length of flannel bandage and placed a couple of clove hitches around the ankle over the boot, one on the inner side and one on the outer to apply an even pull. He then tied the clove hitches round the bottom of the splint, being sure that he secured them tightly to maintain strong traction on the limb and checked that the top of the splint fitted snugly at the groin. 'Right, that's the splint on. You can stop pulling on the boot now', he said to his colleague. He made a Spanish Windlass to permit tightening of the traction if required. The stretcher bearers applied two or three pads beneath the patient's thigh to control rotation and a triangular bandage round the knee to secure the limb to the splint. They were as ready as they ever would be to take the casualty to the RAP and onward to the casualty clearing station. They were quite happy that nothing more was necessary till he underwent surgery at the CCS. All they had to do now was avoid being blown to bits by Fritz or by their own people on the way back to their front line.

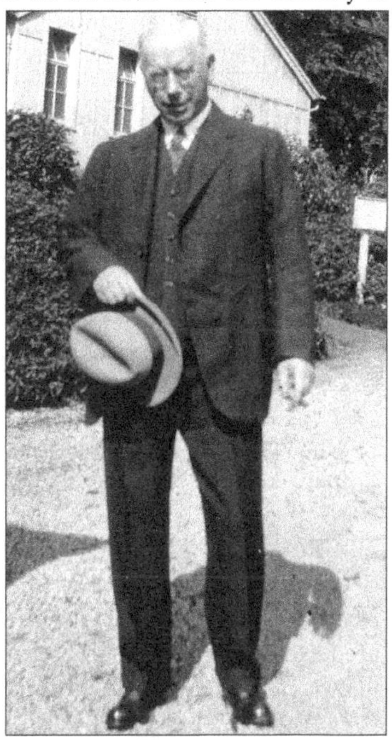

Figure 7.16 Sir Henry Gray (1870-1938). This photograph was taken in Aberdeen some years after the war. (Courtesy Dr Ian Levack)

Henry Gray (1870-1938)

Henry Gray was one of the most capable surgeons to work in France during the Great War. He was born in Aberdeen, the son of a prosperous wholesale provision merchant, and after going to Merchiston Castle School in Edinburgh, he returned to Aberdeen to join his father's business. After two years, he realised a business life was not for him and decided to become a doctor. He enrolled in the Faculty of Medicine at the University of Aberdeen in 1891 and graduated in 1895. He became a Fellow of the Royal College of Surgeons of Edinburgh in 1902 and. in 1904 was appointed consultant surgeon to Aberdeen Royal Infirmary.

Following the outbreak of war in 1914, Gray at first joined a Red Cross unit in France, but the work was not sufficiently challenging. After a brief return to the United Kingdom, he went back to France in November 1914, where he spent the next three and a half years, the first two in charge of a group of base hospitals in Rouen, before becoming Consulting Surgeon to the British Third Army in 1917. His work over three and a half years earned him the C.B. in 1916, the C.M.G. in 1918, and the K.B.E. in 1919. He was mentioned in despatches five times. In 1924, the University of Aberdeen awarded Gray the honorary degree of LLD for his outstanding contributions to war surgery.

Gray applied the important surgical principles of wound excision which he described in 1915 (Chapter 4) to all wounds affecting the musculoskeletal system, including compound gunshot fractures of the femur, which were amongst the deadliest of wounds during the first two years of the war. Gray documented a percentage mortality of around 80 percent for compound fractures of the femur in 1914 and 1915.[51] These were particularly serious wounds because there was always a great deal of muscle damage and the loss of at least a couple of pints of blood. The size of the wound with many possible recesses predisposed to foreign bodies lying undetected within its depths. Pieces of shrapnel and contaminated clothing created the ideal setting for the proliferation of dangerous bacteria and the development of major wound infections. Frequently the muscles had been so badly damaged that there were areas deprived of a blood supply and therefore of oxygen, giving the bacteria responsible for gas gangrene an opportunity to thrive.

The splint most commonly employed to immobilise femoral fractures in the first two years of the war was called the Rifle Splint which was not fit for purpose.[52] It failed to immobilise the fracture, and this resulted in the uncontrolled movement of the broken bone ends during transport of patients causing excessive blood loss. Consequently, the wounded frequently arrived at casualty clearing stations in surgical shock and quite unfit to withstand the wound excision necessary to save their limbs and lives.

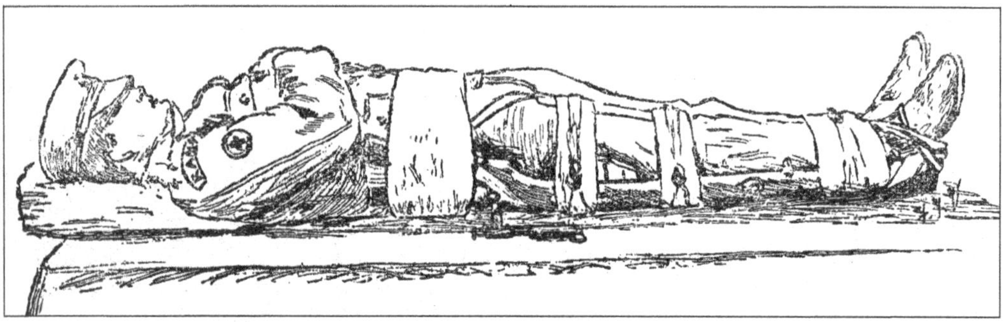

Figure 7.17 Rifle Splint; this diagram was taken from Royal Army Medical Handbook, 1911. The Rifle Splint consisted of a Lee-Enfield service rifle bound to the patient's leg. It was completely ineffective.

During the Battle of Arras, which commenced on 9 April 1917 and continued into late May, Gray ensured that a splint introduced by his good friend Robert Jones (Chapter 9) was used exclusively to immobilise casualties with compound fractures of the femur. It was called a Thomas Splint, and it had been invented by Jones' uncle by marriage, Hugh Owen Thomas, a

51 Watson, F., *The Life of Sir Robert Jones* (London: Hodder & Stoughton, 1934), p. 158.
52 Gray, H.M.W., *The Early Treatment of War Wounds* (London: Henry Frowde and Hodder & Stoughton, 1919), p. 59.

surgeon whose practice was in Nelson Street in Liverpool close to the docks. Thomas initially designed the splint to immobilise knee joints affected by tuberculosis, but soon found that it was very effective for treating fractures of the femur (Figure 7.18). Stretcher bearers retrieving wounded from no man land were instructed in its use and every regimental aid post had a plentiful supply. The Thomas Splint immobilised fractures much more effectively than the Rifle Splint, restricting movement at the fracture site and reducing bleeding, so that the great majority of patients arrived at casualty clearing stations in good clinical condition and fit to undergo wound excision.

Wound excision of compound gunshot fractures of femur

Field dressings and Thomas Splints which had been applied by stretcher bearers in no man's land or by the regimental medical officer in his RAP were left undisturbed before transferring patients urgently to a designated casualty clearing station. Once the wounded arrived at the clearing station, they were immediately prepared for theatre, and were anaesthetised using nitrous oxide, oxygen and ether. Patients who were in surgical shock were first resuscitated in a resuscitation ward, where they were first seen by personnel experienced in dealing with surgical shock (Chapter 6). Field dressings were taken off in theatre to expose the wound, which was first cleaned with an antiseptic agent before beginning wound excision. Skin edges were excised first, and the wound extended proximally and distally for several inches to provide good visibility within the wound. Dead fat was removed and every bit of dead or doubtfully viable

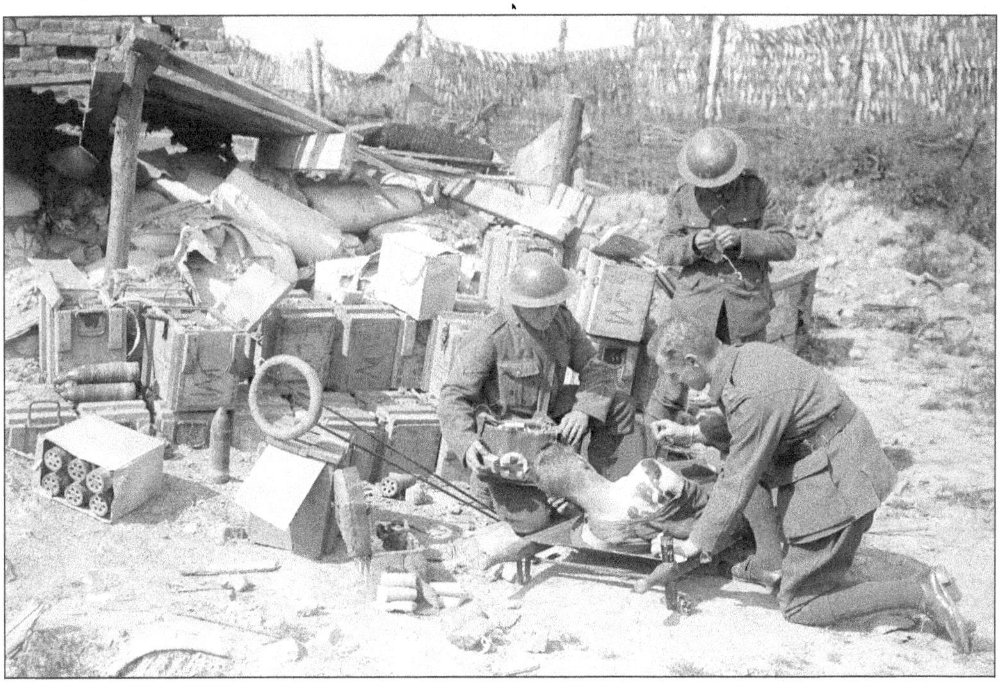

Figure 7.18 Regimental medical officer in his aid post; note the Thomas Splint. (Courtesy Imperial War Museum, Q005916)

muscle was resected. Often this amounted to an entire muscle compartment or more. Muscle resection continued until only pink, viable, bleeding muscle was seen everywhere. Bone holding forceps were used to grab hold of the upper end of the femur above the fracture site and deliver it to the surface of the wound, removing all debris, foreign material and loose pieces of bone without a blood supply from its jagged margin. The same was then done for the lower end of the femur. Every possible recess for foreign bodies was explored with the examining finger, before washing out the wound with sterile saline. If an experienced surgeon was satisfied that the wound was clean, then it could be closed primarily by stitching the skin back together. Such a course of action, however, would only have been safe if performed early, within twelve hours of wounding, by the most experienced surgeons exercising sound clinical judgement as to whether it was, or was not safe, to employ primary closure. If any dead muscle had been left behind at the completion of surgery, then the operation would have been inadequate, and the likely outcome would have been loss of limb or life from the effects of gas gangrene, which could develop and become apparent within a few hours.

Delayed primary closure was the preferred option if there was doubt about the completeness of removal of devitalised tissue. This meant that the wound was left open at the conclusion of the procedure and a salt pack inserted to encourage lymph flow, helpful in combating infection (Chapter 4). At completion of the procedure, a Thomas Splint was reapplied using skin traction kept in place by glue to stick it to the skin (Figure 7.19), and the patient was transferred to a designated base hospital where the wound was inspected after 48 hours. If everything looked healthy it was sutured.

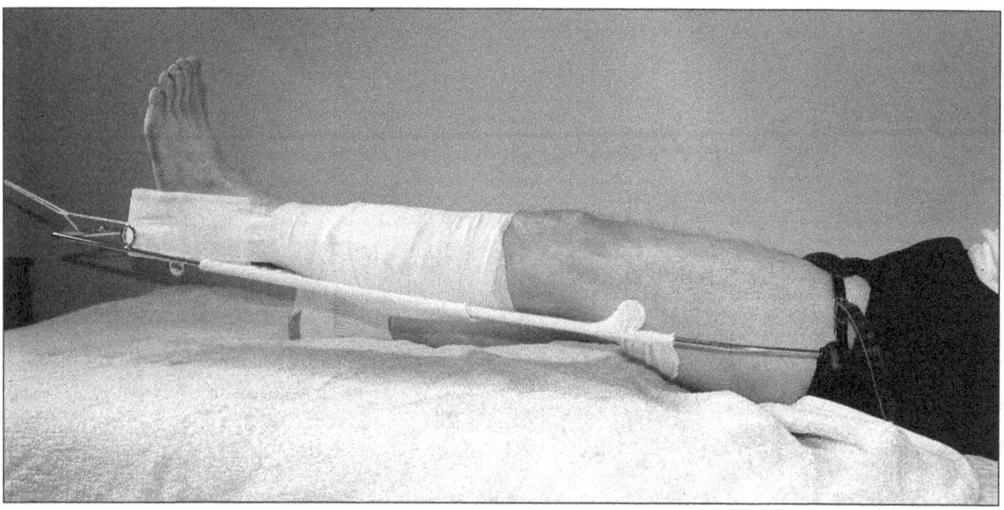

Figure 7.19 Thomas Splint; skin traction was employed during the Great War, using glue to prevent the traction apparatus coming off. It must have been painful to have it removed when the fracture was united. (Author's photograph)

Patients generally remained in France in a designated general or stationary hospital for six weeks, to allow the fracture to become sticky. Clinical examination to confirm this state was achieved by attempting to wiggle the bone ends at the fracture site. If the examiner could not move the fracture, it was deemed sticky and at very low risk of subsequent shortening or angulation. It was then safe to transfer the patient to the United Kingdom without loss of position. The patient could then continue in traction in the Thomas Splint until his fracture went on to firm bony union some six to eight weeks later.

In cases where initial treatment had been delayed and the wound was infected from the outset, secondary closure after approximately a fortnight or leaving the wound open to slowly close spontaneously by secondary intention over a period of several weeks or months were the conservative options available. These patients all first underwent surgery to resect obviously infected or dead tissue before employing antiseptics as an adjuvant to help control the infection. Amputation was the treatment of choice for major infections which were unresponsive to or not appropriate for other measures.

Gray insisted that no patient with a compound femoral fracture was ever sent back to base hospital without first having surgery. Occasionally, a wound might appear so innocuous as to make it seem that the patient could safely wait for definitive surgery at the base, but the damage was always worse than it appeared at first sight. He reported on the outcome of 1,009 cases of compound fracture of the femur during the Battle of Arras, in which the Thomas Splint had been used exclusively. Table 7.5 summarises Gray's results, comparing them with outcomes before the Thomas Splint was used routinely.

Table 7.5 Comparison of outcome of compound fractures of the femur before Arras using the Rifle Splint and at Arras using the Thomas Splint

Prior to Arras	During Arras
Variety of splints based on Rifle Splint	Thomas Splint used exclusively
Majority of cases reached CCS in shock due to blood loss and unfit for wound excision	Only 5% of patients reached CCS in shock due to blood loss; majority fit for wound excision
Mortality in CCS 50%; many died before reaching CCS. Total mortality 80%	Mortality 15.6% in CCS
There was a school of thought that all compound fractures of the femur should be treated by amputation, as patients were so moribund – a brief whiff of gas and an amputation gave the only chance of survival	Gray's amputation rate at Arras was 17.2%. These patients had often lain in a shell hole for many hours and were beyond limb salvage.

Gray, H.M.W., *The Early Treatment of War Wounds* (London: Henry Frowde and Hodder & Stoughton, 1919), pp. 59-60.

By 1916, Gray was regarded as the leading authority in the management of fractures. In the official New Zealand History of the Great War, Lieutenant Colonel AD Carberry stated:

> Surgery, especially that of the front line was a specialty of the 3rd Army, who's Consulting Surgeon, Colonel H.M.W. Gray, was noted since 1916 for his work in the treatment of compound gunshot fractures. His memoranda, issued by the Third Army in 1917, formed the basis of the frontline surgical practice of this and other armies. His well-known book, *The Early Treatment of War Wounds*, published at the end of 1918, epitomised the advancing knowledge of that period. His lectures given at Louvencourt were attended by all our medical officers in turn: the problems of shock prevention at the RAP and ADS, the best

> method of splinting fractures and the demonstration of the regulation set of splints now carried in racks by each motor ambulance, formed the basis of these lectures.[53]

Following the 1919 publication of *The Early Treatment of War Wounds* – based on a series of scientific papers written and published during the war – Gray crossed swords with Sir Anthony Bowlby when the latter attempted to discredit the evidence for the very high mortality rate of compound fractures of the femur in the early years of the conflict, declaring it to have been only 16 percent at casualty clearing stations during 1915.[54] Gray issued an extremely robust response in the *British Medical Journal*, which criticised the inaccurate and misleading figures Bowlby had employed in arriving at the mortality rate of 16 percent.[55] He pointed out that Bowlby's figures had been based on data in admission books at casualty clearing stations. The diagnoses entered in these books were frequently inaccurate, especially during battle periods. At the three casualty clearing stations used by Bowlby in his series, only 141 cases of fractured femur were recorded. There were 23 deaths, giving a mortality of 16 percent. This was a much smaller number of fractures than would have been expected to occur during the period, given the total number of casualties admitted. The accepted incidence of the wound was one case per 50 to 60 admissions. Bowlby should have had an additional 500 cases on which to base his mortality assessment. Gray concluded that Bowlby's figures were extremely flawed, having been based on inaccurate data and he had probably missed 500 cases which should have been included. Gray had assessed his mortality percentage on a careful study of all cases.

Gray went on to say that it was a pity Bowlby had attempted to diminish appreciation of the excellent progress which had been made in the handling of such cases:

> Had his remarks gone unchallenged, then those who had not given serious consideration to the matter would receive a wrong impression of the appalling seriousness of this injury, especially in the early years of the war.[56]

In a subsequent publication Bowlby contradicted himself when he claimed that during the German Spring Offensive of 1918, French soldiers with inadequately splinted fractures had arrived at British casualty clearing stations in a state of severe shock and many had died, while British casualties with effectively splinted fractures arriving at the same medical facilities were in a much better clinical condition thanks to effective immobilisation of fractures using Thomas Splints.[57]

Gray often failed to get on with his contemporaries, which may have hampered the general acceptance of his innovative measures. He was undoubtedly admired by young surgeons working

53 Carberry, A.D., *The New Zealand medical Services in the Great War* (Auckland: Whitcombe and Tombs Ltd, 1924), p. 399.
54 Bowlby, A., The Mortality of Cases of Fractured Femur, *British Medical Journal* 1: 3030 (25 January 1919), p. 112.
55 Gray, H.M.W., The Mortality of Cases of Fractured Femur. *British Medical Journal* 1:3031 (1 February 1919), p. 142.
56 Gray, *British Medical Journal* 1919; No. 1, p. 142.
57 Bowlby, A., Gunshot fractures of the femur, *British Medical Journal*, 1: 3079 (3 January 1920), pp. 1-4.

in casualty clearing stations because he was a great support to them, but he often antagonised his contemporaries by being very outspoken and confrontational.

In 1921, Gray delivered an address in Dundee entitled "*The application of the professional lessons of the war to civil work*," in which he said that his experience during the war led him to conclude that improvements in medical education were necessary to enable doctors to deal with war wounds more adequately in future conflicts.[58] With a better education, the average Scottish medical student would have 'greater prowess in the medical arenas of the world'. He conceded that he himself 'belonged to the ultimate division in the Sassenach classification of those north of the Tweed- the Scotsman, the damned Scotsman and the Aberdonian!'

For their part, prominent members of the surgical establishment did not hold Gray in high esteem. As one London professor observed:

> They wouldn't raise any flags for Gray in London. His support in the army had come from younger men. Gray found it difficult to get on with colleagues; he was too arbitrary; too impulsive; too dictatorial.[59]

Gray may well have been arbitrary, impulsive and dictatorial, but probably that was exactly what was needed to get things done when there were hundreds of casualties awaiting treatment. His junior staff looked to him for firm direction and advice and he was always to be found in the thick of things, getting on with the work and encouraging his younger colleagues, much to the displeasure of some of his contemporaries, it would seem.

After the war, Gray returned to Aberdeen but never settled. Then, in 1923, he was approached by Sir Henry Vincent Meredith, President of the Royal Victoria Hospital in Montreal, inviting him to take up the position of Surgeon-in-Chief at the RVH. Meredith also wanted Gray to be appointed to the Chair of Surgery at McGill University and to that end Meredith approached General Sir Arthur Currie, Principal and Vice-Chancellor at McGill to seek Currie's agreement to his proposal. Currie, who had led the Canadian Corps most successfully during the last 18 months of the war, was having none of it. He did not think Gray was a suitable candidate for the Chair of Surgery and made his position very clear. Gray became embroiled in bitter political infighting between Meredith and Currie and was eventually forced to resign from his position at RVH on 29 September 1925. He ended his career working in private practice in Montreal where he died on 7 October 1938.

Conclusion

A great deal of progress was made in the surgical management of all types of wounds during the four years of the Great War. Soldiers with musculoskeletal wounds, wounds of the skull and brain and penetrating wounds of the chest and abdomen stood a much better chance of survival by 1918. Early wound excision played a vital role in reducing the incidence of major

58 Gray, H.M.W., An address on the application of the professional lessons of the war to civil work, *British Medical Journal*, 1:3134 (22 January 1921), pp.109-14.

59 Scotland, T., Boyer, A., *Henry Gray: Surgeon of the Great War: Saving lives in a theatre of destruction* (Edinburgh: Capercaillie Books, 2015), p. 118.

wound infections and death from overwhelming sepsis, while arrest of life-threatening haemorrhage was of utmost importance in saving lives by helping to prevent surgical (wound) shock. As techniques in resuscitation improved, cases presenting late at casualty clearing stations in a collapsed state and suffering from wound shock were first taken to a resuscitation ward before going to the operating theatre. Warmth, absolute rest, sedatives such as omnopon, a derivative of morphine and transfusion of Gum Arabica and/or blood were employed to resuscitate and stabilise the wounded. Sisters for the resuscitation ward were specially selected for their experience. Without restoration of blood pressure, the probability of surviving the anaesthetic and surgical procedure would be very low.[60] In 1918, Australian Medical Services established Field Ambulance Resuscitation Teams to deliver life-saving medical care at main or even at advanced dressing stations of field ambulances and this is discussed in the next chapter.

60 Gray, H.M.W., *The Early Treatment of War Wounds* (London: Henry Frowde and Hodder & Stoughton, 1919), pp. 73-79.

8

The response of Australian Medical Services to the restoration of mobile warfare in 1918: the triumph of Field Ambulance Resuscitation Teams

Sounds by Night
I hear the dull low thunder of the guns
Beyond the hills that dose uneasily,
A sullen doomful growl that ever runs
From end to end of the heavy freighted sky:
A friend of mine writes squatted on the floor,
And scrapes by yellow, spluttering candlelight.
'Ah hush! He breathes and gazes at the door,
That creaks on rusty hinge in pale affright!
No word spoke he, nor I, for well we knew
What rueful things these sounds did tell.
A pause–I hear the trees sway, sighing thro'
The gloom, like dismal moan of hollow knell.
Then out across the dark and startling me
Burst forth a laugh, a shout of drunken glee.
Roderick Watson Kerr, MC (1893-1960)

At 0440 on 21 March 1918, the Germans began an overwhelming artillery barrage from the Hindenburg Line between Cambrai in the north and St Quentin in the south which lasted for five hours. It was directed against the British Third Army to the north and Fifth Army to the south, the latter occupying a front of 42 miles. This was the start of the Kaiserschlacht, the Kaiser's Battle, codenamed Operation Michael, and was the brainchild of General Erich Ludendorff, First Quartermaster General of the German Armies. His aim was to smash through the British lines and bring a speedy conclusion to the war before the United States of America had mobilised sufficiently to bring an unlimited supply of men and materials to the Western Front.

The British Fifth Army was in a much-weakened state because of heavy losses sustained during the Third Battle of Ypres in 1917 and consisted of only 12 divisions. There were three German Armies, the 17th in the north near Cambrai, the 2nd in the centre and the 18th in the south around St Quentin. At 0940 the German infantry attacked. The southern flank of the German 2nd Amy and the German 18th Army attacked the British Fifth Army and broke

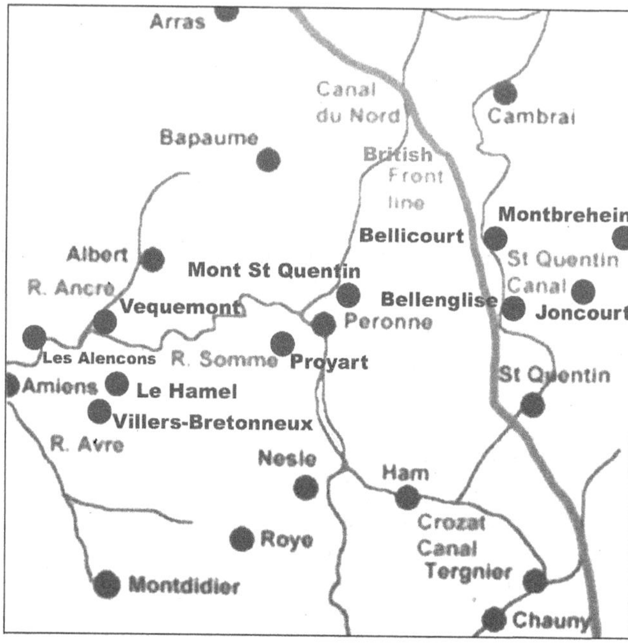

Figure 8.1 Map of River Somme and its associated canals; the British front line on 21 March 1918 is represented by the heavy line running approximately north to south. The St Quentin Canal to its immediate east was an integral part of the Hindenburg Line. (With thanks to Stuart King)

through its Forward Zone positions with ease and were quickly well inside or across the Battle Zone. Matters were made more difficult because at the start of the attack there was dense fog, enabling German storm troops to overwhelm British positions before the defenders realised what was happening.

Casualty Clearing Station 5 (Chapter 7) was at the village of Tincourt roughly midway between Péronne and the Hindenburg Line and was in the path of the attacking German hordes. A young machine gun officer with the rank of temporary major called Lionel Whitby was admitted to CCS 5 with a very severe lower limb wound caused by shellfire. His general condition was poor and Major Gordon-Taylor gave him a life-saving blood transfusion prior to performing a very high thigh amputation. This was the start of a life-long friendship between the two men. Whitby mastered his serious physical disability and studied medicine after the war. He became a pathologist, specialising in haematology. At the outbreak of the Second World War, Whitby was invited to organize the Transfusion Service for the British Army and he established its headquarters at the Army Blood Supply Depot at Bristol. He supplied ¾ million units of blood. His outstanding achievement was summed up by a quotation in his obituary in the Journal of the Royal Army Medical Corps taken from *History of the Second World War-Surgery*:

> One outstanding reason for the greatly improved results of treatment of casualties in the war of 1939-45 was the fact that the restoration of the general condition of the wounded man was made possible by the ready availability of blood (or its derivatives) which could be transferred into the circulation of the patient.[1]

1 Obituary, Lionel Ernest Howard Whitby, C.V.O., M.C., M.A., M.D., F.R.C.P., Hon.D.Sc. (Toronto), Hon.LL.D.(Glasg.), -Hon.M.D.(Louvain), D.P.H., *Journal Royal Army Medical Corps*, Vol. 103 (1 April 1957), pp. 102-03.

In 1945, Lionel Whitby became Regius Professor of Physic at Cambridge University and was knighted. He was Vice-Chancellor of the University from 1951 to 1953 and bestowed an Honorary Doctorate of Science on Gordon-Taylor, the surgeon who saved his life.

Casualty Clearing Station Number 5 soon made ready to pull back because the Fifth Army was forced to withdraw to the rear zone which was practically non-existent. By the end of the day, General Sir Hubert Gough, Commanding Officer of the Fifth Army ordered a withdrawal to behind the River Somme and Crozat Canal.

To the north around Cambrai, the German 17th Army was less successful and was slowed down and sometimes brought to a standstill in front of Third Army Battle Zone positions. Ludendorff's original plan was for the 2nd and 17th Armies to break through and turn north, rolling up the British line, while the 18th Army to the south prevented any French intervention, but things did not go according to plan. The failure of the right wing of Michael near Cambrai meant there was no rolling up of the British line by the 2nd Army as anticipated. On the following day, 22 March, Ludendorff instructed his right wing to carry on battering against Third Army defences, while in the south the 18th Army continued to smash its way forwards against the British Fifth Army while at the same time separating the British from adjacent French forces. The Germans had created a forty-mile-wide breech in the Fifth Army defences, but instead of exploiting this gap to the full, Ludendorff continued to make the 17th Army slog in the direction of Arras against stiff resistance, while the northern flank of his 2nd Army advanced in the direction of Albert. Only the successful 18th Army continued to push the British Fifth Army back and drive a wedge between it and the French to the south. Instead of employing one axis of attack, Ludendorff persevered with three, and in so doing lost his opportunity to destroy the British Fifth Army. The Germans of the 18th Army sustained many battle casualties which progressively weakened their ability to continue their attack and a contributory factor to their impending failure was the discovery that captured British positions had large food stores. In contrast, they had such meagre rations. What's more, the finding made them acutely conscious of the fact that their wives and children back in Germany were short of food and in some cases were starving to death. The overwhelming German destructive power of 21 March began to fade and with it loomed the failure of Operation Michael.[2] While the Germans weakened, the British began to stabilise their positions and were holding on.

By 25 March, only the 18th Army made progress towards Amiens. The 17th Army was exhausted and was at a standstill while the 2nd Army could get little further than Albert. Thanks to the timely arrival of the Australian 3rd and 4th Divisions, Field Marshal Sir Douglas Haig was confident of holding his ground north of the Somme, but the territory to the south of the river was a source of great anxiety. It had to be held at all costs to protect the vital railway junction of Amiens a few miles to the west.

Ludendorff himself was now under severe strain. The poor performance of the German 17th Army had ruined Operation Michael, and this enraged Ludendorff. By 27 March, the 17th Army had ground to a complete standstill and Ludendorff launched Operation Mars against Arras, while Operation Michael shrank to the capture of Amiens.[3] After heavy fighting on 4-5

2 Barnett, C., *The Sword Bearers: Studies in supreme command in the First World War* (London: Eyre and Spottiswoode, 1963), pp. 306-23.

3 Barnett, *The Sword Bearers*, p. 328.

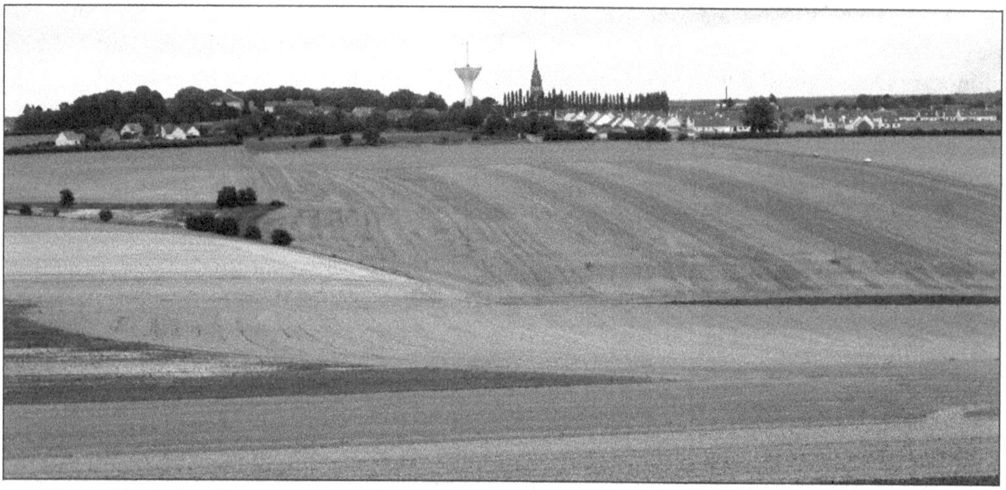

Figure 8.2 Villers-Bretonneux; the German advance along the Somme basin towards Amiens was brought to a standstill in front of this small town after heavy fighting 4-5 April 1918. Villers-Bretonneux stood between the Germans and Amiens fifteen miles beyond. (Author's photograph)

April 1918, the German 18th Army was stopped east of Villers-Bretonneux, a small town which stood between the Germans and Amiens fifteen miles beyond. Operation Michael was dead.

Ludendorff opened the second of his spring offensives, Operation Georgette, on 9 April 1918. This was directed against the British Second Army on Messines Ridge, with the aim of driving them off the ridge and then sweeping on to the railway junction of Hazebrouck twenty miles beyond. It too failed.

There were indications by 17 and 18 April that a German attack against Villers-Bretonneux was imminent as they continued with their efforts to capture Amiens beyond. The entire area around the town was drenched in mustard gas as the Germans prepared. It was around this area that Manfred von Richthofen, Germany's most famous flying ace, was killed, probably by a shot from the ground fired by an Australian machine gunner from a position near Corbie. On 24 April, the Germans attacked Villers-Bretonneux, using tanks for the second time in the war. A few had been used previously on 21 March 1918 to mop up remnant pockets of enemy soldiers.[4] The tanks smashed through British positions in dense fog and German infantry overwhelmed the defenders. Villers-Bretonneux fell to the Germans who began digging in on the precious heights beyond the town overlooking Amiens.

At 2200 on 24 April 1918, Australians from the 4th and 5th Divisions counter-attacked the Germans in Villers-Bretonneux in a pincer movement. The 4th Division went around the southern margin and the 5th Division round the northern margin of the town. By the following day they had surrounded Villers-Bretonneux and recaptured the town, although house to house fighting continued for another couple of days to clear out the last of the German occupants. The 2nd and 3rd Australian divisions transferred from positions north of the Somme, changing places with British III Corps which went north of the river. Four of the five Australian

4 Bean, C.E.W., *Anzac to Amiens* (Canberra: Australian War Memorial, 1946), pp. 430-31.

Divisions of the Australian Corps were now in position south of the Somme. Only their 1st Division for the time being was fighting with the British Second Army in the north five miles from Hazebrouck, although it would soon re-join the Corps on the Somme for the Battle of Amiens on 8 August 1918.

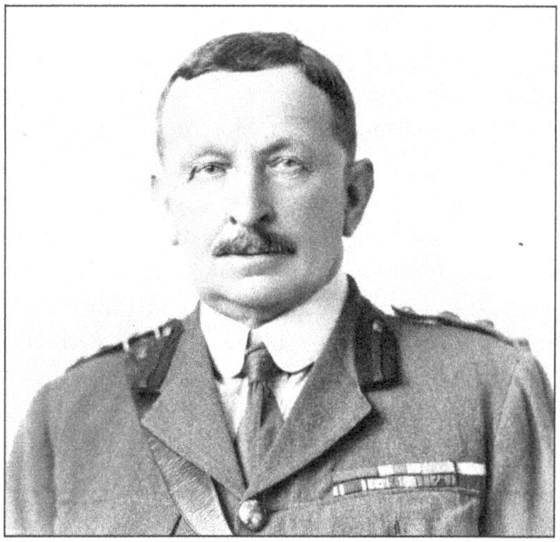

Figure 8.3 Colonel George Walter Barber (1868-1951), Deputy Director Medical Services for Australian Forces. (Courtesy Australian War Memorial, Canberra, Ref H 19364)

Colonel George Walter Barber (1868-1951) was appointed to the position of Deputy Director of Australian Medical Services on 8 April 1918 and was responsible for organising the Australian Medical Services for the five Australian Divisions in France. He had access to and was advisor to the Australian Corps Commander on medical matters and was answerable to General Sir Neville Howse VC, Director General of Army Medical Services for the Australian Imperial Force. When Barber was first appointed, General Birdwood was in command of the Australian Corps, but Birdwood was appointed to lead the British Fifth Army after General Sir Hubert Gough was sacked after being judged to be responsible for the Fifth Army's precipitous retreat in the face of Operation Michael. Lieutenant General Sir John Monash became commander of the Australian Corps on 1 June 1918.[5]

Barber was born in Lancashire, England, and graduated in medicine from London in 1891. He emigrated from England to Australia in 1895. In October 1914 he was appointed major in the Australian Imperial Force and served in Egypt and Gallipoli. He was promoted to Lieutenant-Colonel in January 1916 and went to France as Assistant Director of Medical Services to the 4th Australian Division. He served with distinction at Pozières and Mouquet Farm during the Battle of the Somme. He remained with the 4th Division in 1917 and served at Bullecourt, Messines Ridge and Passchendaele, being mentioned in dispatches three times.[6]

Barber's skills as an administrator were most fully appreciated when trench warfare gave way to mobile warfare during the spring of 1918, when Barber realised that mobile warfare was there to stay, and he prepared to institute whatever measures were necessary to ensure the smooth and rapid evacuation of casualties. He declared:

> It seemed obvious that we had done with stationary warfare and that we should be engaged in mobile warfare-advance or retreat. It was therefore urgently necessary to make arrangements in preparation.[7]

5 Serle, G., *Monash, Sir John (1865-1931)*, Australian Dictionary of Biography, Vol. 10, (MUP), 1986.

6 Land, W., *Barber, George Walter (1868-1961)*, Australian Dictionary of Biography, Volume 7, (MUP), 1979.

7 Butler, A.G., *Official History of the Australian Army Medical Services, 1914–1918 Volume II – The Western Front* (Canberra: Australian War Memorial, 1940), p. 653.

Barber's preparations included the co-ordination of medical services to make them more mobile and flexible and better able to combat the long distances to casualty clearing stations. His administrative staff had a very good working relationship with the executive units, they being the Regimental Medical Establishment, the Field Ambulances and the Sanitary Sections. Barber encouraged an exchange of ideas, so that administrative and executive units felt free to discuss matters and develop initiatives. He paid particular attention to the organisation of the Sanitary Sections and he altered their status to make them more effective in combating disease, thereby reducing non-battle casualty wastage, dysentery in particular. Between 21 March and 7 May 1918, the Australians had sustained 15,083 battle casualties and 14,000 non-battle casualties. By the end of May, recruiting in Australia had reduced to less than 2,000 per month and Australian depots in Britain were unable to keep pace. Three battalions were disbanded and there was a threat that others would follow. It was therefore essential to keep numbers up and Barber recognised that Sanitary Sections had a vital role to play in minimising losses from disease. Over some considerable time, Sanitary Sections had become mere technicians and were suppliers and installers of sanitary appliances, which was a waste of their skills. Their role should have been an advisory one to instruct executive officers in good practice, leaving others to do the physical labour. Barber ensured that this happened, and also that Sanitary Sections advanced with the infantry units and were not stuck miles behind the front line. The following standing order was issued:

> To rectify a prevailing misapprehension, a Sanitary Section is not responsible for, and is not in a position to carry out, the provision and distribution of the various sanitary appliances that are necessary in an area. Every unit must be able to maintain satisfactory sanitation with improvised appliances until more permanent structures can be supplied.[8]

Partly as a result of the efforts of the Sanitary Sections to minimise non-battle casualty losses, the Australians did not have to disband any more battalions. Barbour's skills as an administrator are reminiscent of those of Sir James McGrigor during the Peninsular War, who as a result of his successful efforts to reduce wastage from disease during the winter of 1812-13, enabled Sir Arthur Wellesley (later Duke of Wellington) to continue to wage war against the French. No other British figure during the 19th century had McGrigor's outstanding administrative abilities.

Three major problems concerning the treatment of wounded were identified which required to be addressed following the resumption of mobile warfare in 1918 and innovative measures were introduced to solve them. The first was that dressing stations which were suitable for static warfare were simply no longer fit for purpose. Figure 8.4 is Essex Farm Advanced Dressing Station on the Ypres to Yser Canal near Ypres, which dealt with wounded during the Third Battle of Ypres in 1917. Set in concrete to protect medical personnel and wounded, it was quite obviously useless for mobile warfare.

Australian medical personnel developed a standardised advanced dressing station (Figure 8.5). Work on the design began in May 1918 and was completed by July. It was easily reproducible and was made in pre-fabricated sections which could be quickly assembled and disassembled. When the infantry attacked, the advanced dressing station became the main dressing station, and a new advanced dressing station was transported forward using three lorries. Just as infantry brigades leapfrogged one another as they attacked, so too did the advanced dressing stations to

8 Butler, *Official History Vol. II*, p. 654.

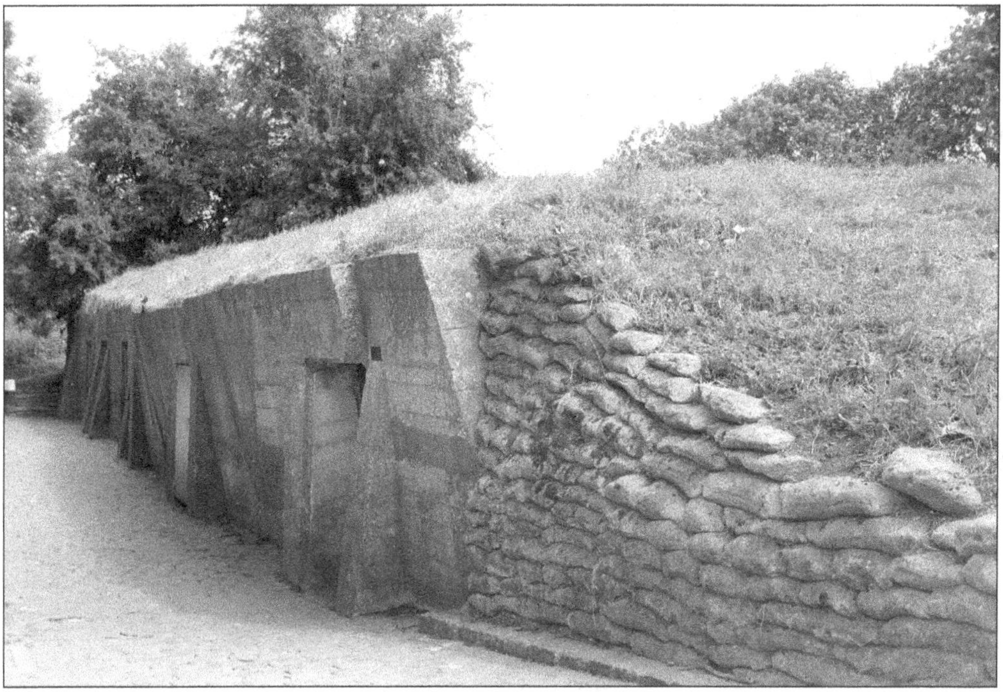

Figure 8.4 Essex Farm Advanced Dressing Station situated on Ypres to Yser Canal approximately two miles from Ypres. (Author's photograph)

remain in contact with their respective brigades. The prototype standardised advanced dressing station was on a very exposed section of road and had been built into a hillside with considerable effort. It was decided this was unnecessary for general purposes, and all that was required was to rivet the walls with sandbags up to half way to counter the effect of 'daisy cutters', which were high explosive shells used frequently by the Germans in 1918 and which sent shrapnel flying out horizontally as the name suggests.

There was a spacious operating theatre within the dressing hut, which as you will soon discover was used by the Field Ambulance Resuscitation Teams (see below) to resuscitate badly wounded patients and to carry out limb and life-saving surgery.

Looking first towards the right of Figure 8.5, there was a rectangular stretcher shelter, an entrance and a tented receiving room. The patient then went to the left along a covered way to a large dressing hut. When there, he had appropriate treatment administered, before he continued his journey to the left and out of the dressing hut. There was a reciprocating windlass at each end of the dressing hut which helped with the admission and discharge of patients. On the far left of the ADS was an evacuation room, from where patients were loaded onto ambulance wagons and taken on their way along the evacuation pathway. A gas treatment room had to be added since there were many gassed cases in 1918:

> On the night of July 16th-17th the enemy threw about 6,000 gas shells on the 2nd Division's front, producing some 200 casualties; again, on July 22nd-23rd about 9,000 shells caused

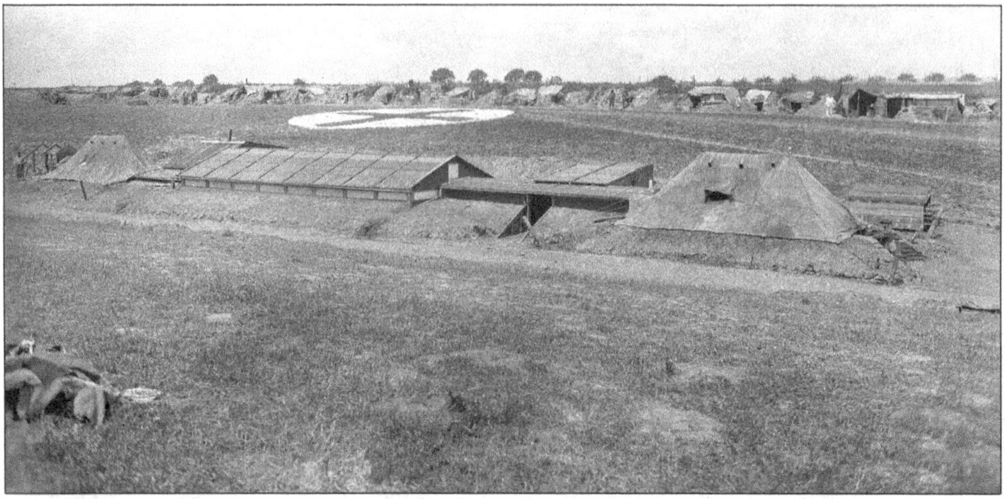

Figure 8.5 Australian Standardised Advanced Dressing Station developed in response to restoration of mobile warfare. It could be transported forwards in three transport lorries and quickly assembled in a suitable location close to the new front line. (Courtesy Australian War Memorial, Canberra, Ref EO 3904)

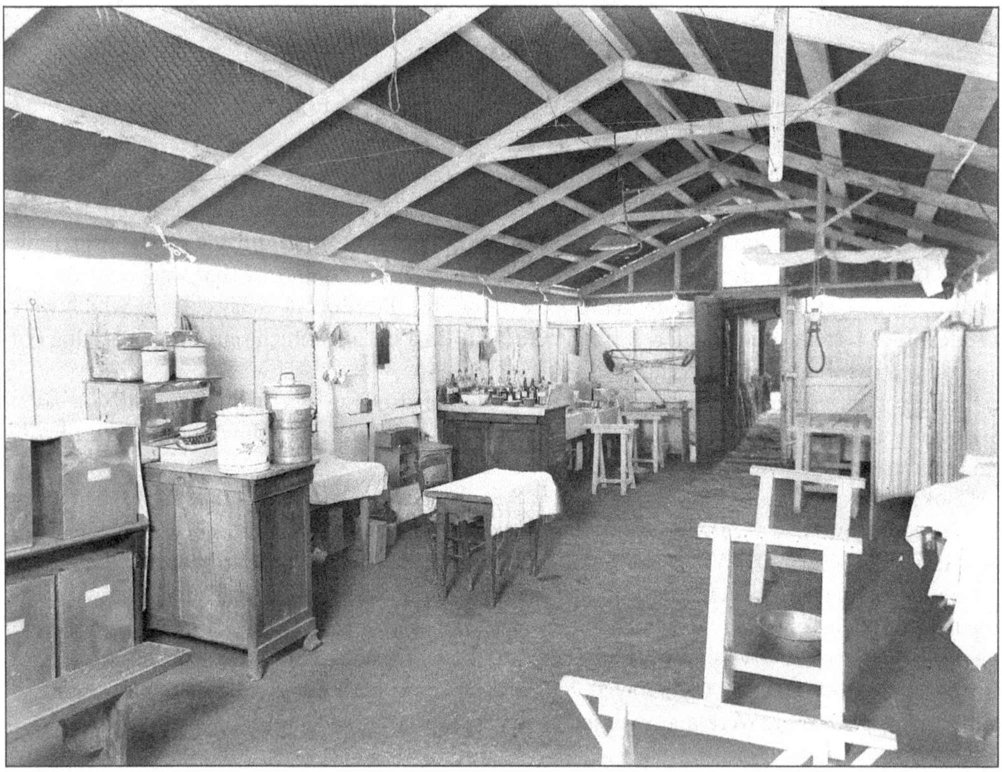

Figure 8.6 Operating theatre within the dressing hut of the Standardised Advanced Dressing Station; this facility was used frequently to carry out urgent surgical procedures between July and September 1918. (Courtesy Australian War Memorial, Canberra, Ref EO 2771)

> some 450 casualties. In each case a few "Blue Cross" shells were first thrown in order to cause sneezing and deaden the sense of smell, and they were followed by "Yellow Cross" containing dichlorethyl-sulphide ("mustard gas"). The nights selected were slightly wet, and misty.[9]

Table 8.1 summarises gassing casualties for 1918. The figures come from the Official History of the Australian Medical Services.[10]

Table 8.1 Australian admissions with acute gas poisoning 1918.

	Total number admitted	**Died**	**Percentage mortality**
Australian gas poisoning admissions during 1918	12,025	221	1.8

Butler, A.G., *Official History of the Australian Army Medical Services, 1914–1918, Volume III – Special Problems and Services,* (Canberra: Australian War Memorial, 1943), p. 896.

The second major problem confronting the medical services was one of distance. During almost four years of static warfare, experience had shown that there were only sufficient ambulance wagons to transport stretcher cases to main dressing stations and casualty clearing stations. Walking wounded had made their way back on foot, which was only possible because of the short distances involved. Any rapid, significant advance meant that the distance to casualty clearing stations in the rear was too great for walking wounded to manage on foot. To deal with this problem, full advantage was taken of returning empty ammunition wagons to transport the walking wounded back towards the casualty clearing stations. Where ammunition convoy routes separated from casualty evacuation pathways, an ambulance depot was established where the routes diverged. These depots were christened Corps Relay Posts. Each was run by one tent subdivision of a field ambulance. Corps Relay Posts were too far in the rear to be administered by an Assistant Director of Medical Services (ADMS) and Barber in his capacity as DDMS was responsible for them. They often functioned effectively as a main dressing station for walking wounded. As Barber later observed:

> Full advantage was taken of returning ammunition transport but, as the ammunition railheads did not coincide with the location of the Casualty Clearing Stations, it was found necessary to establish ambulance posts where the routes diverged: one ambulance post each for the right and left sectors. These were christened Corps Relay Posts, and had establishment of one tent sub-division, with transport; they were administered by the DDMS, as they were too far in rear of their respective ADMS. Walking wounded were debussed here (removed from the lorries) and proceeded to Casualty Clearing Stations by lorries or buses obtained from the Army and kept at the Post for this purpose; this plan worked very well.[11]

9 Butler, *Official History Vol. II*, p. 676.

10 Butler, A.G., *Official History of the Australian Army Medical Services, 1914–1918 Vol. III – Special Problems and Services* (Canberra: Australian war Memorial, 1943), p. 896.

11 Butler, *Official History Vol. II*, pp. 657-58.

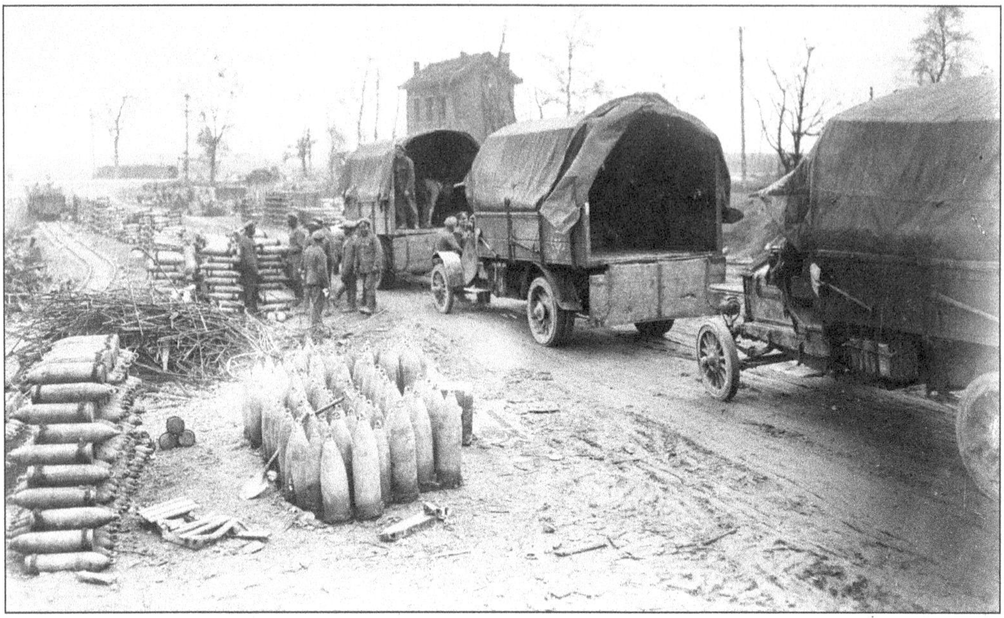

Figure 8.7 Transport wagons at ammunition dumps; Australians used empty returning wagons to transport walking wounded to Corps Relay Posts which were strategically positioned where evacuation pathways for the wounded diverged from routes to ammunition railheads. (Courtesy Imperial War Museum, London, Ref Q010451)

The purpose of the Corps Relay Posts was to evacuate the less severely walking wounded back to casualty clearing stations for surgery as quickly as possible. Just because they were less severely wounded did not exclude them from getting into trouble and their wounds had to be dealt with quickly and efficiently to minimise the risk of infection.

The third major problem was also one of distance, since the German advance on 21 March 1918 had resulted in many casualty clearing stations being located much further behind the lines than they might otherwise have been and consequently it took far too long to reach them. At the same time, there was a growing awareness of the importance of early resuscitation and surgery to significantly reduce the probability of many of the limb and life-threatening pyogenic infections (streptococcal and staphylococcal) and anaerobic infections (gas gangrene and tetanus) seen all too often in the earlier years of the war. There was a clear need for effective resuscitation and expert surgical care to be delivered by personnel of field ambulances, providing life saving treatment much sooner than was currently available.

Dr Alan Worsley Holmes à Court (1887-1957) was born in Brisbane in 1887. He studied medicine at Sydney University from where he graduated in 1911. During the war, Holmes à Court served as a captain with the Australian Army Medical Corps in the hospital ship, *Karoola* between1916 and 1917. He was then posted to the 2nd Australian General Hospital in France and promoted major on 28 January 1918. In May 1918, he transferred to the 4th Australian Field Ambulance at a time when mobile warfare had been restored.

Towards the end of June 1918, Holmes à Court was influential in improving the management of patients in field ambulances when he introduced a Field Ambulance Resuscitation Team.

He was inspired after he visited the nearby British Third Army Casualty Clearing Station No 3 at Gézaincourt, where Consulting Surgeon Henry Gray had established a shock centre in 1917. Gray had a great deal of knowledge about the clinical aspects of shock as a result of his extensive experience in dealing with compound fractures of the femur and was on the MRC Shock Advisory Committee, which consisted of clinicians, physiologists and scientists whose aim was to gain a better understanding of the aetiology and management of wound shock. As discussed in Chapter 6, the day to day running of the shock centre at Gézaincourt was in the hands of Captain Kenneth Walker, and thanks to Walker it became a Mecca for front line medical officers, including a number from the near-by Australian Corps attached to the British Fourth Army.[12]

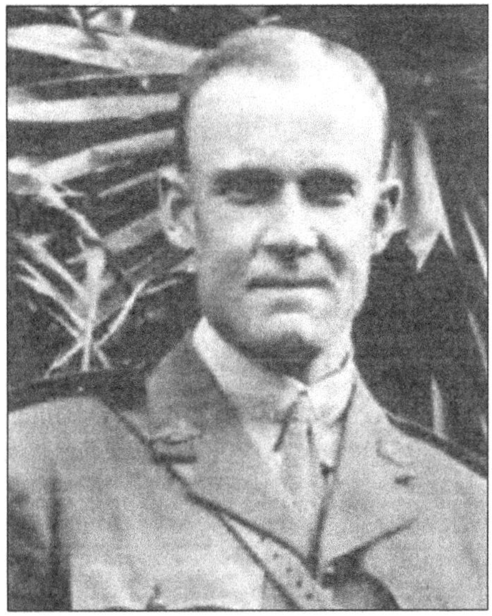

Figure 8.8 Dr Alan Worsley Holmes à Court (1887-1957). (Private collection)

Captain Walker possessed a tremendous enthusiasm for his work which inspired others. He felt it was a joy to see a badly wounded man revive miraculously after a blood transfusion and to watch him regain consciousness as he 'came back to life'. At first, back in 1915, life- saving transfusion was only performed at base hospitals, then by 1917 at casualty clearing stations. Surely it should be made available in more forward positions too.[13]

The American, Dr Oswald Hope Robertson spent time at CCS 3 and provided invaluable aid to the shock centre at Gézaincourt with his experience and expertise in the administration of blood transfusion using preserved blood. Within a short time, a small blood bank was established where a number of bottles of Group IV (Group O) blood were prepared and stored in a cool dugout at CCS 3 and ready for emergencies. All that was required when a patient required immediate transfusion was to take the necessary steps described in Chapter 6 to bring the suspension back to the original volume of the blood from which the red corpuscles had been derived. Walker noted:

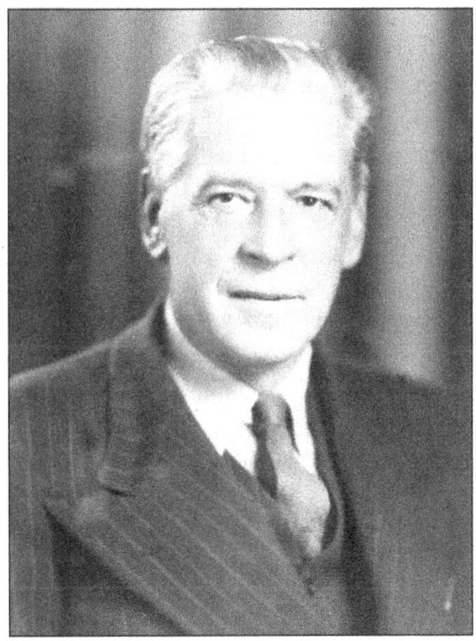

Figure 8.9 Kenneth Walker (1882-1966) in later life. (Courtesy Wellcome Library, London)

12 Butler, *Official History Vol. II*, pp. 662-63.
13 Walker, K., *The Story of Blood*, (London: Herbert Jenkins Ltd., 1958), pp. 144-45.

> Transfusion for us had now become almost as simple a procedure as the injection of a normal saline solution into a vein and opened up all sorts of wonderful new possibilities. An ambitious scheme began to take shape in the writer's mind, namely, that of pushing transfusion right forward into the trenches. There was no reason why many badly wounded men should not thereby be saved. I had a wooden box constructed capable of accommodating two large jars of preserved corpuscles and this could be slung by means of a broad leather strap from my shoulders.[14]

Walker decided it would be an excellent idea to present himself in front line trenches with his preserved blood at the time of trench raids. He spoke to a friendly and accommodating Brigadier about his idea and was furnished with the necessary authority and information. From time to time, messages would appear for Walker at CCS 3 saying 'For the attention of Captain KM Walker; tea party at 2000, Thursday 15 October, plenty of spoons and mugs will be required'. There would be an attached map reading and Walker would know where and when to report with the blood. He would set off on the appointed day, at first by ambulance wagon and then on foot, calling at battalion headquarters on the way. Trench raids nearly always took place at night and finding his way in the fading light was not always straightforward. Sometimes he even fell in with the men who were going on the raid, their faces and hands blackened in preparation for what was to come. Walker would stay with them in the trench as they waited till it was time to go over. All regimental badges and other identifying features were removed. There were always wounds to be treated when the survivors came back, whether or not transfusion was needed. Walker said that the physical impact of transfusion was less than he had hoped for, because he only transfused corpuscles, there being no facilities to make up the volume of blood with saline. The psychological benefit, on the other hand, was notable. News of his arrival spread rapidly round the trench and had an excellent effect on the morale of the raiding party: "There's a bloke arrived from GHQ who pumps blood into you and brings you back to life, even after you're dead."[15]

Walker took his idea of blood transfusion with preserved blood to the Shock Committee in London (Chapter 6). He took a bottle of blood from CCS 3 in a cool box with him. The journey took 48 hours, and the red blood corpuscles reached London in good condition. Walker declared that a transfusion service was a necessary step to improve the management of the severely wounded. He suggested that a public appeal could be made for donors. Even King George V might consider donating a pint, as might Miss Gladys Cooper, Walker's favourite stage actress. Their respective contributions would set great examples to the general public:

> And think, I said, waxing enthusiastic, think of the thrill of the wounded officer who awakes from shock knowing that the blood of Gladys Cooper is coursing through his veins.[16]

The Royal Air Force (RAF), formed on 1 April 1918 by the amalgamation of the Royal Flying Corps and the Royal Naval Air Service, could transport the preserved blood in cool boxes to

14 Walker, *The Story of Blood,* p. 148.
15 Walker, *The Story of Blood,* p. 148.
16 Walker, K., *I talk of Dreams: An experiment in autobiography* (London: Jonathan Cape, 1946), p. 198.

France. This idea, however, was never put into practice because the German Spring Offensive began just as Walker returned to France and the British Fifth Army was thrown back towards Amiens. Other matters took priority and Walker's ambitious concept of a large blood bank based in Britain had to be put on hold indefinitely. It would be the next generation of enterprising clinicians in World War II who would establish blood banks on such a grand scale.

It is little wonder that Henry Gray referred to Walker in glowing terms in his book *The Early Treatment of War Wounds.* There were so many young medical officers who had made so many outstanding contributions to the treatment of the wounded, that it would be impossible to name them all. Gray continued:

> I am sure no one will take umbrage when I make an exception by mentioning Captain K.M. Walker, whose work in the forward areas has been of such a pioneer kind, so good, so unassuming and so helpful to wounded men and medical officers alike.[17]

It is very easy to understand why Holmes a Court found Captain Walker to be such an inspirational figure and returned to his unit after visiting Walker at CCS 3, full of ideas about what he might do to develop and improve the management of wounded soldiers by the Australian Medical Services.

On 24 June at Daours, there was an incident which acted as a catalyst for the formation of a Field Ambulance Resuscitation Team, when the Assistant Director of Medical Services (ADMS) of the 4th Australian Division, Colonel AH Mosely, was wounded in the leg by a fragment of high explosive shell which severed his posterior tibial artery, one of three major vessel supplying blood to the leg and foot. His wound bled profusely, and a tourniquet was applied to stop the haemorrhage and to prevent exsanguination of the patient. He was evacuated to the main dressing station at les Alençons, where unfortunately the surgical expertise to expose and tie off the bleeding vessel was not available, and Mosely was evacuated to a casualty clearing station at Crouy 11 miles away with the tourniquet still inflated. The journey was over rough and overcrowded roads and it took several hours. It has already been pointed out that many casualty clearing stations were further back than they otherwise might have been because British medical authorities were very cautious after the rapid German advance during Operation Michael which forced casualty clearing stations to stop work, pack up and then fall back to new and safer locations. The capture of CCS 37 by the Germans on 27 May 1918 made authorities even more nervous (Chapter 3). By the time the tourniquet was eventually removed several hours later it was too late to save Colonel Moseley's leg, which had had the circulation cur off for so long that it required an amputation.[18]

Evidence was also emerging that serious delay in reaching casualty clearing stations was having a major adverse impact on the general condition of some of the patients. For 85% of the wounded reaching the CCS, there was no adverse effect. These men arrived in good clinical condition and were able to proceed with surgery straight away. However, 10% of patients reached the CCS in reversible shock and had to be resuscitated with intravenous gum or with blood transfusion before proceeding with surgery. Furthermore, 5% reached the CCS in irreversible

17 Gray, H.M.W., *The Early Treatment of War Wounds* (London: Henry Frowde, Hodder and Stoughton, 1919), p. xi.

18 Butler, *Official History Vol. II*, pp. 662-663.

shock, which meant that despite all measures taken to try and improve their general condition and to raise their blood pressure by transfusion, nothing worked, and they all died. [19]

Table 8.2 Impact of a 6-9 hour journey to a casualty clearing station on the general condition of the wounded.

Condition of Patient	Percentage
A No Appreciable Hardship	85
B Reversible Shock	10
C Irreversible Shock	5

Butler, A.G., *Official History of the Australian Medical Services, 1914-1918, Volume II, – The Western Front* (Canberra: Australian War Memorial, 1940), pp. 956-57.

Group B patients would have benefitted from earlier intervention and some of Group C patients might have survived.

It is very likely that had resuscitative measures been instituted sooner, all the patients in the reversible shock group would have benefitted from earlier intervention and some of those in irreversible shock might have survived, because had they been seen sooner, the shock might still have responded to resuscitative measures including blood transfusion. The length of time a patient is in shock is critical, and if the blood pressure remains low for too long, it fails to respond to all resuscitative measures and the patient goes into a state of irreversible multiple organ failure and dies.

Following the unfortunate incident with Dr Mosely, an unofficial Field Ambulance Resuscitation Team was established, mainly as a result of the drive of Holmes à Court. Much of the equipment necessary for the successful operation of the team was supplied by Captain Walker at CCS 3, including serum for the typing of donors, gum and glucose solutions. The scheme was approved by General Howse, Director General of Army Medical Services for the Australian Imperial Force and ratified by Lieutenant-General Monash. The Senior Consulting Surgeon to the BEF, Sir Anthony Bowlby was very supportive of the idea, as were Major George Gask and later Major Gordon Gordon-Taylor, Consulting Surgeons to the British Fourth Army, both of whom were helpful in overcoming official inertia in the matter of army supplies. The first official Field Ambulance Resuscitation Team was ready to go into action at the Battle of Hamel on 4 July 1918.

The Battle of Hamel: a triumph for early resuscitation and surgery

The Battle of Hamel was a limited engagement and the first commanded by Lieutenant General Sir John Monash. His force was originally composed of Australians from the 2nd, 4th and 5th Divisions and 10 companies of the American 33rd Division. Unfortunately, General Pershing, the American Expeditionary Force (AEF) commander, had not been

19 Butler, *Official History Vol. II*, pp. 956-957.

informed about the proposed attack and had not given his permission for American soldiers to take part. Six American companies were withdrawn on 3 July, but because it was too late to withdraw the remaining four, they were allowed to go forward with the Australians.[20] The Battle of Hamel was fought along a front of 6,000 yards and penetrated to a maximum depth of 4,000 yards. Sixty tanks took part and they advanced immediately behind the artillery barrage alongside the leading waves of infantry, who also had air support from the RAF. The attack began at 0310 and by 0500 Australian soldiers had reached the final line to the east of le Hamel (Figure 8.10).

Figure 8.11 demonstrates the same position to the east of le Hamel today. Villers Bretonneux is just beyond the hill on the skyline to the left of the photograph

Holmes à Court's Field Ambulance Resuscitation Team was based at the main dressing station at les Alençons (Figure 8.1). The team consisted of one medical officer proficient in war surgery and blood transfusion and a second expert in the administration of nitrous oxide/oxygen anaesthesia and general resuscitation. There was an NCO and three orderlies who had been specially trained for the work. Operative work was restricted to urgent surgical procedures, such as ligation of bleeding major vessels and amputations of mangled and unsalvageable limbs.[21] Resuscitation was begun by infusion of glucose solution, Gum Acacia (Arabica) and sodium bicarbonate. Blood transfusion could be administered in three ways. Fresh blood could be obtained by using donors who were lightly wounded casualties or preserved blood could be employed, although Holmes à Court found the complicated mechanism involved to make it ready for transfusion was rather awkward in the bustling environment of a busy dressing station. He much preferred using stored citrated blood, which was prepared an hour or two before by removing blood from a typed donor and transferring it directly into a bottle containing an isotonic sodium citrate solution. The preparation did not involve any complex reconstitution to make it available, and provided the blood was used within two hours it fulfilled its role very well.[22] Equipment included appropriate surgical instruments, gas-oxygen apparatus, blood transfusion sets including grouping apparatus and six Kimpton Brown Flasks for fresh blood transfusion (Figure 8.12). A Kimpton Brown Flask consisted of a glass tube with a cannula drawn out at one end. This could be inserted into the donor's vein and placed in such a position that blood would run into it and then lain so that the blood would not escape. When inserted into the recipient's vein and held upright the blood would then enter the circulation. The flasks were autoclaved for sterility and liquid paraffin was used to lubricate the inside of the tube and prevent blood from clotting.

Holmes à Court devised a much simpler method to prevent blood clotting. He dissolved flakes of wax in ether, which was then poured into the flask. When the ether evaporated there was a thin coating of wax on all the surfaces of the flask.[23]

20 Bean, *Anzac to Amiens*, pp. 460-61.
21 Butler, *Official History Vol. II*, p. 954.
22 Holmes à Court, A., Intravenous Injections in the treatment of haemorrhage and shock, *The Medical Journal of Australia*, Vol. II, No. 3 (17 July 1920), pp. 49-56.
23 Westhorpe, R., The introduction of a mobile resuscitation service-1918, in Fink, B.R., LE Morris L.E. and Stephen, C.R (eds.), *The History of Anaesthesia: Third International Symposium* (Illinois: Wood Library, Museum of Anaesthesiology, 1992), pp. 438-438.

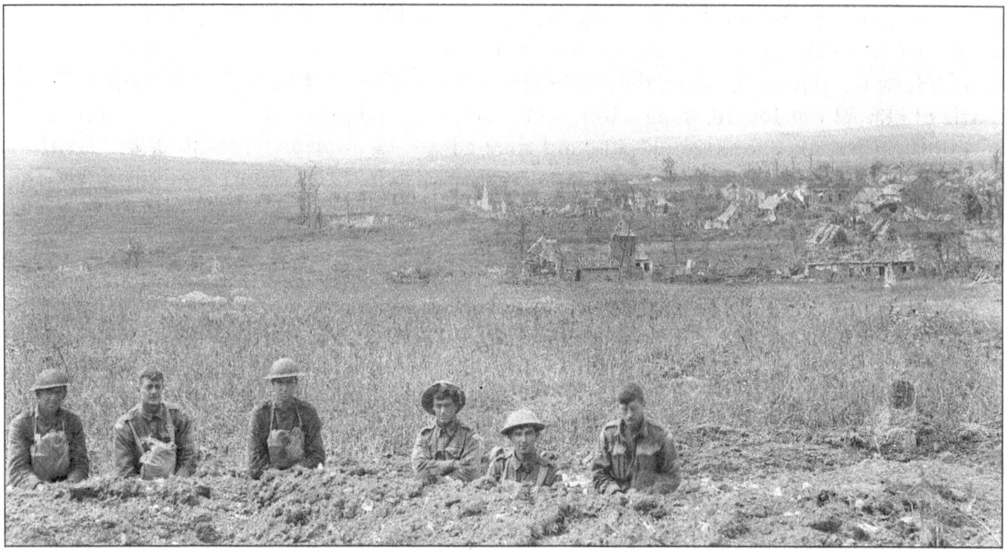

Figure 8.10 Australian soldiers at their final positions following the Battle of Hamel on 4 July 1918. The ruins of the village of le Hamel are behind them. Their starting line was level with the ruins of Villers-Bretonneux, which cannot be seen, but are beyond the hill on the left of the photograph. (Courtesy Australian War Memorial, Canberra, Ref EO 2844A)

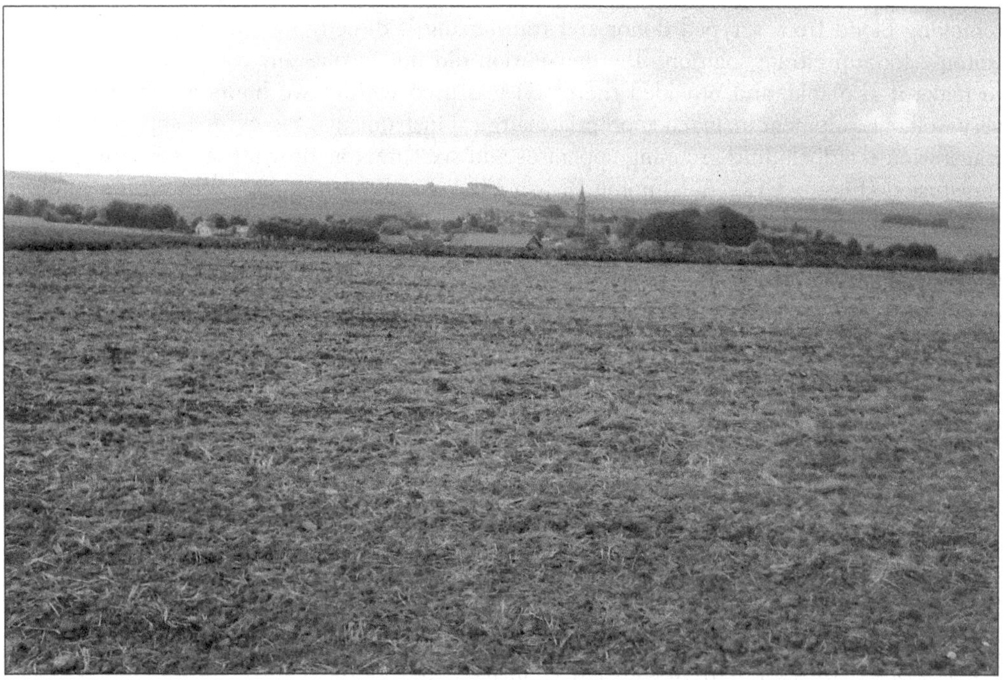

Figure 8.11 The village of le Hamel in 2016; the photograph is taken from a similar position to that in Figure 8.9. (Author's photograph)

There was also one Robertson Bottle and citrate for the preparation of preserved blood for transfusion, gum infusion sets including 18 doses of gum for reconstitution and infusion, and miscellaneous surgical equipment. All equipment was packed in a Field Ambulance Service Pannier. A motor ambulance wagon was provided should there be a need to move personnel and equipment to an advanced dressing station, but as it happened, the Field Ambulance Resuscitation Team remained in Les Alençons throughout the day on 4 July.

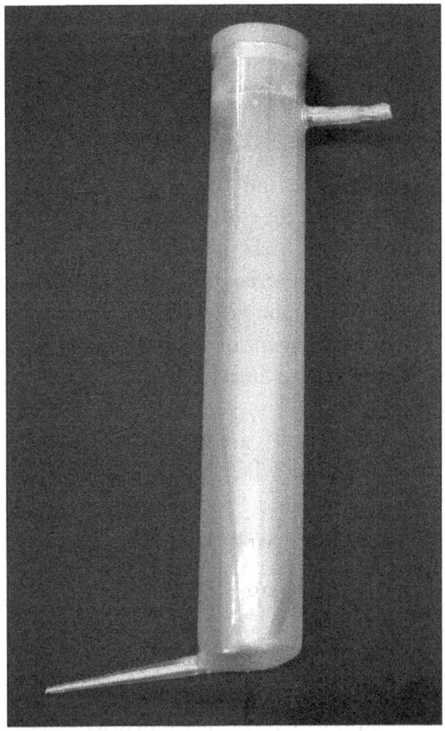

Figure 8.12 Kimpton Brown Flask. (With thanks to Dr Rod Westhorpe, formerly Honorary Curator, Geoffrey Kaye Museum of Anaesthetic History, Melbourne, Australia)

According to Butler, *Official History Australian Medical Services Volume II*, casualties began to arrive at the MDS at 0600. Four hundred and ten stretcher cases passed through between 0600 and 2100, of which 30 (7.3 percent) demanded immediate surgical intervention. The commonest indication for surgery was the completely shattered limb requiring amputation. These cases often had multiple fractures with irreparable damage to nerve, blood vessels, muscle and skin. Patients were cold and clammy with a rapid and barely perceptible pulse and low blood pressure. The slightest movement would have been excruciatingly painful as exposed nerves were subjected to inadvertent traction which worsened the patient's general condition. Many of these cases were just the sort encountered in 1915 by Marshall at CCS 17 at Remy Siding, except that Marshall's cases were suffering from the systemic effects of severe blood loss with the addition of major sepsis, their wounds having been inflicted many hours before. His patients requiring lower limb amputations above mid-thigh experienced a mortality of 90 percent because of the delay. On 4 July 1918, the Field Ambulance Resuscitation Team dealt with its cases very soon after the infliction of wounds, which made a great difference to the outcome. One of the most convincing arguments for early amputation came in 1813 when George James Guthrie documented a significant difference in operative mortality between wounded soldiers undergoing early compared with late amputation. Guthrie recorded 147 patients who had an early amputation in the field, of whom nineteen (14.8 percent) died. His series of cases also included 404 individuals who underwent a delayed amputation, of whom 149 (58 percent) died (Chapter 2). Guthrie's operative procedures were of course, performed without anaesthesia, which did not exist at the time.

Holmes à Court employed nitrous oxide and oxygen anaesthesia to perform the surgery. A local anaesthetic agent could be injected into the exposed nerves and into the skin to supplement the gaseous anaesthetic. The amputation stump could then be loosely opposed using a few sutures, and the patient sent back to base hospital for further management, bypassing the casualty clearing station and leaving the latter free to deal with compound fractures of the femur as well as chest and abdominal wounds. Henry Gray stressed the importance of early amputation, pointing out that in general it was performed considerably less frequently than indicated. It is to the great credit of the Field Ambulance Resuscitation Team that they tackled this problem head on:

> When the limb has been so badly damaged that its subsequent amputation is a matter of certainty, the earlier it is removed the better it is for the patient. The splinting of these badly damaged limbs is a difficult and painful process, and, as they are frequently associated with haemorrhage, conservative treatment becomes still more difficult. Early amputation is called upon far more frequently than it is performed. Not only is it the safest treatment from the point of view of shock, it is also the easiest treatment from the point of view of the medical officer.[24]

The other type of case which was ideally suited to the skills of the Field Ambulance Resuscitation Team was one where there was severe bleeding from a major vessel in a limb. Colonel A.H. Mosely's case is a good example to use as an illustration. Mosely sustained a wound in his leg when a piece of shrapnel severed his posterior tibial artery and caused profuse bleeding. Because the surgical expertise was not available to stop the bleeding at the main dressing station, a tourniquet was applied, and he was sent back to the casualty clearing station. By the time he got there, it was too late, and he required an amputation. Henry Gray observed:

> When an important artery or vein has been divided in the depths of a wound, the operation required in order that it may be tied may present great difficulties. If, however, the casualty clearing station is some distance away and there is no alternative but that of despatching the patient with a tourniquet that must of necessity remain in position many hours, these difficulties must be faced. In arriving at a decision as to whether to operate or to trust to a tourniquet, it is worth remembering that about 80% of limbs whose blood supply has been cut off by a tourniquet for a period of three hours or thereby eventually come to amputation.[25]

Had the Field Ambulance Resuscitation Team existed at the time of Mosely's wounding, his leg would probably have been saved. A tourniquet would only have been applied for the duration of the operation and the wound in Mosely's leg extended by making a longitudinal incision from both ends of it to provide better access, enabling the surgeon to see what was going on. Any damaged muscles would have been excised, working down to the damaged vessel lying deep within the leg, everything made visible by the relatively bloodless field provided by the tourniquet. The damaged posterior tibial artery would have been seen and ligated at both ends, as described by Guthrie 100 years before (Chapter 2), and any other obvious smaller bleeding vessels likewise tied off. The tourniquet would then have been released to ensure that haemostasis had been achieved before closing the wound. The entire procedure would probably have taken less than one hour. There would have been no danger to the limb in applying a tourniquet for this short period of time.

24 Gray, H.M.W., *The Early Treatment of War Wounds* (London: Henry Frowde, Hodder and Stoughton, 1919), p.86.
25 Gray, *The Early Treatment of War Wounds*, pp. 44-45.

The surgical results achieved by the Field Ambulance Resuscitation Team at the Battle of Hamel were felt to be so impressive that it was recommended that every Australian Division should have a similar team in the forthcoming weeks and months. The motor ambulance wagons provided for their use gave the resuscitation teams mobility, which enabled them to work either from the main dressing station or from an advanced dressing station, although the latter was much less likely. Their equipment could easily be loaded onto the wagons. The design of the dressing stations was standard, so there was no difficulty in orientation experienced by transferring work to a new location.

The Battle of Hamel was a dress rehearsal for the Battle of Amiens which began on 8 August 1918. Preparations were made in complete secrecy. The British Fourth Army under General Sir Henry Rawlinson advanced both north and south of the River Somme. British III Corps attacked to the north of the river, while the Australian Corps attacked to the south. The Canadian Corps attacked south of the Australians. The tactics were the same as those employed by Monash at the Battle of Hamel, with comprehensive artillery, tank and air support. The 2nd and 3rd Australian Divisions took their first objectives before the 4th and 5th divisions leapfrogged through to seize the next. The appropriate field ambulances leapfrogged with their brigades to maintain close contact. The British Fourth Army advanced eight miles on an eight-and-a-half mile-front. The ever-widening distance between the front and the casualty clearing stations caused much congestion on the roads. Australian divisional transport had to be employed to transport the wounded from the main dressing stations to the casualty clearing stations to the detriment of forward evacuation. Next day, the casualty clearing stations dealing with Australian wounded were brought forward from Vignacourt and Crouy to Vequemont, some five miles from Villers-Bretonneux, and this relieved the situation. The Battle of Amiens continued on 10 and 11 August, by which time German resistance was stiffening and the territory gained progressively diminished. Australian casualties between 9 and 11 August amounted to 5,991 killed, wounded and missing. The total number of admissions to Fourth Army casualty clearing stations, British, Australian and Canadian casualties inclusive, were 15, 588. There were also 1,914 German casualties who required treatment.

On 30 August 1918, the 2nd Australian Division, which had advanced along the Somme basin to the south of the river, crossed the Somme close to where the river makes a right- angled bend, changing from west-east to north-south direction opposite Mont St Quentin before going past Péronne (Figure 8.1). The following day depleted brigades of the 2nd Division captured German positions at the summit of Mont St Quentin and consolidated these positions over the next couple of days. At the same time, the 5th Australian Division captured Péronne. The Germans had thought Mont St Quentin was unassailable but were wrong. They were left with no option but to withdraw to the Pre-Hindenburg (Hindenburg Outpost) Line less than a mile from the Hindenburg Line itself.

Once the Australians had advanced to reach the Somme opposite Péronne and Mont St Quentin, there was a considerable distance from their front line to advanced dressing stations in the rear. Brigades were also functioning on an unusually wide frontage, so that transport had to move from side to side as well as from front to back. Light ford ambulance wagons proved to be very useful, because they could run right up to regimental aid posts and transport casualties to the advanced dressing stations. The main dressing stations continued to be the base for Field Ambulance Resuscitation Teams, while Casualty Clearing Station No 5 opened at Proyart, enabling Gordon-Taylor and his colleagues to deal expeditiously with compound fractures of the femur and wounds of the chest and abdomen. Soldiers whose wounds fell within the remit of Field Ambulance Resuscitation Teams went to the designated main dressing station from advanced dressing stations. Once again, there were some patients who required immediate amputation for shattered extremities and others who needed bleeding vessels tied off to avoid the use of limb threatening tourniquets. Patients in urgent need of resuscitation were also dealt with by Field Ambulance Resuscitation Teams in the main dressing stations, where they were transfused before being sent back in better clinical condition to the casualty clearing stations. It has already been noted that Field Ambulance Resuscitation Teams assumed the responsibility of carrying out resuscitation, since they were able to deal with the problems of wound shock sooner. They also became responsible for teaching inexperienced medical officers how to resuscitate shocked patients.

The Germans were forced to move back rapidly to the Hindenburg Outpost Line, closely pursued by the Australians of Rawlinson's Fourth Army. On 18 September 1918, the 4th Australian Division captured that part of the Hindenburg Outpost Line on a prominent ridge overlooking the village of Bellenglise, where the 4th Division Memorial stands today (Figure 8.13).

The most significant problem experienced by Australian Medical Services during this attack was the depth of penetration of enemy positions, which put stretcher bearers under particular strain. In an attempt to help matters, stretcher bearer sections of field ambulances were put under the direct command of brigade to better ensure the speedy evacuation of casualties.

It can be appreciated that different phases of the advance since the Battle of Amiens on 8 August presented Australian Medical Services with different problems, which were solved by ensuring close cooperation between Barber's administrative medical staff, executive medical units and senior military officers. Lieutenant General Monash was extremely supportive of medical personnel and their methods of dealing with the wounded. All the measures adopted helped to ensure that casualties were kept moving as quickly as possible in order to receive appropriate treatment as soon as possible.

If one looks from the 4th Australian Division Memorial in an easterly direction, one can see the village of Bellenglise behind the trees which obscure the St Quentin Canal (Figure 8.14).

The village of Bellicourt is 3.2 miles north of Bellenglise and there the St Quentin Canal goes under a tunnelled section for three and a half miles. Monash was confident he could smash through the Hindenburg Line north of Bellicourt, since he would be able to use tanks over the tunnelled section. He had the 3rd and 5th Australian Divisions and American 27th and 30th Divisions at his disposal for his assault on the Hindenburg Line. General Rawlinson gave Monash the go ahead, but he realised that Monash's proposed attack was over too narrow a front. He had learned that much at least from his experience on the Somme in 1916. The British 46th (North Midland) Division would lengthen the front to be attacked by forcing a crossing of the St Quentin Canal between Bellenglise and Bellicourt, the assault being centred on the Bridge of Riqueval (Figure 8.15).

The Fourth Army attacked the Hindenburg Line on 29 September 1918 but despite being able to advance over the tunnelled section, part of Monash's Australian and American force was held up due to a combination of factors which left his attack at a distinct disadvantage and in partial disarray. The American 30th Division and 5th Australian Division

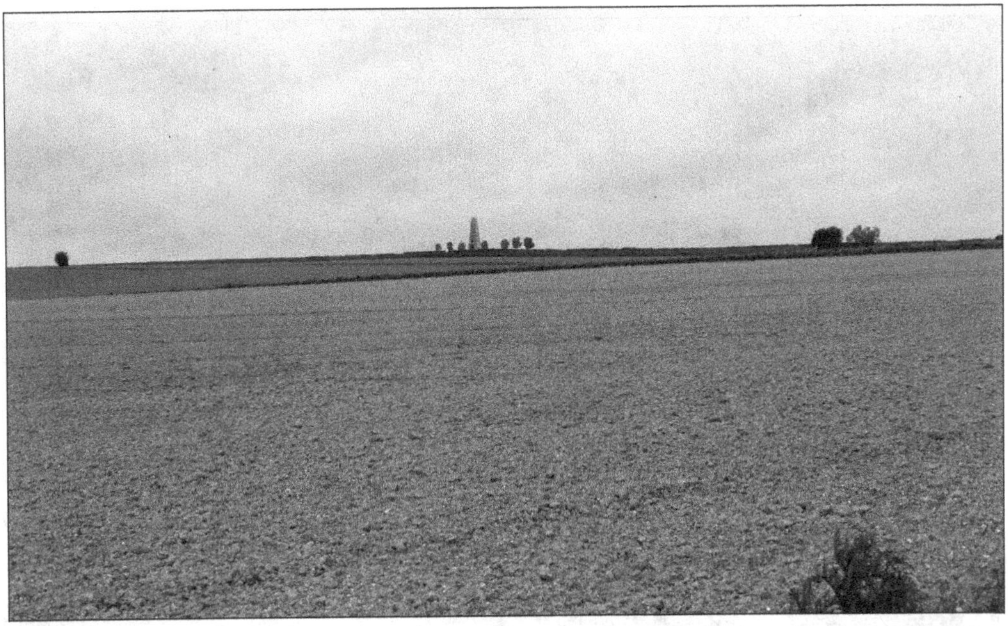

Figure 8.13 4th Australian Division Memorial on the Pre-Hindenburg Line on ridge overlooking Bellenglise; the Pre-Hindenburg Line was captured by the division on 18 September 1918. (Author's photograph)

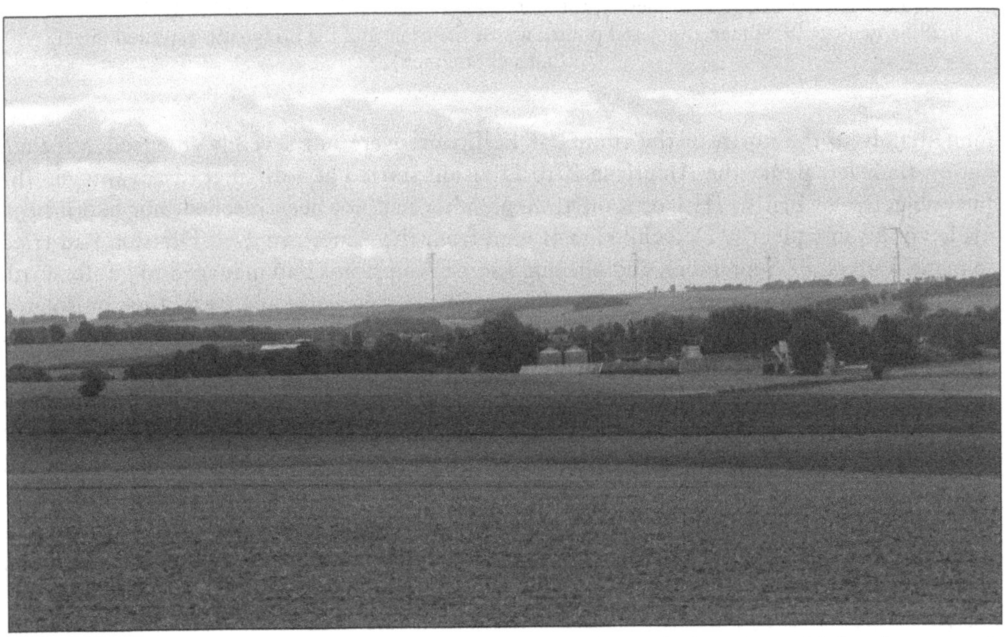

Figure 8.14 Looking from 4th Australian Division Memorial towards the village of Bellenglise, most of which is obscured by trees. The St Quentin Canal skirts round the near side of the village. Both the canal and Bellenglise were integral parts of the Hindenburg Line. (Author's photograph)

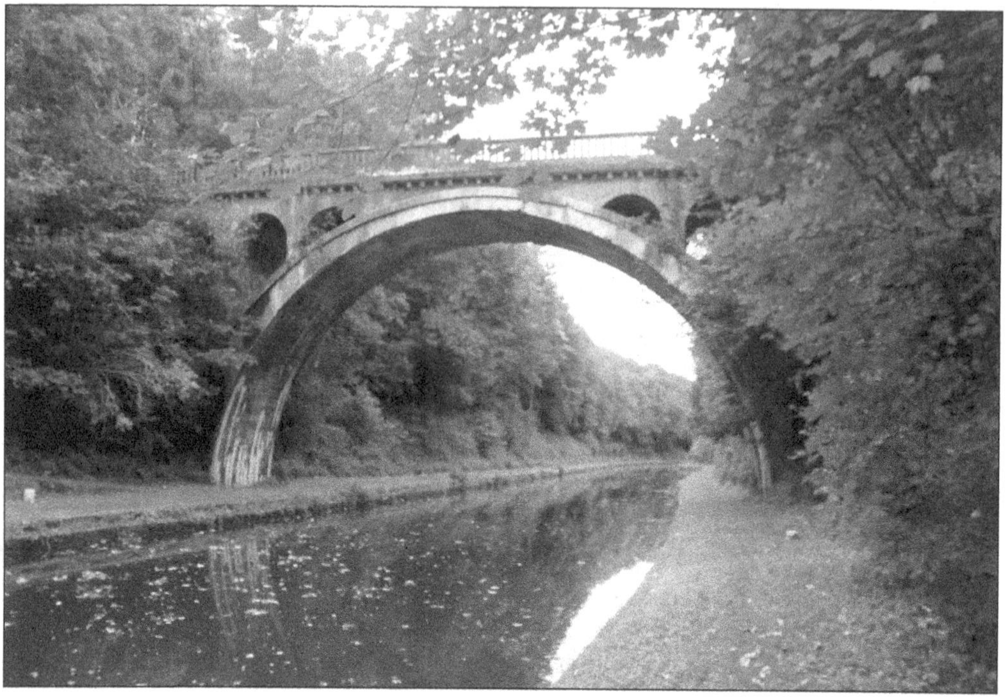

Figure 8.15 The Bridge at Riqueval, captured by men of the 46th (North Midland) Division on 29 September 1918; men swam and punted across the canal and the bridge was captured intact. (Author's photograph)

immediately to the north of the tunnel at Bellicourt were not severely adversely affected, but on their left flank, the American 27th Division started at a distinct disadvantage. The final objective of British III Corps on 18 September had not been reached, nor had it been made good subsequently. Detachments of men from the American 27th Division had tried to make it up on 27 September, and although some Americans had managed to get forward, they failed to mop up German positions due to their inexperience and were stuck in isolated positions surrounded by enemy forces. Fearing that there were pockets of American outposts ahead, the artillery barrage for the assault on the Hindenburg Line on 29 September went in where it would have done had the proper starting position for the 27th Division been reached. This was 1,000 yards ahead of their actual position. Consequently, the Americans advanced without the aid of an effective barrage and were cut to pieces. When the 3rd Australian Division attacked with a view to leapfrogging through, it too ran into heavy machine gun fire from German strong points. There followed a very confused period and an inevitable delay. Without a firm, driving platform to facilitate the evacuation of casualties, their removal from the battlefield was adversely affected, and one Australian Medical Officer was moved to write:

> The American 27th Division jumped off 1,000 yards behind line of the barrage; cut to blazes; our 3rd division came in for a lot of machine-gun fire. Things generally mixed. Evacuation awful[26]

The 4th Australian Division Field Ambulance Resuscitation Team under Major Holmes à Court was put at the disposal of the American 27th Division. Because of the chaotic situation, no forward movement of advanced dressing stations on the Australian/American front was possible for the first 24 hours after the start of the attack on 29 September. Conditions were extremely difficult both close to the front for stretcher bearers and to the rear for the mechanised transport of wounded due to fierce German shellfire:

> The congestion of troops and artillery on the roads leading to Bellicourt, when the Yanks were held up, was awful, and all under observation from Fritz. Naturally he shelled the roads heavily … The bearers attached to the battalions, and the others, following closely on behind, experienced a nerve-racking time.[27]

American and Australian stretcher bearers pooled resources to collect the wounded and to transport them back to the advanced dressing stations as quickly as they could. Only by the night of 30 September/1 October did the roads clear sufficiently to allow transport to get through to Bellicourt and a new advanced dressing station was finally established, and order was restored.

Meanwhile the 46th (North Midland) Division crossed the St Quentin Canal between Bellicourt and Bellenglise on 29 September. Some men punted across the canal on canvas boats and some swam across using life jackets taken from troop ships. Others captured the Bridge at Riqueval intact. Having crossed the canal and broken through the Hindenburg Line, they advanced another couple of miles to a tiny village called Magny la Fosse, before the 32nd Division leapfrogged through in preparation for the next attack on the village of Joncourt. The successful crossing of the St Quentin Canal and breach of the Hindenburg Line by the 46th Division was one of the most remarkable achievements of the war.

After capturing their section of the Hindenburg Line, the Australians fought on until the evening of 5 October 1918, when their 2nd Division captured the village of Montbrehein. The five Australian Divisions had been taking turns during the advance and had been fighting without respite since the Battle of Amiens on 8 August. When they left exhausted, their war on the Western Front was over. They would never return.

Casualties sustained by the 3rd and 5th Australian Divisions during the heavy fighting around the Hindenburg Line between 29 September and 2 October 1918 were as follows: Killed: 391; died of wounds: 91; died from effects of gas: 9; gassed and survived: 310; wounded and survived: 1,792; total casualties 2,593.[28]

26 Butler, *Official History Vol. II*, p. 740.
27 Butler, *Official History Vol. II*, p. 745.
28 Butler, *Official History Vol. II*, p. 763.

From the Line

Have you seen men come from the Line?
Tottering, doddering, as if bad wine
Had drugged their very souls;
Their garments rent with holes
And caked with mud
And streaked with blood
Of others, or their own;
Haggard, weary-limbed and chilled to the bone,
Trudging aimless, hopeless, on
With listless eyes and faces drawn
Taut with woe?

Have you seen them aimless go?
Bowed down with muddy pack
And muddy rifle slung on back,
And soaking overcoat,
Staring on with eyes that note
Nothing but the mire
Quenched of every fire?

Have you seen men when they come?
From shell-holes filled with scum
Of mud and blood and flesh,
Where there's nothing fresh
Like grass, or trees, or flowers,
And the numbing year-like hours
Lag on – drag on,
And the hopeless dawn
Brings naught but death, and rain –
The rain a fiend of pain
That scourges without end,
And Death, a smiling friend?

Have you seen men when they come from hell?
If not – ah, well
Speak not with easy eloquence
That seems like sense
Of 'War and its Necessity'!
And do not rant, I pray,
On 'War's Magnificent Nobility'!

If you've seen men come from the Line
You'll know it's Peace that is divine!
If you've not seen the things I've sung –
Let silence bind your tongue,
But, make all wars to cease,
And work, and work for Everlasting Peace.

Roderick Watson Kerr, MC
(1893-1960)

The clinical activity of the Field Ambulance Resuscitation Teams during the months of August and September 1918 is summarised below. It excludes cases requiring general resuscitative measures.

- Operations 948
- Blood transfusions 52
- Gum and other infusions 62

Many limbs were saved by the removal of tourniquets and many lives saved by the early amputation of mangled limbs. Severely shocked patients were significantly improved and arrived in casualty clearing stations in much better condition than they otherwise would.

Major Gordon Gordon-Taylor, who became Consulting Surgeon to Fourth Army on 27 September 1918, was in no doubt about the valuable contributions made by the Australian Field Ambulance Resuscitation Teams:

> Several months' experience in the Casualty Clearing zone behind the Australian Corps has enabled me to form an estimate of the excellent work of the resuscitation teams of that

> Corps. There can be no room for doubt that very many lives have been saved by the work of Major Holmes à Court and the members of the other resuscitation teams. Their experience in the Dressing Stations coincides with that of the Casualty Clearing Hospitals that in blood transfusion we have the most remarkable and valuable means of treating cases of severe shock and haemorrhage. Their results conclusively prove the value of these methods of resuscitation in the Field Ambulances.[29]

Following the war, Holmes à Court returned to Australia and wrote his MD thesis based on his wartime experience with the Field Ambulance Resuscitation Team. He published the results of a series of 60 shocked patients who had been treated by his unit. Of the 60 patients, 11 or 18 percent died. The remaining 49 were passed on in good condition and their subsequent history followed whenever possible. Given the huge numbers being dealt with, Holmes à Court regarded the percentage mortality as low. Here are two examples from his series:

Case XXXIV

Condition – (a) General: extreme shock and severe haemorrhage; local: both legs shattered below knee; observed four hours after injury; very collapsed; radial pulse imperceptible.

Treatment – Réchauffement; blood transfusion; 700c.cm. (citrated blood); condition improved; pulse now palpable, 136 per minute, very thready; blood pressure, 80 mm. Hg; operation one and a half hours later under N_2O and O_2 anaesthesia; the left leg was amputated at the junction of the upper and the middle third. The right leg was placed on a splint. Conditions now became very critical; blood transfusion, 600 c. cm.

Result --- One hour later the condition showed improvement; the pulse rate was 114 and the blood pressure 98 mm. Hg. Thirty-six hours later, progressing well.

Case XLI

Condition – (a) General: severe haemorrhage; collapse; (b) local: shell wound of the left side of the neck; left common carotid artery severed; observed one and a half hours after injury. Patient had fainted from loss of blood; the wound was plugged with temporary clot. *Treatment* – Left common carotid artery was ligatured above and below the injury. The foreign body was removed. Gum infusion, 750 c. cm.

Result – Pulse became stronger (previously imperceptible); rate, 96 per minute; blood pressure, 120 mm. Hg.; subsequent recovery.[30]

29 Butler, *Official History Vol. II*, p. 955.
30 Holmes à Court, A., *The Medical Journal of Australia*, 17 July 1920, pp. 49-56.

Holmes à Court drew the following conclusions:

- Life can be maintained after a loss of five-sixths of the total blood, so long as the blood volume is rapidly restored.
- Restoration of the circulation is most effectively achieved by blood transfusion.
- Citrated blood appears to be as effective a whole blood and is more convenient to handle when working under adverse conditions.
- Preserved blood may be used in cases where no blood donors are readily available, provided adequate facilities exist for the preservation and storage of the blood cells.
- Infusion of Gum Acacia is effective in restoring the circulation so long as the loss of haemoglobin has not been excessive. This method is particularly suitable for patients suffering from haemorrhage of moderate degree.
- Saline infusions, both isotonic and hypertonic can affect only a transient restoration of blood volume, a fall in blood pressure occurring within twenty to thirty minutes after intravenous injection. Salt solutions are therefore of little use in acute haemorrhage.

Gordon-Taylor's association with surgeons from Australia and New Zealand

During the time he served on the Western Front, Gordon-Taylor became one of the best known and most respected surgeons working in the casualty clearing stations. He became acquainted with many young surgeons from Australia and New Zealand and was very supportive of them. At various times during the war, personnel from CCS 5 were transferred to 'hot spots' where there was heavy fighting and where their clinical skills were much needed. One young New Zealand surgeon, Francis Gordon Bell MC, first met Gordon-Taylor on the Somme in 1916 and their paths frequently crossed thereafter in the casualty clearing stations. Bell's affection and regard for Gordon-Taylor steadily grew as the former subsequently attested:

> During the Passchendaele fighting of 1917, I was attached to a forward group of clearing stations at Brandhoek where visiting surgical teams included Ernest Miles, C.J. Fagge, Rock Carling and Gordon-Taylor...... and of them all, Gordon-Taylor stood pre-eminent, partly because of his surgical distinction and partly because of his innate kindliness, sympathetic understanding and appreciative attitude towards the younger men...no British surgeon was better known to us and none could have provided a happier link between the old and the new. The key to his supremacy lay, as it did in those far distant war days in his obviously genuine sympathy and understanding of the problems of younger men, and no one was quicker to give praise when due.[31]

When Gordon-Taylor was appointed Acting Consulting Surgeon to the Fourth Army, his close working association with Australian medical personnel in the closing months of the war helped to forge lasting friendships. After the war, Gordon-Taylor kept up these friendships and in

31 Obituary, Sir Gordon Gordon-Taylor, K.B.E., C.B., M.D., Hon. L.L.D., Hon. D.Sc., M.S., F.R.C.S., Hon. F.R.C.S. Ed., Hon. F.R.C.S.I., Hon. F.A.C.S., Hon. F.R.C.S.(Canada), *British Medical Journal*, 2:5203 (24 September 1960), pp. 947-948.

1934 he travelled to Australia as an examiner in Anatomy for the Primary Fellowship. He made five subsequent visits in this role and his reputation as a friend, colleague and surgical ambassador grew ever stronger. The Australasian College honoured him in 1949 by founding the Gordon Taylor prize for the best candidate in their Primary examination, and Fellows of the Australasian College commissioned a portrait by James Gunn in August 1960 as an acknowledgement of their strong bonds of friendship and respect.

The portrait by Gunn was painted shortly before Gordon-Taylor's death. He was knocked down by a car on 3 September 1960 outside Lord's Cricket Ground and died in the Middlesex Hospital.

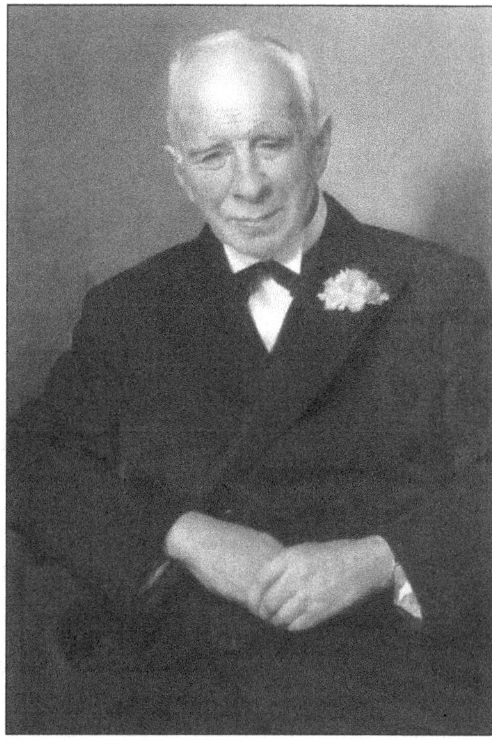

Figure 8.16 Portrait of Sir Gordon Gordon-Taylor. (Courtesy Royal Australasian College of Surgeons)

9

The surgical legacy of the Great War: A missed opportunity

This chapter sets out to show that while many significant advances were made in surgery during the Great War, it did not necessarily follow that these advances would be subsequently employed in civilian practice after the conflict was over. In the case of orthopaedic surgery, quite the opposite was the case and progress in fracture management in Great Britain was delayed by a general surgical establishment which sought to prevent orthopaedic surgeons being recognised as specialists best able to deal with fractures. It required the determination and perseverance of dedicated individuals to overcome this stern opposition and it took many years to do so.

In Britain before the war, most surgeons were 'general' surgeons who could turn their hand to any and every procedure. Some had a particular interest in problems of the musculoskeletal system, and this was reflected in the types of cases they saw and operated on. These surgeons were breaking away from their traditional roots and moving towards specialisation. The surgical establishment consisted of generalists in the broadest sense, individuals who were opposed to specialisation and whose power base was centred in London.

Between 1914 and 1918 there were 2.7 million battle casualties on the Western Front and just over one quarter were never seen by the medical services. These were men who had been killed, were missing (presumed dead) or were prisoners of war. Just under three quarters of the casualties were seen and were treated, of whom 151,356 died from the wounds they had sustained.

Table 9.1 Battle casualties France and Flanders 1914-18.

	Total	Percentage	Total Percentage
Casualties not treated by the Medical Services			
Killed	381,261	14.2	
Missing	144,896	5.4	26.1
Prisoners of war	174,926	6.5	
Casualties treated by the Medical Services			
Died of wounds	151,356	5.6	73.9
Wounded and survived	1,837,613	68.3	

Mitchell, T.J., Smith, G.M., *History of the Great War, Medical Services, Casualties and Medical Statistics,* (London: His Majesty's Stationery Office, 1931).

In 48,290 cases admitted to casualty clearing stations, the distribution of wounds on different sites of the body was as follows: 65.6 percent musculoskeletal; 15.96 percent head, face and neck; 4.48 percent chest, front and sides; 3.18 percent abdomen, front and sides; 1.54 percent eyes; 9.22 percent multiple.[1] Wounds of the musculoskeletal system in isolation and associated with multiple system involvement accounted for the largest group by a long way and required the attention of surgeons with orthopaedic experience.

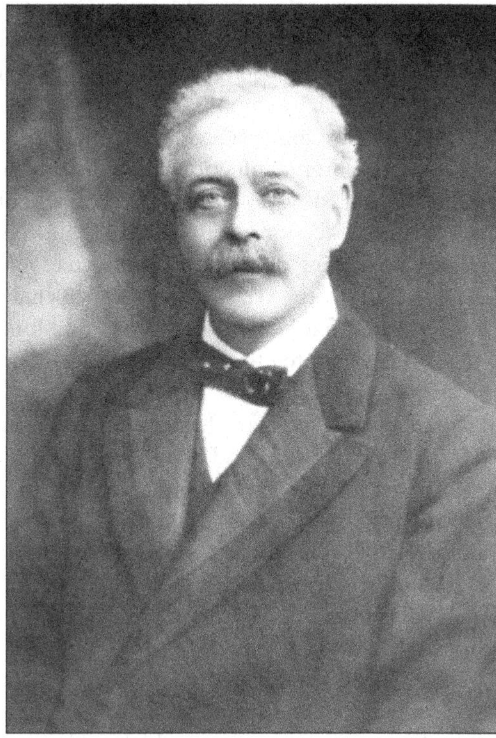

Figure 9.1 Robert Jones (1857-1933). (Courtesy Wellcome Library, London)

In the latter part of the 19th century and early 20th century clinicians who had a declared interest in orthopaedic surgery dealt mostly with established deformity in crippled children. They did not look after fractures, which were in the hands of general surgeons and general practitioners. There was a short-lasting British Orthopaedic Society which was founded in 1894, but it wasn't until the first decade of the 20th century that orthopaedics began to make noticeable progress. The Royal National Orthopaedic Hospital, London, opened in 1909 with five consultants, two of whom practised orthopaedic surgery exclusively. They were Mr E Muirhead Little and Mr Evan Laming Evans.[2] There was another very important figure, Robert Jones from Liverpool, who although from a general surgical background was quite unique, since he had attained international recognition as an orthopaedic surgeon and was elected President of the Orthopaedic Section of the International Congress of Medicine which met in London in 1913.

Robert Jones (1857-1933)

Robert Jones was born in Liverpool. He studied medicine at Liverpool University, graduated in 1878, and subsequently became a Fellow of the Royal College of Surgeons of Edinburgh. He was appointed Surgeon-Superintendent to the Manchester Ship Canal, work on which was begun in 1887 and completed in 1894. Around 20,000 workmen were employed on its construction, and

1 Mitchell, T.J., Smith, G.M., *History of the Great War Medical Services Casualties and Medical Statistics* (London: His Majesty's Stationery Office 1931), p. 41.

2 Platt, H., British Orthopaedic Association: First Founders Lecture, *Journal of Bone and Joint Surgery*, Vol. 41B, No 2, (May 1959), pp. 231-236.

Jones treated more than 3,000 injuries in strategically built hospitals close to the construction sites. He had to deal with over 200 major injuries during this time, including fractures of the femur (thigh bone).[3] He employed a splint first invented by his uncle by marriage, Hugh Owen Thomas (1834-91), to immobilise fractures of the femur. Thomas originally designed this splint to deal with knee joints which were affected by tuberculosis. Normally one associates tuberculosis with a chronic infection of the lungs which frequently caused death, but TB can affect most tissues including bones and joints. The Thomas Knee Splint immobilised tuberculous knee joints very well, allowing them to heal up in the best possible position after the joints had been disrupted to varying degrees by the tuberculous disease process. Jones' clinical experience with the injuries from the Manchester Ship Canal established him as a leading authority in the management of fractures, which later stood him in good stead during the Great War.

Jones was appointed to the position of Honorary Surgeon to the Southern General Hospital in Liverpool in 1889, where Agnes Hunt, who had a little hospital for crippled children in the village of Baschurch near Oswestry, first brought patients to Jones for consultation. Soon, he paid visits to Baschurch, and established regular Sunday clinics there, which he continued doing until the outbreak of the war in 1914. Today, the Robert Jones and Agnes Hunt Hospital in Oswestry is a world-famous orthopaedic unit.

As already explained, Jones became an internationally recognised expert in bone and joint surgery and he forged close ties with American orthopaedic surgeons, many of whom crossed the Atlantic to the port of Liverpool and spent time watching Jones at work in his clinics and operating theatre. On one of his operating lists, there were 22 patients, twenty of whom were orthopaedic cases covering a wide range of procedures in adults and children. There were two non-orthopaedic cases, positioned at numbers 21 and 22 on the list, which were surgery for a cleft palate and a nephropexy, which is the surgical fixation of a floating kidney.[4] Cleft palate today is considered to be so specialised that there are very few centres in Britain which have sufficiently experienced surgeons to deal with it. Visiting surgeons from the United States were unanimous in their appreciation of Jones' work. The medical profession in the United States, unlike in Britain, had recognised that orthopaedics was a distinct specialty and an American Orthopaedic Association had been established in 1887.[5]

Following the outbreak of war, Jones joined up as a captain in the reserve and was soon promoted to the rank of major. One of his duties was to inspect the hospitals of Western Command. He noted that there were many wounded soldiers with major problems caused by badly treated fractures and drew this to the attention of Sir Alfred Keogh, Director General of Army Medical Services. Jones had a very influential friend and colleague who held him in the highest esteem and who would provide him with a great deal of help and support throughout the war and after. His name was Sir Berkeley Moynihan (1865-1936).

Moynihan was a surgeon who did his undergraduate training in Leeds but took his final exams at the University of London. As a newly qualified doctor he was determined to be on an equal footing with London graduates, who were conditioned to believe themselves superior to clinicians from elsewhere. Moynihan spent his life working at Leeds Infirmary and became its

3 Watson, F., *The Life of Sir Robert Jones* (London: Hodder and Stoughton Ltd, 1934), p. 63.

4 Waugh, W., *A History of the British Orthopaedic Association* (London: British Orthopaedic Association, 1993).

5 Cooter, R., *Surgery and Society in Peace and War* (Basingstoke: MacMillan Press Ltd., 1993), p. 26.

first Professor of Clinical Surgery in 1909. He soon acquired an international reputation and was knighted in 1912. He went on to become Professor of Surgery at Leeds in 1925 and was President of the Royal College of Surgeons of England between 1926 and 1931.

As far as London surgeons were concerned, any clinician who was not from the Capital was regarded as a 'country cousin'. In 1909, this prompted the 'provincial' Moynihan to send a letter to 28 surgeons who worked all round Britain, inviting them to join a new surgical society which he named the Moynihan Chirurgical Club. Naturally surgeons who worked in London were excluded from joining. Amongst those Moynihan invited were Robert Jones, Harold Stiles from Edinburgh and Henry Gray from Aberdeen. Moynihan's aim was quite clear:

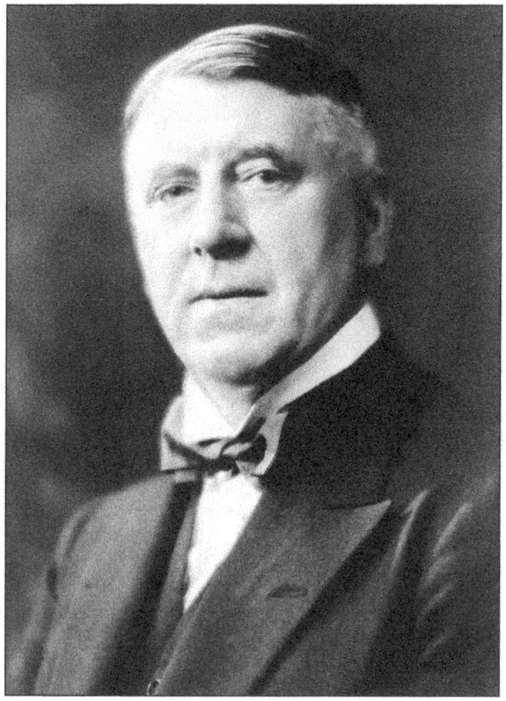

Figure 9.2 Sir Berkeley Moynihan (1865-1936). (Courtesy Wellcome Library, London)

> The activities of the Club shall be directed towards the advancement of surgery by visiting centres of surgical activity at home and abroad and by a free and informal interchange of ideas on the work seen.[6]

There was another very important reason for establishing the club, which was to demonstrate to London surgeons that surgical development could take place perfectly well out with the metropolis. Moynihan declared in an air of effortless superiority: "I wish it to be understood that I am not in competition with my London colleagues."[7]

Moynihan's intention was quite the opposite, of course, and he intended to be very much in competition with his London colleagues. Figure 9.3 is an early photograph of the Moynihan Chirurgical Club, with Moynihan seated near the centre at the front. Moynihan was President of the club in 1909 and again from 1911-13, so the photograph was presumably taken at a meeting during one of those years.

Moreover, in the photograph are Robert Jones (seated far right), Henry Gray (standing far left in the second row) and Harold Stiles (seated third from left). Robert Jones was President of the club between 1913 and 1914. An important point to stress as far as orthopaedic surgery is concerned, is that Moynihan, Jones and Gray all played very important roles in the development

6 Platt, H., Moynihan; The Education and Training of the Surgeon. Eleventh Moynihan Lecture delivered University of Leeds 25 May 1961, *Annals of the Royal College of Surgeons of England*, 4 (30 April 1962), pp. 220-28.

7 Platt, Moynihan; The Education and Training of the Surgeon.

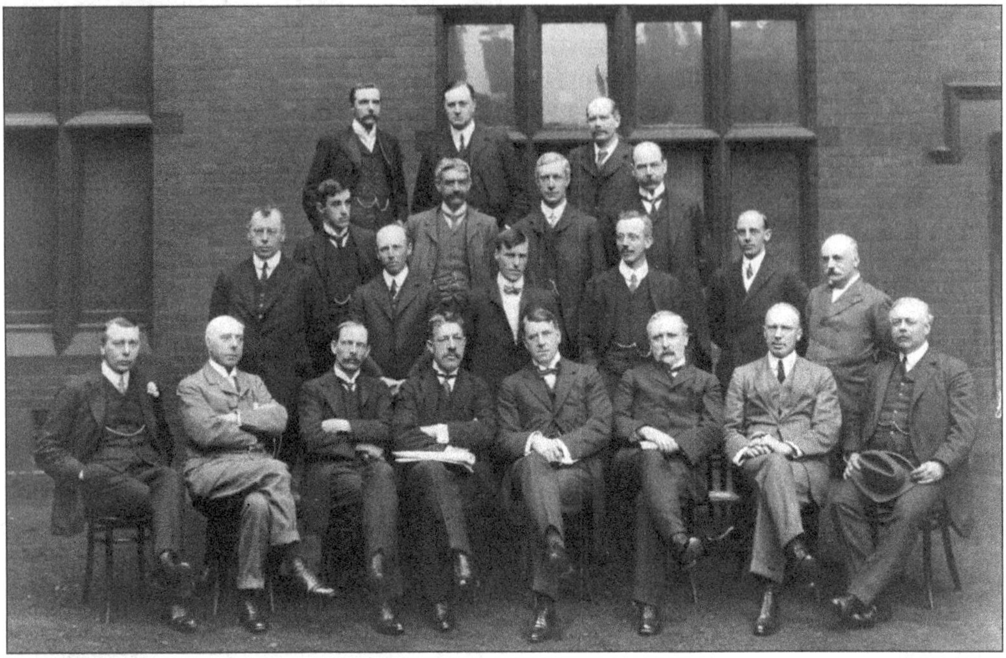

Figure 9.3 Moynihan Chirurgical Club.
From Left to Right
Back Row Mr Burgess Mr F Macrea Mr Bond
Third Row Mr Grey Turner Mr Hogarth Pringle Mr Walter Thomson Dr T Wardrop Griffith
Second Row Mr Henry Gray Mr JF Dobson Professor J Kay Jamieson Mr T Thomas Mr LR Braithwaite Mr S Bishop
Front Row Mr Willis Mr Jalland Mr Harold Stiles Mr WB Coley Mr BGA Moynihan Mr Rutherford Morrison Mr Alexis Thomson Mr Robert Jones
(Courtesy Professor Jimmy Hutchison and the Moynihan Chirurgical Club)

of orthopaedic surgery during the Great War. Gray spent all his time in France and his achievements in dealing with casualties from the Western Front have been dealt with elsewhere in Chapters 4, 6 and 7. Jones made outstanding contributions to orthopaedics in Great Britain and Ireland, but his activities did not go unnoticed by general surgical establishment figures in London who disapproved of the prominent position he came to occupy (see below).

After Robert Jones' very critical comments about the appalling treatment of fractures to Sir Alfred Keogh, Moynihan, who had been commissioned temporary Colonel RAMC, visited hospitals in France between December 1914 and March 1915. Upon his return to Britain he met Keogh and declared that the treatment of compound fractures was deplorable and that the country would soon be 'flooded by men doomed to deformity and crippling'. If Keogh did not do something about it, a scandal would break over his head.[8] Partly as a result of pressure applied by Moynihan and Jones, Keogh directed Jones to open an experimental orthopaedic unit at Alder

8 Platt, Moynihan; The Education and Training of the Surgeon.

Hey Hospital in Liverpool, segregating patients with orthopaedic wounds for the first time and providing them with the best possible treatment, both in terms of surgery and rehabilitation. Jones was allocated two hundred and fifty beds which quickly became five hundred and sixty.[9]

So successful was the Alder Hey experiment that orthopaedic services soon expanded to meet the clinical demand. In March 1916, Jones became responsible for providing surgical care and rehabilitation to soldiers with orthopaedic wounds in the first orthopaedic centre in the country, opened on the site of the Hammersmith Workhouse in Shepherd's Bush, London. Soon there would be other centres round the entire country, all having teams of surgeons with the expertise to deal with late orthopaedic problems, such as mal-union or non-union of fractures, as well as nerve repairs or tendon transfers. Orthopaedic centres also had a curative workshop where soldiers undergoing rehabilitation were put to work and given an occupation. Jones maintained that simply exercising a stiff joint repetitively was tedious and demoralising, but movement in association with an occupation was productive, good for morale, and restored function at the same time. [10]

In the same month that Shepherd's Bush was opened, Jones became Director of Military Orthopaedics, thanks again to the influence of Sir Berkeley Moynihan, who used all his powers of persuasion to pressurise Keogh into appointing Jones to the position, by first declaring to Keogh that the war was one of orthopaedic surgery and that Keogh ought to appoint a Director of Military Orthopaedics.[11]

Keogh allegedly replied:

> Yes, Sir Berkeley, I know what you mean; you want me to appoint Robert Jones. I would like to do so, but I dare not appoint him. If I did, the London surgeons would have my head on a charger.[12]

Moynihan retorted that if Keogh would not appoint Jones, then he, Moynihan, would resign, so Jones was duly appointed and orthopaedic centres soon opened in other parts of the country, staffed by surgeons with previous orthopaedic experience who were able to plan a complete course of treatment for every patient. There were also surgeons, who though not yet specialising, were interested in orthopaedics and only required experience to enable them in turn to take charge of other new centres. Clinical staff in the centres helped to train young medical officers destined to go overseas. Unfortunately, there were major staff shortages and as more orthopaedic centres opened, these staffing problems became more difficult to deal with. The War Office was faced with the insistent demand that more able-bodied men, including medical officers, should go to France. In June 1916 there was an urgent call for five hundred doctors overseas. The medical profession as a whole was against any exceptions and many young medical officers who were being trained in orthopaedic centres were ordered to France, sometimes to be killed or wounded on the Western Front.

9 Watson, *The Life of Sir Robert Jones*, pp. 148-49.
10 Jones, R., *Notes on Military Orthopaedics* (London, New York, Toronto and Melbourne: Cassel and Company Ltd., 1917).
11 Platt, Moynihan; The Education and Training of the Surgeon.
12 Platt, Moynihan; The Education and Training of the Surgeon.

The general surgeons in London viewed developments in orthopaedics with growing concern and suspicion. Most wounds inflicted in France and Flanders were musculoskeletal and now orthopaedic surgeons were proposing to take away all fracture cases from the hands of the general surgeons who felt they had to put a stop to this new trend without delay. A formal objection to Jones' appointment as Director of Military Orthopaedics was lodged with the President of the Royal College of Surgeons of England. The Council of the College at first seemed ready to rescind Jones' appointment. Delivering the Eleventh Moynihan Lecture in Leeds on 25 May 1961, orthopaedic surgeon Sir Harry Platt described how Moynihan, supported by John Lynn-Thomas and Ernest Hey Groves, successfully argued the case for Jones to remain in post. John Lynn-Thomas (1861-1939) had a particular interest in fractures and dislocations and was Jones' Deputy Inspector of Orthopaedics in Wales. He was also a founding member of the Moynihan Chirurgical Club. Ernest Hey-Groves (1872-1944) was another general surgeon with a particular interest in orthopaedics. He was a good friend of Moynihan and in 1914 was Hunterian Professor at the Royal College of Surgeons of England and delivered a lecture on the operative treatment of fractures.[13]

Moynihan was powerful enough to keep the general surgical establishment under control, allowing Jones to use his energies to open orthopaedic centres in Manchester, Leeds, Newcastle, Oxford, Reading, Cardiff, Birmingham, Bristol, Bath, Dublin, Belfast, Edinburgh, Glasgow and Aberdeen.

Figure 9.4 depicts Scottish General Hospital Number 1 in Aberdeen, one of three orthopaedic centres in Scotland. Known before the war as Oldmill Hospital, it opened on 15 May 1907 as a Poor Law Institution, and was one of the last poorhouses to be built in Scotland. During the First World War the institution was taken over as a Military Hospital from 24 May 1915 to 1 June 1919.[14]

Figure 9.5 is one of the restorative workshops in Scottish General Hospital Number 1 and shows men repairing fishing nets for the deep-sea fishing industry, one of Aberdeen's main employers at that time. This activity encouraged stiff finger, wrist and shoulder joints to regain movement and also helped to restore morale, which may well have been at low ebb, because many of these men had been moved from pillar to post for many weeks or months before being dealt with effectively in an orthopaedic centre.

Jones' longstanding association with surgeons from North America became of great importance when the United States declared war on Germany in April 1917. One of the first things American clinicians did following the outbreak of hostilities was to send orthopaedic surgeons to train and work with Jones in the United Kingdom, which helped to alleviate his staffing problem. Led by Joel Goldthwaite, whose distinguished career had earned him the position of Chief of Orthopaedics at the Massachusetts General Hospital, the first batch of 20 orthopaedic surgeons arrived the following May. Paid by the United States Military, they were put at the disposal of Robert Jones and deployed as he saw fit. Goldthwaite returned to America and brought over another 42 surgeons. Only the presence of American surgeons made it possible for orthopaedic centres in Britain to survive and expand. Ultimately, more than 400 American

13 Groves, Ernest William Hey, *Plarr's Lives of the Fellows Online*, Royal College of Surgeons <https://livesonline.rcseng.ac.uk/biogs/E004298b.htm>.

14 Historic Hospitals, Oldmill Military Hospital (now Woodend Hospital, Aberdeen <https://historic-hospitals.com/2016/01/16/oldmill-military-hospital-now-woodend-hospital-aberdeen/>.

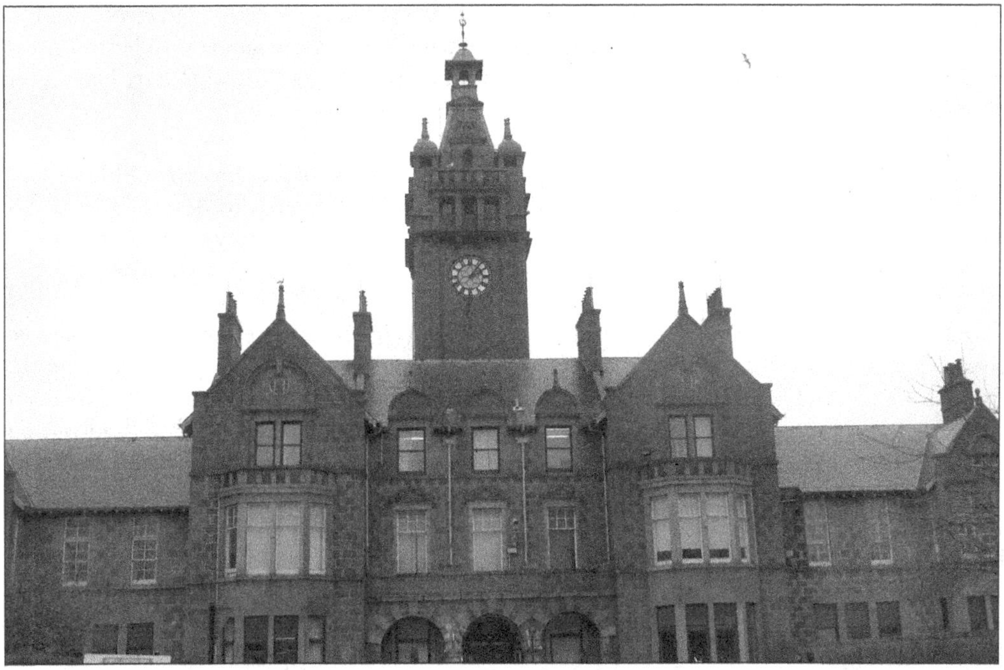

Figure 9.4 Old Mill Hospital (Scottish General Hospital Number 1). (Author's photograph)

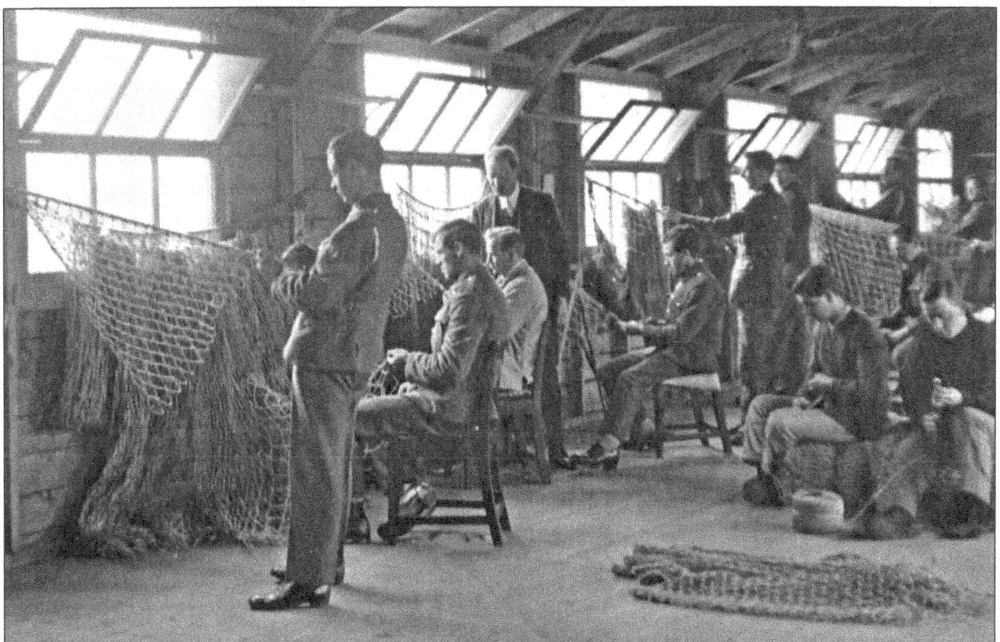

Figure 9.5 Restorative workshop, Scottish General Hospital Number 1. (Courtesy Aberdeen Medico-Chirurgical Society)

surgeons passed through the orthopaedic centres. Most were there for three or four months, but the original 20 places were kept filled with replacements.[15] American surgeon Robert Osgood from Boston arrived in Britain on 22 May 1917 and met with his old friend Robert Jones after disembarking at Liverpool:

> It was a wonderful meeting, almost too much for the tired nerves of the Director of Military Orthopaedics of Great Britain, who had been struggling with entirely inadequate help to care for the maimed and halt and palsied victims alike of the German war and of hasty ill-considered surgery.[16]

Osgood became Jones' Deputy and went around all the orthopaedic centres where his fellow countrymen were working to see what they were doing and to advise, help and train them. In Scottish General Hospital Number 1 in Aberdeen, for example, there were three American surgeons called Francisco, Billington and Langworthy. The hospital had 500 beds and was on the outskirts of the city. The British Officer in charge was Colonel Marnoch, Regius Professor of Surgery at the University of Aberdeen. Osgood was particularly impressed by the restorative workshop and commented on the beneficial effect that repairing deep sea fishing nets had on hand and shoulder function. Apart from curative workshops there was a well-equipped gymnasium, hydrotherapy and electrotherapy facilities and excellent operating rooms (theatres). [17]

A close working relationship developed between the American orthopaedic surgeons and their British counterparts. As already stated, the Americans had formed an American Orthopaedic Association in 1887, and a publication called *Transactions of the American Orthopaedic Association* appeared two years later. It was renamed the *American Journal of Orthopaedics* in 1903. Osgood was a key figure in persuading the British to form an orthopaedic association similar to the American model before he departed to devote his time to the organisation of the rapidly expanding Medical Services of the United States Army. It was Osgood and Osgood alone who persuaded interested parties to meet at the Café Royal on 28 November 1917 to set things in motion. The inaugural meeting of the British Orthopaedic Association took place at Queen Mary's Convalescent Auxiliary Hospital, Roehampton on 2 February 1918 with twenty of the founding members in attendance. Robert Osgood was an invited guest and Figure 9.6 shows twelve of the new members with Osgood standing on the far left.

Whilst all this was happening, opposition from the general surgical establishment did not go away, and on 18 June 1918, Robert Jones wrote to his friend Joel Goldthwaite of the American Medical Service:

> Orthopaedics is doing well in this country, with the exception of attacks in the open and attacks which are insidious. The last attack which I shall have to meet is on the part of the Royal College of Surgeons (of England). Apparently, a strong letter has been written, stating that orthopaedics are depriving the civil hospitals of their best teaching materials and the surgeons of their best work; and appealing to the Royal College of Surgeons to put

15 Cooter, *Surgery and Society in Peace and War*, pp. 125-26.
16 Osgood, R., The Orthopaedic Centers of Great Britain and their American Officers, *Journal of Bone and Joint Surgery, American*, s2-16 (1918), pp. 132-40.
17 Osgood, The Orthopaedic Centers of Great Britain and their American Officers, 1918.

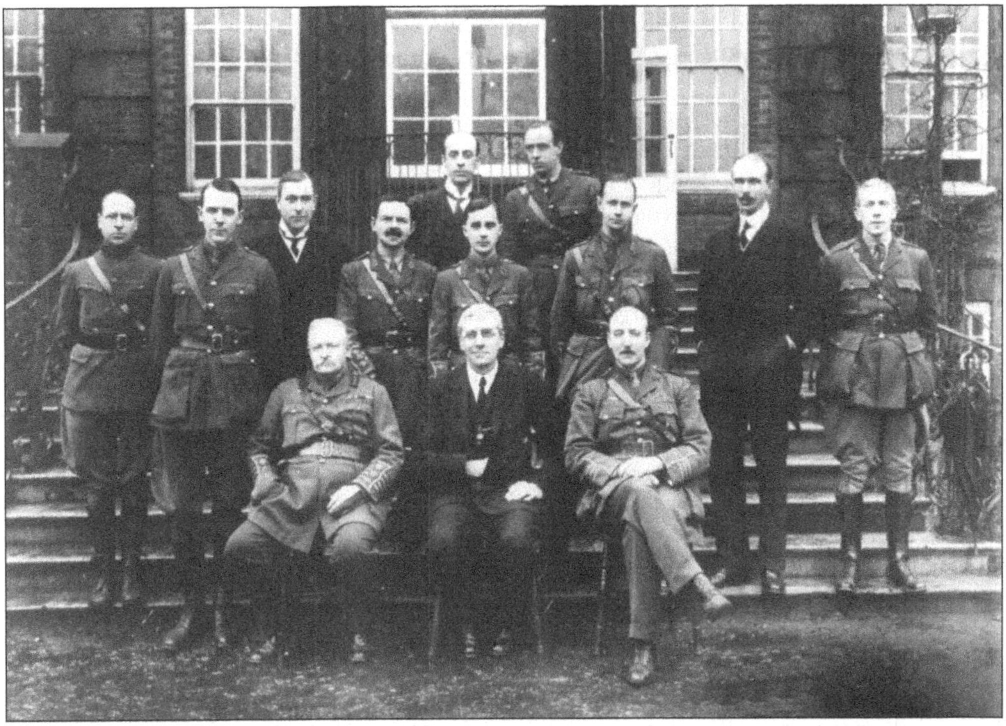

Figure 9.6 Inaugural meeting of British Orthopaedic Association, 2 February 1918. (Courtesy British Orthopaedic Association for granting permission to use image and Courtesy University of Manchester for providing image)
Left to right, with ranks held at the time
Seated Col TH Openshaw Mr E Muirhead Little Captain WE Bennett
Standing Major RB Osgood Captain TP McMurray Mr ASB Bankart Captain D McCrae Aitken Captain H Platt Major RC Emslie Mr E Laming Evans Captain Naughton Dunn
At the back Mr WH Trethowan Captain WR Bristow

> things on a proper basis. The result is that a sub-committee has been formed on the part of the Royal College of Surgeons to discuss the question and there will be a meeting of the Director General and myself to lay down propositions. This, as you can see, is a strong body to placate, but I will do the best I can. One feels with the tremendous amount of work we are doing, that these worries, when the success of our scheme is assured, act as a depressant.[18]

This was the last thing Jones needed, and it is little wonder that he felt depressed by the perpetual sniping by jealous general surgeons when there was a war being fought and so much work to be done. Be that as it may, in July 1918, Jones was compelled to withstand an attempt by a

18 Watson, *The Life of Sir Robert Jones*, pp. 219-21.

committee of the Council of the Royal College of Surgeons of England to circumscribe orthopaedics. Presided over by George Makins, President of the College, the committee observed:

> [It was] regarded with mistrust and disapprobation the movement in progress to remove the treatment of conditions always properly regarded as the main portion of the general surgeon's work from his hands, and place it in those of the 'Orthopaedic Specialists'; and thus to educate the layman to the belief that the British surgeon is incapable of dealing with the majority of the most serious injuries the body may sustain.[19]

Writing in the *British Journal of Surgery*, Makins also observed:

> We find a specialist for the treatment of fractured jaws; another for fractures of the thigh; and strange inconsistency, we meet with a third department, that of orthopaedics—for which a special course of a few months in some instances suffices to qualify—claiming almost the whole field of the surgery of injuries.[20]

Makins continued:

> From an administrative point of view, in dealing with the huge accumulation of the casualties of war, the convenience of such a system may be allowed, as also that it has been attended with a considerable measure of success and benefit to the soldier. On the other hand, when the peculiar conditions of war are ended, the segregation of patients scattered over the entire United Kingdom to such a degree is impractical and its continuance is undesirable as well from the administrative as other points of view.[21]

Makins' myopic and blinkered perspective set the scene for the next quarter of a century or more. After the war was over, instead of the specialty of orthopaedics flourishing and orthopaedic surgeons applying lessons learned during the war to civilian practice, they found further progress blocked by surgical establishment figures who continued to manage (or mismanage) fractures, which they considered part of their Empire.

In complete contrast, American orthopaedic surgeons went home after the war in a much stronger position. They had arrived in Britain as members of a relatively minor specialty but having played a very large part in military orthopaedic surgery, they returned to America claiming the right to deal with the surgery of all bone and joint cases. Eliot Brackett from the Massachusetts General Hospital was Chief of the Division of Orthopaedic Surgery for the American Expeditionary Force from August 1917 and he dictated exactly how soldiers with orthopaedic wounds should be dealt with from the moment of being wounded right through to conclusion of treatment, which included rehabilitation in the United States for those in need:

19 Royal College of Surgeons, Minutes of Council, 16 July 1918, in Cooter, *Surgery and Society in Peace and War*, pp.159-60.

20 Makins, G.H., Introductory, *British Journal of Surgery*, Vol. 6, No. 21 (1918), pp. 1-11.

21 Makins, Introductory, *British Journal of Surgery*, 1918.

> Arrangements have been made for orthopaedic care of soldiers to begin at time of injury and to be carried on continuously until the soldier is returned to duty, or, disabled, is returned to industrial life.[22]

Whilst Jones never had the freedom to do precisely as he thought fit thanks to the surgical establishment seeking ways to prevent the expansion of orthopaedics, the General Medical Board of the Council of National Defense for America made no objection to Brackett's all-encompassing plan. In January 1918, a bill was drafted for the provision of vocational rehabilitation in the United States which would have major implications for the benefit and subsequent development of orthopaedic surgery.[23]

The Great War had been a major catalyst for surgical progress in fracture management as new treatments were sought to improve the appalling outcomes and avoidable deaths of many wounded soldiers, particularly in the opening months of the conflict. Massive numbers of casualties meant that new methods of treatment were evaluated quickly and if such methods were shown to be effective, management regimes could be changed without delay. The specialty of orthopaedic surgery began to take firm shape as growing numbers of dedicated clinicians in France and Britain focussed on ways aimed at improving operative results of fractures and patient outcomes. In France, Henry Gray's experience and expertise with musculoskeletal wounds was particularly notable and he became recognised as the leading authority in fracture treatment on the Western Front. Meanwhile in Britain, Robert Jones had established centres of orthopaedic excellence throughout the length and breadth of the country.

When the conflict came to an end, it seemed entirely reasonable to suppose that the surgical lessons learned during the war both in France and in Britain could be modified and applied to civilian orthopaedic practice. The management of fractures had made great progress between 1914 and 1918. Sir Harold Stiles (1863-1946), Regius Professor of Surgery at the University of Edinburgh from 1919, and founding member of the Moynihan Chirurgical Club, was very clear when he wrote in 1919 about his experience in the war. He had been Jones' Deputy Director in Scotland and had acquired expertise in the management of wounds affecting the peripheral nerves while in charge of the orthopaedic centre of Scottish General Hospital Number 2 at Bangour near Edinburgh.[24] Stiles emphasised the evolution of the technique of early wound excision as a prophylaxis against sepsis in war surgery, and how it could be used in the treatment of industrial injuries. The Thomas Splint, such an advance in the treatment of fractures of the femur during the war, should become an essential part of the armamentarium of the post-war treatment of fractures of the femur.[25] Stiles declared:

> The surgery of the war has been the surgery of young men-men with keen and receptive brains, men who have been trained in the fundamental medical sciences and who have been able to apply their knowledge not merely to the improving of old methods of treatment, but also to the devising of new methods to meet the new conditions they had to deal with and

22 Cooter, *Surgery and Society in Peace and War*, p. 129.
23 Cooter, *Surgery and Society in Peace and War*, p. 130.
24 Stiles, H.J., Forrester-Brown, M.F., *Treatment of Injuries of the Peripheral Spinal Nerves* (London: Henry Frowde and Hodder and Stoughton, 1922).
25 Stiles, H., Surgical Training, *British Medical Journal*, 2: 3068 (October 18, 1919), pp. 487-89.

> the new environment in which they found themselves. It is largely due to the teamwork by younger men that great advances have been made, not only in wound treatment, but in the early and late treatment of fractures, especially fractures of the femur, in wounds involving joints, in injuries to the nerves, and in military orthopaedics generally.[26]

Harold Stiles was one of the few surgeons who had made his name in bone and joint surgery before the war. He was a good friend of Robert Jones whom he knew well, both men sharing a common interest in orthopaedic surgery and both being founding members of the Moynihan Chirurgical Club in 1909. During the 1920s and 1930s, Stiles played an active role in establishing Scotland's first orthopaedic hospital for crippled children, the Princess Margaret Rose, in Edinburgh and in founding the Chair of Orthopaedic Surgery in Edinburgh.[27]

Sadly, Stiles' success in promoting orthopaedic surgery after the war was the exception rather than the rule and generally speaking there was a great deal of opposition to the development of orthopaedics, partly as a result of jealousy and partly as a result of entrenched views held by powerful general surgeons who had looked after fractures before the war and saw no reason why there should be any change after the conflict.

Post-war fracture movement

Harry Platt (1886-1986)

Harry Platt was born in Lancashire and as a child had tuberculous arthritis of one of his knees. This precluded him from taking part in sport and he suffered a permanent disability of his knee. He was a patient of Robert Jones, for whom he developed a great affection. Given his sickly childhood, it is interesting to note that Harry Platt lived to be one hundred years old. He studied medicine at the University of Manchester and graduated in 1909. He trained in orthopaedics in London at the Royal National Orthopaedic Hospital before spending a year working at the Massachusetts General Hospital in Boston with Eliot Brackett and Robert Osgood. Upon his return to Britain in 1914, he became Honorary Consulting Surgeon in Orthopaedics to Ancoats Hospital in North Manchester, with one third of the surgical beds. On the outbreak of the war he became a Captain in the Royal Army Medical Corps and was one of the founding members of the British Orthopaedic Association in 1918. Platt is standing in the centre of the second row in Figure 9.6. By the time this photograph was taken, Platt was Consulting Surgeon in charge of an orthopaedic centre at Grangethorpe, Manchester, where he acquired considerable experience in treating nerve injuries and in applying the techniques of bone grafting to assist in the healing of fractures which had failed to unite (delayed union). Figure 9.7 is a portrait of Platt painted many years later which hangs in the Royal College of Surgeons. Platt went on to be knighted in 1948 and was President of the Royal College of Surgeons of England between 1954 and 1957.[28]

26 Stiles, Surgical Training, *British Medical Journal*, 1919.
27 Cooter, R., *Surgery and Society in Peace and War*, pp. 42-43.
28 Platt, Sir Harry, (1886-1986), *Plarr's Lives of the Fellows Online*, Royal College of Surgeons <https://livesonline.rcseng.ac.uk/biogs/E000232b.htm>.

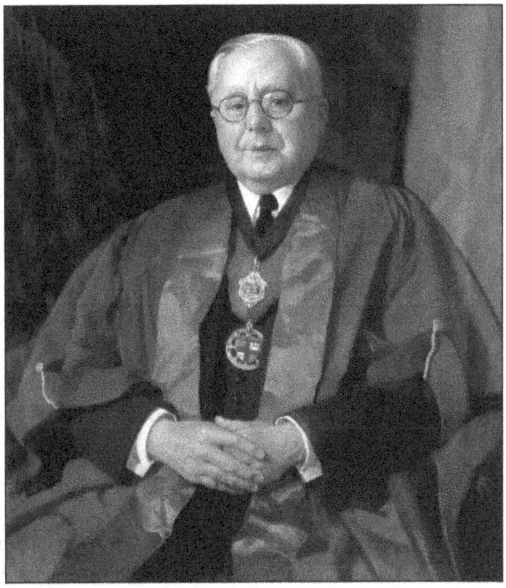

Figure 9.7 Sir Harry Platt (1886-1986). (Courtesy Royal College of Surgeons of England)

After the war, Platt returned to Ancoats Hospital where he carried into civilian practice the lessons learned from wartime, namely segregation of fractures, teamwork, continuity of care and expert follow up. He established the first dedicated fracture service under orthopaedic control and became one of the main driving forces behind the fracture movement, which was an attempt by orthopaedic surgeons to persuade the entrenched surgical establishment that a dedicated facture service run by orthopaedic surgeons was the way forward.

Another strong supporter of the fracture movement was Rowley Bristow (1883-1947), who is standing in the back row on the right in Figure 9.6. Bristow was Consulting Surgeon to the flagship orthopaedic centre at Shepherd's Bush with the rank of Major, RAMC, and continued to hold the post between 1919 and 1923 after the hospital passed under the charge of the Ministry of Pensions. Between 1916 and 1918, he was also Assistant Inspector of Military Orthopaedics working under Robert Jones, whom Bristow found to be an inspirational figure. After the war, Jones was appointed Director of the Orthopaedic Department of St Thomas's Hospital, London and Bristow was his deputy, although the running and direction of the department was very much in Bristow's hands.[29]

When hostilities were over, Jones viewed Shepherd's Bush as a citadel for the future of orthopaedics and the restoration of disabled soldiers. It had been a centre of orthopaedic excellence from 1916 and there was a great opportunity for Shepherd's Bush to remain the permanent home of British orthopaedics. But it was not to be, even though it had handled nearly 4,000 inpatients with 2,494 operations and 101, 596 outpatient attendances in 1921. It closed on 11 April 1925. Jones' biographer, Frederick Watson noted:

> To him (Jones) the matter was vital. There must remain one concrete example, one teaching hospital, as a national centre of orthopaedics. But Shepherd's Bush he could not save, and the blow was a bitter one. A hospital of the greatest war in history, equipped in staff, operating theatres and workshops-a model for the technique of which he was the master, was fated to be handed back to a body of Guardians for a purpose as dreary as it was insignificant. Seldom has Bumbledom secured a more preposterous triumph. The sole claim of Shepherd's Bush for a place in the eternal struggle of mankind against disease and suffering had been tossed on one side.[30]

29 Bristow, Walter Rowley (1882-1947), *Plarr's Lives of the Fellows Online*, Royal College of Surgeons <http://livesonline.rcseng.ac.uk/biogs/E003905b.htm>.

30 Watson, *The Life of Sir Robert Jones*, pp. 215-16.

Jones hits out against the general surgical establishment

On 12 May 1925, Robert Jones delivered a lecture before an audience at the University of Liverpool entitled *Crippling due to fractures: Its prevention and remedy.* The lecture was published subsequently in the British Medical Journal.[31] Jones began by saying that while considerable progress had been made in surgery as it affected the brain, the chest and the abdomen, there had been a deplorable inertia in the surgery of fractures. The treatment of fractures in 1925 had become 'tragic' because most fractures, whether treated conservatively or operatively, had been badly handled with resultant major disability.

Jones reflected on events during the Great War and noted the remarkable improvement that had occurred in the management of fractures, particularly those affecting the femur. In the first two years of the conflict fractures of the femur were associated with a very high percentage mortality of around 80 percent. Most deaths occurred on the way to, or at, the casualty clearing stations. The Thomas Splint was scarcely known about in 1914, and yet once its use became established, the prognosis of femoral fractures improved greatly. Jones mentioned the work of Henry Gray, Consulting Surgeon to the British Third Army, who employed the Thomas Splint exclusively at the Battle of Arras in order to immobilise fractures of the femur, reducing the mortality to around 20 percent. George Washington Crile of the Fourth American Base Hospital, and an expert in the treatment of shock, said that the Thomas Splint had done more than any other single measure to prevent death from wound shock.

The segregation of patients with fractured femurs at base hospitals was also very important and Jones highlighted the work of Major Maurice Sinclair in Boulogne, who was the first to segregate these fractures. Patients treated in Sinclair's unit came back to Britain with scarcely any shortening and with excellent alignment. Unfortunately, until orthopaedic centres were well established throughout Britain, many soldiers with fractured femurs were sent to the nearest convenient place for transport and often splints were taken off too soon before the fracture had united sufficiently, with the result that length and alignment of fractures were lost by people who did not know what they were doing. Orthopaedics required segregation, teamwork and expertise to get good results.

Jones continued by saying that unfortunately lessons learned by orthopaedic surgeons during the war were often ignored by surgeons in the 'big teaching hospitals' where standards were very poor. Outpatient fractures were looked after by unsupervised junior medical staff without any links to senior staff in the wards. Errors of omission or commission were common and there was no one to supervise their work or to instruct them in the correct way to treat fractures. Junior staff stayed a short time only and new ones came along and made the same mistakes. Inpatient fractures were 'looked after' by the house-surgeon, who was the most junior doctor covering the ward, and the consultants generally took no part in the management of patients with fractures. As a rule, consultants resented the presence of orthopaedic 'bed-blockers' in whom they had no interest and who cluttered up valuable surgical beds and prevented more important cases getting in. Their sole aim was to get orthopaedic cases out as quickly as possible, and the easiest way to achieve this was to put plaster casts on them all and discharge them forthwith. Patients with

31 Jones, R., Crippling due to fractures: its prevention and remedy, *British Medical Journal,* 1:3359 (16 May 1925), pp. 909-13.

fractures of the femur mismanaged this way developed major limb shortening of several inches as a result of powerful muscles in the thigh going into spasm causing the fractures to telescope and overlap. Given that the majority of fractures occurred in fit young adults, this meant that many fracture patients never worked again:

> To a surgeon who takes pride in his work, the full recovery from a bad fracture should be a thrilling achievement, while malunion, stiffened joints and wage-earning disabilities, should, as correspondingly, fill him with remorse. To the patient, it is inconceivable that a hospital with a worldwide reputation should give him anything but the very best.[32]

Jones was particularly concerned by the effect this disorganisation was having on the education of medical students, which was generally deplorable. Brought up in an environment where the treatment of fractures was in a subsidiary role and poorly taught, the student only realised how ill-informed he was after he qualified and how badly equipped, he was to deal with fractures. Orthopaedic mistakes could not be hidden, and a poorly treated fracture resulting in a malunion might condemn the recently qualified doctor and cause him to 'strike camp and move further afield' where neither he nor his bad orthopaedic result was known about. The author would like to point out that the great majority of medical graduates in the 1920s were men, unlike today.

Jones makes recommendations

Jones observed that more progress had been made in the management of fractures during the four years Great War than in an entire generation of the big teaching hospitals thanks to segregation and team work. Certain general principles had to be followed to optimise their treatment.

- Segregation of in-patient fractures into wards under specialist surgical unit;
- Creation of special out-patient fracture facilities which were run by the same surgeon or surgeons responsible for the wards;
- Surgeon in charge of department should be a consultant whose practice and teaching were committed to orthopaedic surgery throughout his entire career to ensure continuity of care.

There should be fracture teams consisting of the following personnel:

- One or more consultants including the orthopaedic consultant;
- An experienced senior assistant, in the service of all consultants, responsible for the day to day running of the unit and provision of student teaching;
- Experienced physiotherapist;
- Specially trained sister in charge of the orthopaedic ward.

32 Jones, Crippling due to fractures, *British Medical Journal,* 1925.

Student teaching

Jones believed that student teaching was particularly important, because students were the consultants of the future. All senior students should attend fracture clinics at least once or twice a week. Rather than formal lectures, a series of clinical demonstrations would be much more useful. Jones believed the X-ray department should be in close touch with the orthopaedic ward and the fracture clinic. Students should be taught never to lose an opportunity to obtain an X-ray to check the position of a fracture and to derive instruction in interpreting it. According to Jones writing in 1900:

> The advent of X-rays has added immensely to the accuracy of our knowledge and to the classification of our cases and has saved our patients from much unnecessary and often aimless manipulation. We must, however, beware that we do not paralyse our diagnostic facilities from pure inanition. The Roentgen rays should not usurp every other means at our disposal.[33]

Jones' lecture and subsequent paper inevitably created strong feelings amongst many surgeons, some of whom were in favour of specialisation and others who were against. The British Medical Association met in Bath in August 1925 and a special session on Surgery and Orthopaedics was chaired by Moynihan. Professor George Gask was one of the principal opponents of specialisation.

As previously stated, Gask qualified in medicine from St Bartholomew's in 1898 and by 1914 he was an established consultant. He went to France in 1916, was mentioned in despatches four times and won the DSO in 1917. He was appointed Consulting Surgeon to the British Fourth Army in 1918 and was created CMG in 1919 for his outstanding services. He was particularly well known for his work on the surgical treatment of wounds of the chest and lungs. The West London Medico-Chirurgical Society awarded him its gold medal for his part in this work. In 1919, Gask became Professor of Surgery at the University of London with his clinical unit at St Bartholomew's Hospital. He was a very thoughtful individual and was moved by a deep sense of mission to improve student education.[34] This made him a very unusual opponent of orthopaedic specialisation, since Jones had made a very strong case for specialisation in the context of student teaching. Gask opposed the idea that greater division of labour would lead to greater efficiency. Half the fractures were looked after by general practitioners in cottage hospitals and Gask argued that greater division of labour hardly applied to the manufacture of good GPs. Conversely, orthopaedic surgeons were not concerned with the education of GPs and partly linked bad fracture treatment with management by GPs in cottage hospitals. They felt that GPs should not be responsible for looking after fractures. Orthopaedic surgeons did not wish to pursue this line further, however, since they depended on GPs for patient referrals and their income. For their part, GPs had no objection to specialisation. They were mindful of their patients' desire for specialist care and were also mindful of the legal and professional risks for orthopaedic cases that went wrong, such as malunion of

33 Jones, Crippling due to fractures, *British Medical Journal,* 1925.
34 Gask, George Ernest (1875-1951), *Plarr's Lives of the Fellows Online*, Royal College of Surgeons, <https://livesonline.rcseng.ac.uk/biogs/E004155b.htm>.

fractures. General practitioners in fact regarded themselves and the orthopaedic surgeons as underdogs fighting against the general surgical establishment.[35]

The surgical establishment continued to oppose orthopaedic specialisation and unsurprisingly nothing happened. A damning report by Sir Dawson Williams, editor of the BMJ between 1896 and 1928 appeared in the British Medical Journal in 1927:

> One of the stock arguments used by the opponents of specialisation is the fear that by transferring any department of surgery from the general surgeon to the specialist the student might become indifferent to the specialty and cease to receive instruction in it. This might possibly be true of some special departments already existing, but it is, in our judgement, a baseless fear as regards the treatment of fractures. The plain fact is that, as things are at present in London, the student gets little instruction in the treatment of fractures of the upper extremity and no experience in the treatment of the much more important fractures of the lower extremity, for the simple reason that such cases are not usually admitted to the wards of the great teaching hospitals. The demand for beds in these institutions is so urgent that acute diseases and conditions affecting the cavities of the body have preference; and abdominal sections, which can be sent to convalescent institutions or to their own homes a fortnight after operation, occupy the beds instead of fracture cases, which would probably on the average require at least six weeks' treatment.[36]

In 1935, a decade after Jones delivered his controversial lecture in Liverpool, a British Medical Association Committee on Fractures which had been set up in 1933 published its report. The committee's remit was to consider existing methods of treatment of fractures and to make recommendations for possible improvements.[37]

British Medical Association, report of committee on fractures

The committee reported that in most instances, patients with fractures were still being looked after by surgeons with no particular interest in orthopaedics in a general ward or by general practitioners. There were no organised fracture services for these patients and in a high proportion of cases, fractures remained unreduced because no effort had been made to improve the position of the fracture or check its reduction by radiographic examination. It would be 1938 before X-rays were used routinely to assist with the management of fractures. Fractures were not checked regularly, and clinics were so infrequent that by the time a fracture was found to be in a poor position it was too late to do anything about it because by then the fracture was well on the way to malunion. Sometimes as a result of ignorance a plaster cast was removed too soon before the fracture had healed, and the position of the broken bone was lost as the un-united fracture re-displaced. Joints adjacent to the fracture often became stiff because important instruction in

35 Cooter, *Surgery and Society in Peace and War*, pp. 180-87.

36 Williams, D., The Treatment of Fractures, *British Medical Journal*, 2: 3484 (15 October 1927), p. 695.

37 British Medical Association, Report of Committee on Fractures, *Supplement to the British Medical Journal*, 1:3867 (16 February 1935), S57-S68.

joint exercise had never been given to the patient. Table 9.2 shows the average incapacity period for adult patients treated in a non-organised setup.

Other patients were treated by personnel working in an organised and dedicated fracture service. Harry Platt's unit at Ancoats Hospital was cited as one such example. Platt had 25 of the 75 beds for orthopaedic cases. There was a minor fracture clinic every day run by the resident surgical officer and a major fracture clinic every week. Plaster technicians and splint teams attended every clinic and 100 patients could be seen in a clinic lasting three hours in an ideal setting for undergraduate and postgraduate teaching. Cases of special interest were discussed at regular meetings. Table 9.3 demonstrates the average incapacity period for adult patients treated in an organised setup.

The average duration of disability was three times shorter in the organised compared with the non-organised group. There was an overall permanent disability of 1 percent in the organised group and 37 percent in the non-organised group. One of the most difficult fractures to deal with was the fractured femur because strong muscles in the thigh contracted in spasm, resulting in telescoping of the broken bones with resultant shortening of the limb. Permanent disability was found to be 9 percent in the organised group and 61 percent in the non-organised group.

Recommendations

The committee made four recommendations.

- Segregation of orthopaedic cases into a dedicated unit where they can be looked after by a specially trained and experienced staff;
- Continuity of care; successive stages of treatment should be closely related as an integral part of the whole; once discharged from the ward, patient continues to be cared for by the same team;
- Good aftercare essential to restore function as much as possible; active exercise, not passive massage, vital to restore function;
- Unity of control of care; all stages of treatment under control of a designated surgeon.

These recommendations would have made any resultant service remarkably similar to the organisation of fracture treatment during the Great War, which had ended seventeen years previously. As things stood, however, orthopaedics in civilian practice had simply not moved on. Henry Gray's excellent management of acute fractures in casualty clearing stations on the Western Front and Maurice Sinclair's segregation of femoral fractures at base hospitals in France had counted for nothing, while Robert Jones' orthopaedic centres in Great Britain and Ireland had simply disappeared.

Four years after the publication of the Report of the Committee on Fractures, the Second World War began and with it hopes that orthopaedic surgery would get a welcome and much-needed boost. It was, however, not to be and orthopaedic surgery was relegated to a side show status, even though orthopaedic facilities were required for both military and civilian casualties. There was nothing ground-breaking or contentious about the re-opening of orthopaedic centres, and in any case, it had all been done before. Meanwhile, as the Battle of Britain raged in the skies over the fields of Southern England, Archibald McIndoe established a plastic surgical

Table 9.2 Average period of incapacity for adults not treated in organised clinics.

Site of fracture	Number of cases	Average disability period	Number of cases permanently incapacitated
Colles	38	29	9
Scaphoid	65	46	38
Clavicle	20	22	1
Femur	31	60	19
Patella	18	57	8
Tibia and Fibula	60	62	15
Ankle	44	47	14

British Medical Association, Report of Committee on Fractures, *Supplement to the British Medical Journal,* 1:3867 (16 February 1935), S57-S68.

Table 9.3 Average incapacity periods for adults treated in organised fracture clinic.

Site of Fracture	Number of cases	Average disability period in weeks	Number of cases permanently incapacitated
Colles (just above wrist)	452	7	2
Scaphoid (bone in wrist)	132	11	2
Shaft radius and ulna	40	14	0
Clavicle (collar bone)	85	5	1
Femur (thigh bone)	45	37	4
Patella (kneecap)	29	26	1
Tibia and fibula (leg bones)	155	21	1
Ankle	193	11	0

British Medical Association, Report of Committee on Fractures, *Supplement to the British Medical Journal,* 1:3867 (15 February 1935), S57-S68.

unit at East Grinstead to deal with badly burned pilots of the RAF and plastic surgery captured the limelight.

In Aberdeen, where the author spent his working life as an orthopaedic surgeon, it remained debatable until the establishment of the National Health Service in 1948 whether there would 'ever be a living here for a specialised orthopaedic surgeon'.[38] It would be 1953 before general surgeons finally relinquished the treatment of fractures at Aberdeen Royal Infirmary, so it wasn't only the London general surgeons who opposed orthopaedic expansion. When the author was appointed as a consultant to Aberdeen Royal Infirmary in 1983, there were six orthopaedic surgeons. At the time of writing this book in 2018 there are now 26.

38 Levack, I., Dudley, H., *The Aberdeen Royal Infirmary: The People's Hospital of the North-East* (London and Philadelphia, 1992), p. 139.

Orthopaedic surgery, which had made such important advances during 1914-18, was stopped in its tracks in Britain at the end of the war by the surgical establishment. This was a missed opportunity which should never have happened. It put British orthopaedic surgeons far behind their North American counterparts and it took them many years to catch up. American surgeons had derived so much valuable experience working with Robert Jones in his orthopaedic centres that they returned home after the war ready and able to take on the challenge of looking after all bone and joint surgical cases. They, at least, knew a good thing when they saw it and unlike British surgeons, they derived great benefit from the surgical advances made on the Western Front and in Britain.

Bibliography

Books

Bamji, A., *Faces from the Front: Harold Gillies, The Queen's Hospital, Sidcup and the Origins of Modern Plastic Surgery* (Solihull: Helion and Company, 2017).
Barnett, C., *The Sword Bearers: Studies in Supreme Command in the First World War* (London: Eyre and Spottiswoode, 1963).
Bean, C.E.W., *Anzac to Amiens* (Canberra: Australian War Memorial, 1946).
Bell, John, *The Principles of Surgery in Two Volumes* (Edinburgh: T. Cadell & N. Davies; T.N. Longman & O. Rees & others, 1801).
Bliss, M., *Harvey Cushing, A Life in Surgery* (Oxford, New York: Oxford University Press, 2005).
Butler, A.G., *Official History of the Australian Army Medical Services, 1914–1918 Vol. II – The Western Front* (Canberra: Australian War Memorial, 1940).
Butler, A.G., *Official History of the Australian Army Medical Services, 1914–1918 Vol. III – Special Problems and Services* (Canberra: Australian War Memorial, 1943).
Cantlie, N., *A History of the Army Medical Department, Vol. 2* (Edinburgh: Churchill Livingston, 1974).
Carberry, A.D., *The New Zealand Medical Services in the Great War* (Auckland: Whitcombe and Tombs Ltd., 1924).
Clayton, A., *Chavasse: Double VC* (Barnsley: Pen and Sword, 1992).
Cooter, R., *Surgery and Society in Peace and War* (Basingstoke: MacMillan Press Ltd., 1993).
Cooter, R.M., Harrison, M., Sturdy, S., *War, Medicine and Modernity* (Stroud, Gloucestershire: Sutton Publishing Ltd., 1998).
Gordon-Taylor, G., *The Abdominal Injuries of Warfare* (Bristol: John Wright and Sons, 1939).
Gray, H.M.W., *The Early Treatment of War Wounds* (London: Henry Frowde, Hodder and Stoughton, 1919).
Guthrie, G.J., *Commentaries on the Surgery of the War in Portugal, Spain and the Netherlands* (Philadelphia: J.B. Lippincott, 1862).
Guthrie, George James, *A Treatise on Gunshot Wounds: On Inflammation, Erysipelas, And Mortification, On Injuries of Nerves* (London: Burgess and Hill, 1827).
Hennen, John, *Principles of Military Surgery 3rd Ed.* (London: John Wilson, 1829).
Hudson, Roger (Editor), *William Russell, Special Correspondent of the Times* (London: Folio Society, 1995).
Jones, R., *Notes on Military Orthopaedics* (London, New York, Toronto and Melbourne: Cassel and Company Ltd., 1917).

Land, W., *Barber,* George Walter (1868-1961), *Australian Dictionary of Biography*, Vol. 7, (MUP), 1979.

Larrey, D.J., *Memoirs of Military Surgery of Campaigns of the French Army Vol. I Translated by RW Hall* (Baltimore: J. Cushing, 1814).

Letterman, J., *Medical Recollections of the Army of the Potomac* (New York: D. Appleton and Company, 1866).

Levack, I., Dudley, H., *The Aberdeen Royal Infirmary: The People's Hospital of the North-East* (London and Philadelphia: 1992).

Longmore, Thomas, *Gunshot Injuries: Their History, Characteristic Features, Complications and General Treatment* (London: Longmans Green and Co., 1877).

Macpherson, W.G., *History of the Great War Based on Official Documents: Medical Services General History Vol. II* (London: MacMillan, 1923).

Macpherson, W.G., *History of the Great War Based on Official Documents: Medical Services General History Vol. III* (London: His Majesty's Stationery Office, 1924).

Marshall, H., *Statistical Report on the Sickness, Mortality, and Invaliding Among the Troops in the West Indies* (London: W. Clowes and Sons, 1838).

McGrigor, James, *Medical Sketches of the Expedition from India to Egypt* (London: John Murray, Fleet Street, 1804).

McGrigor, Mary, Editor, *Sir James McGrigor, The Scalpel and the Sword*; *the Autobiography of the Father of Army Medicine* (Dalkeith: Scottish Cultural Press, 2000).

Miller, D., MacCormick, A., (1856-1947*), Australian Dictionary of Biography*, Vol. 10, 1986.

Mitchell, T.J., Smith, G.M., *History of the Great War: Medical Services Casualties and Medical Statistics* (London: His Majesty's Stationery Office, 1931).

Robertson, A., in Scotland, T., Heys, S., Wars *Pestilence and the Surgeon's Blade: The Evolution of British Military Medicine and Surgery During the 19th century* (Solihull: Helion and Company, 2013).

Robertson, A., in Scotland, T., Heys, S., *War Surgery 1914-18* (Solihull: Helion and Company, 2012).

Royal College of Surgeons, Minutes of Council, 16 July 1918, pp. 159-160, in Cooter, *Surgery and Society in Peace and War* (Basingstoke: MacMillan Press Ltd; 1993).

Scotland, T., Heys, S., *War Surgery 1914-18* (Solihull: Helion and Company, 2012).

Scotland, T., Heys, S., *Wars, Pestilence and the Surgeon's Blade: The Evolution of British Military Medicine and Surgery During the 19th century* (Solihull, Helion and Company, 2013).

Scotland, T., Boyer, A., *Henry Gray, Surgeon of the Great War: Saving Lives in a Theatre of Destruction* (Edinburgh: Capercaillie, 2015).

Serle, G., Monash, Sir John (1865-1931), *Australian Dictionary of Biography*, Vol. 10, (MUP), 1986.

Steinberg, John, *The Russo-Japanese War in Global Perspective, World War Zero,* Vol. 2 (Leiden: Brill Academic Publishers, 2007).

Stevens, J. and C. (eds.), *Unknown Warriors, The letters of Kate Luard, RRC and Bar, Nursing Sister in France* (Stroud: History Press, 2014).

Stevenson, W.F., *Wounds in War: The Mechanism of Their Production and Treatment* (London: Longman Green and Co, 1904).

Stiles, H.J., Forrester-Brown, M.F., *Treatment of Injuries of the Peripheral Spinal Nerves* (London: Henry Frowde and Hodder and Stoughton, 1922).

Van Der Kloot, W, *Great Scientists Wage the Great War* (Stroud: Fonthill Media, 2014).
Walker, K., *I Talk of Dreams, an Experiment in Autobiography* (London: Jonathan Cape, 1946).
Walker, K., *The Story of Blood* (London: Herbert Jenkins Ltd., 1958).
Wallace, C.S., Fraser, J., *Surgery at a Casualty Clearing Station* (London: A&C Black Ltd., 1918).
Wallace, C.S., *War Surgery of the Abdomen* (London: J&A Churchill, 1918).
Watson, F., *The Life of Sir Robert Jones* (London: Hodder and Stoughton Ltd., 1934).
Waugh, W., *A History of the British Orthopaedic Association* (London: British Orthopaedic Association, 1993).
Whitehead, I.R., *Doctors in the Great War* (Barnsley: Leo Cooper, 1999).

Journals

Bennet, J.D., Princess Vera Gedroits: Military Surgeon, Poet and Author, *British Medical Journal*, 305: 6868 (19 December 1992), pp. 1532-34.
Bennett, J.D., Abdominal Surgery in War: The Early Story, *Journal of the Royal Society of Medicine*; 84: 9, (1991), pp.554-57.
Blair, J.S.G., Captain Oswald Hope Robertson, *Journal Royal Army Medical Corps*, 150:4: (1 December 2004), pp. 291-92.
Bowlby, A., The Mortality of Cases of Fractured Femur, *British Medical Journal* 1: 3030 (25 January 1919), p. 112.
Bowlby, A., The Work of the Clearing Hospitals During the Past Six Weeks, *British Medical Journal*, 2:2816 (19 December 1914), pp. 1053-54.
Bowlby, A., The Mortality of Cases of Fractured Femur, *British Medical Journal* 1: 3030 (25 January 1919), p. 112.
Bowlby, A., Gunshot Fractures of the Femur, *British Medical Journal*, 1: 3079 (3 January 1920), pp. 1-4.
Boyle, H.E.G., Nitrous Oxide-Oxygen-ether Outfit, *Lancet*, 1 (1919), p. 226.
British Medical Association, Report of Committee on Fractures, *Supplement to the British Medical Journal*, 1:3867 (16 February 1935), S57-S68.
Cannon, W.B., Acidosis in Cases of Shock, Haemorrhage and Gas Infection, *Journal of American Medical Association*, 70 (23 February 1918), pp. 531-35.
Cushing, H., A Study of a Series of Wounds Involving the Brain and its Enveloping Structures, *British Journal of Surgery*, 5 (April 1918), pp. 558-684.
Cushing, H., Notes on Penetrating Wounds of the Brain, *British Medical Journal*, 1:2982 (February 23, 1918), pp. 221-26.
Evans, Barbara, A Doctor in the Great War: An interview with Sir Geoffrey Marshall, *British Medical Journal*, 285: 6357 (18 December 1982), pp. 1780-83.
Fraser, J., Drummond, H., A Clinical and Experimental Study of Three Hundred Perforating Wounds of the Abdomen, *British Medical Journal*, 1:2932 (March 10, 1917), pp. 321-29.
Gask, G., Gunshot Wounds of the Chest, *British Medical Journal*, 1:4089 (20 May 1939), pp. 1043-45.
Gask, G.E., Wilkinson, K.D., Penetrating Gunshot Wounds of the Chest and Their Treatment, *British Medical Journal*, 2: 2972 (15 December 1917), pp. 781-84.

Gordon-Taylor, G., The abdominal injuries of warfare-II, *British Medical Journal*, 2:4099 (July 29, 1939), pp. 235-38.

Gray, H.M.W., An Address on the Application of the Professional Lessons of the War to Civil Work, *British Medical Journal*, 1:3134 (22 January 1921), pp.109-14.

Gray, H.M.W., The Mortality of Cases of Fractured Femur, *British Medical Journal* 1:3031 (1 February 1919), p. 142.

Gray, H.M.W., The Treatment of Gunshot Wounds by Excision and Primary Suture, *Journal Royal Army Medical Corps*, 24 (June 1915), pp. 551-54.

Gray, H.M.W., Treatment of Gunshot Wounds by Excision and Primary suture, *British Medical Journal* 1915; 2: 2852, (28 August 1915), p. 317.

Gray, T. Cecil, Mitchiner Memorial Lecture: 'Another Side of Mars', *Journal of the Royal Army Medical Corps*, 130 (1984), pp. 3-11.

Guedel, A., Third Stage Ether: A sub-classification regarding the significance of the position and movements of the eyeball, *American Journal of Surgery*, 34, (1920), pp. 53-57.

Guiou, N.M., Blood Transfusion in a Field Ambulance, *British Medical Journal* 1: 2999 (22 June 22, 1918), pp. 695-96.

Helling, T.S., Daon, E., The Great War, Antoine Depage and the Resurgence of Debridement, *Annals of Surgery*, Vol. 228, No 2 (1998), pp. 173-81.

Hepburn, H.H., Notes on Tetanus, *Canadian Medical Association Journal*, 12:5, (May 1922), pp. 312-15.

Holmes à Court, A., Intravenous Injections in the Treatment of Haemorrhage and Shock, *The Medical Journal of Australia*, Vol. II, No. 2, (10 July 1920), pp. 25-30.

Holmes à Court, A., Intravenous Injections in the Treatment of Haemorrhage and Shock, *The Medical Journal of Australia*, Vol. II, No. 2 (17 July 1920), pp. 49-56.

Jones, R., Crippling Due to Fractures: Its Prevention and Remedy, *British Medical Journal*, 1: 3359 (16 May 1925), pp. 909-13.

Lister, J., On the Antiseptic Principle in the Practice of Surgery, *British Medical Journal*, 2: 351 (21 September 1867), pp.246-48.

Makins, G.H., Introductory, *British Journal of Surgery*, Vol. 6, No. 21 (1918), pp. 1-11.

Marshall, G., The Administration of Anaesthesia at the Front, *British Medical Journal*, 1: 2944 (2 June 1917), pp. 722-25.

McGrigor, James, Sketch of the Medical History of the British Armies in the Peninsula of Spain and Portugal during the Late Campaigns, *Medico Chirurgical Transactions*, 6 (1815), pp. 482-86.

Metcalfe, N. H., Military Influence upon the Development of Anaesthesia from the American Civil War (1861-1865) to the Outbreak of the First World War, *Anaesthesia*, 60:12, (2005), pp. 1213-17.

Metcalfe, N.H., The Effect of the First World War (1914-18) on the Development of British Anaesthesia, *European Journal of Anaesthesia*, 24:8 (24 August 2007), pp. 649-57.

Milligan, E.T.C., The Early Treatment of Projectile Wounds by Excision of the Damaged Tissue, *British Medical Journal*, 1: 2843 (26 June 1915), p. 1081.

Mouat, A., Observations on Some Points Connected with the Use of Chloroform in Military Practice, *The Lancet*, 1856, ii: pp.78-81.

Obituary, Sir Gordon Gordon-Taylor, K.B.E., C.B., M.D., Hon. L.L.D., Hon. D.Sc., M.S., F.R.C.S., Hon. F.R.C.S. Ed., Hon. F.R.C.S.I., Hon. F.A.C.S., Hon. F.R.C.S.(Canada), *British Medical Journal*, 2:5203 (24 September 1960), pp. 947-48.

Obituary, Sir Henry Gray, KBE, CB, CMG, LLD, FRCSEd, *British Medical Journa*l, 2: 4058 (15 October 1938), p. 814.

Obituary, Lionel Ernest Howard Whitby, C.V.O., M.C., M.A., M.D., F.R.C.P., Hon.D.Sc. (Toronto), Hon.LL.D.(Glasg.), Hon.M.D. (Louvain), D.P.H.

Journal Royal Army Medical Corps 1957, Vol. 103 (1 April 1957), pp. 102-03.

Osgood, R., The Orthopaedic Centers of Great Britain and Their American Officers, *Journal of Bone and Joint Surgery, American*, s2-16 (1918), pp. 132-40.

Parker, P.J., Commentary in Stevenson, W.F., Surgical Experiences from the Boer War, *Journal Royal Army Medical Corps*, Vol. 1, No. 2 (1903), pp. 89-95.

Platt, H., British Orthopaedic Association: First Founders Lecture, *Journal of Bone and Joint Surgery*, Vol. 41B, No. 2 (May 1959), pp. 231-36.

Platt, H., Moynihan; The Education and Training of the Surgeon. Eleventh Moynihan Lecture Delivered University of Leeds 25 May 1961, *Annals of the Royal College of Surgeons of England*, 4 (30 April 1962), pp. 220-28.

Roberts, J.E.H., Craig, J.G., The Surgical Treatment of Severe Wounds of the Chest, *British Medical Journal*, 2: 2966 (3 November 1917), pp. 576-79.

Robertson L.B., Gordon Watson, C., Further Observations on the Results of Blood Transfusion in War Surgery, *British Medical Journal*, 2:2969 (24 November 1917), pp. 679-683.

Robertson, L. Bruce, The Transfusion of Whole Blood, *British Medical Journal*, 2: 2897 (8 July 1916), pp. 38-40.

Robertson, O.H., Transfusion with Preserved Red Blood Cells, *British Medical Journal* 1: 2999 (22 June 1918), pp. 691-95.

Sargent, P., Holmes, G., Report on the Later Results of Gunshot Wounds of the Head, *Journal of the Royal Army Medical Corps*, Vol. 27, No. 3 (September 1916), pp. 300-11.

Sargent, P., Holmes, G., Preliminary Notes on the Treatment of the Cranial Injuries of Warfare, *British Medical Journal*, 1:2830 (27 March 1915), pp. 537-41.

Stevenson, W.F., Surgical Experiences from the Boer War, *Journal Royal Army Medical Corps*, Vol. 1, No. 2 (1903), pp. 89-95.

Stiles, H., Surgical Training, *British Medical Journal*, 2: 3068 (October 18, 1919), pp. 487-89.

The London Gazette, Supplement, No. 29802, 26 October 1916.

The London Gazette, Supplement, No. 30284, 14 September 1917.

Till, A.S., Gordon-Taylor: War Surgeon and Historian, *Annals of the Royal College of Surgeons of England*, Vol. 54 (1974), pp. 33-47.

Treves, F., The War in South Africa after Spion Kop, *British Medical Journal*, 1: 2045 (10 March 1900), pp. 599-607.

Westhorpe, R., The Introduction of a Mobile Resuscitation Service 1918 in Fink, B.R., LE Morris L.E., & Stephen, C.R. (eds.), *The History of Anaesthesia: Third International Symposium* (Illinois: Wood Library, Museum of Anaesthesiology, 1992), pp. 438-39.

Williams, D., The Treatment of Fractures, *British Medical Journal*, 2: 3484 (15 October 1927), p. 695.

Wright, A.E., Colebrook, L., On the Acidosis of Shock and Suspended Circulation, *Lancet* 1:191 (1 June 1918), pp. 763-65.

Electronic Sources

Bristow, Walter, Plarr's Lives of the Fellows Online, Royal College of Surgeons <http://livesonline.rcseng.ac.uk/biogs/E003905b.htm> (Accessed 12 March 2018).

Gask, George Ernest, *Plarr's Lives of the Fellows Online*, Royal College of Surgeons, <https://livesonline.rcseng.ac.uk/biogs/E004155b.htm> (Accessed 12 March 2018).

Groves, Ernest William Hey, *Plarr's Lives of the Fellows Online*, Royal College of Surgeons, https://livesonline.rcseng.ac.uk/biogs/E004298b.htm accessed 12 March, 2018.

Harvey Cushing <https://allauthor.com/quotes/124386/> (Accessed 12 March 2018).

Historic Hospitals, Oldmill Military Hospital (now Woodend Hospital), Aberdeen <https://historic-hospitals.com/2016/01/16/oldmill-military-hospital-now-woodend-hospital-aberdeen/> (Accessed 12 March 2018).

Lawrence Bruce Robertson, *Dictionary of Canadian Biography* <http://www.biographi.ca/en/bio/robertson_lawrence_bruce_15E.html> (Accessed 12 March 2018).

Makins, Sir George Henry, Plarr's Lives of the Fellows Online, Royal College of Surgeons, https://livesonline.rcseng.ac.uk/biogs/E000223b.htm> (Accessed 12 March 2018).

Pearce, J.M.S., Historical Note Sir Gordon Holmes <http://jnnp.bmj.com/content/75/10/1502> (Accessed 12 March 2018).

Platt, Sir Harry, Plarr's Lives of the Fellows Online, Royal College of Surgeons, <https://livesonline.rcseng.ac.uk/biogs/E000232b.htm> (Accessed 12 March 2018).

Sargent, Sir Percy William George, Plarr's Lives of the Fellows Online, Royal College of Surgeons <https://livesonline.rcseng.ac.uk/biogs/E004573b.htm> (Accessed 12 March 2018).

Wallace, Sir Cuthbert Sydney, Plarr's Lives of the Fellows Online, Royal College of Surgeons <https://livesonline.rcseng.ac.uk/biogs/E000228b.htm> (Accessed 12 March 2018).

Van Der Kloot, W, *William Maddock Bayliss's Therapy for Wound Shock* <http://rsnr.royalsocietypublishing.org/> (Accessed 16 October 2017).

Index

People

Places

Military Units and Formations

General

Medical